Handbook of Laboratory Health and Safety Measures

This Handbook is dedicated to those who work in laboratories

SECOND EDITION

Handbook of Laboratory Health and Safety Measures

Edited by

S.B. Pal

Universität Ulm
Abteilung für Innere Medizin I
D-7900 Ulm (Donau)
Federal Republic of Germany

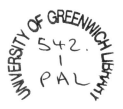

KLUWER ACADEMIC PUBLISHERS
DORDRECHT / BOSTON / LONDON

Distributors

for the United States and Canada: Kluwer Academic Publishers, PO Box 358, Accord Station, Hingham, MA 02018-0358, USA
for all other countries: Kluwer Academic Publishers Group, Distribution Center, PO Box 322, 3300 AH Dordrecht, The Netherlands

British Library Cataloguing in Publication Data

Handbook of laboratory health and safety measures. – 2nd. ed.
  1. Great Britain. Laboratories. Safety aspects
  I. Pal, S. B. (Srikantha Bhushan) *1928–1989*

  ISBN 0-7462-0077-3

Published in the United Kingdom by Kluwer Academic Publishers,
PO Box 55, Lancaster, UK.

Kluwer Academic Publishers BV incorporates the publishing programmes of
D. Reidel, Martinus Nijhoff, Dr W. Junk and MTP Press.

Laserprinter typeset by Martin Lister Publishing Services, Carnforth, Lancs.

Printed in Great Britain by Butler & Tanner Limited, Frome and London

Contents

Preface

During the past two decades, many books, governmental reports and regulations on safety measures against chemicals, fire, microbiological and radioactive hazards in laboratories have been published from various countries. These topics have also been briefly discussed in books on laboratory planning and management. The application of various scientific instruments based on different ionizing and non-ionizing radiations have brought new safety problems to the laboratory workers of today, irrespective of their scientific disciplines, be they medicine, natural or life sciences. However, no comprehensive laboratory handbook dealing with all these hazards, some of which are recently introduced, had so far been available in a single volume. Therefore, it was thought worthwhile to publish this Handbook on safety and health measures for laboratories, with contributions from several experts on these subjects. As this second edition of the Handbook, like the first edition, is a multiauthor volume, some duplication in content among chapters is unavoidable in order to maintain the context of a chapter as well as make each chapter complete.

An attempt has also been made to maintain the central theme, which is how to work in a laboratory with maximum possible environmental safety. Some chapters contained in the first volume have been updated for this second edition, and further chapters added, to make this volume even more comprehensive in dealing with all possible hazards in the laboratory. I am indebted to Dr Peter L. Clarke of Kluwer Academic Publishers, who has undertaken the publication of this volume and Mrs M.R. Lingard-Pal for acting as an honorary editorial assistant.

S.B. Pal
1989

List of Contributors

P. Bowker
Department of Orthopaedic
Mechanics
University of Salford
Salford M5 4WT
UK

C.M. Chaturvedi
Department of Zoology
Banaras Hindu University
Varanasi 221005
India

G.E. Chivers
Centre for Continuing Vocational
Education
University of Sheffield
65 Wilkinson Street
Sheffield S10 2GJ
UK

C.H. Collins
The Ashes
Hadlow
Kent TN11 0AS
UK

B. Czepulkowski
Mediscript
Willow End
Hendon Wood Lane
London NW7 4HS
UK

B.L. Diffey
Regional Medical Physics
Department
Durham Unit
Dryburn Hospital
Durham DH1 5TW
UK

D. Donaldson
Department of Pathology
East Surrey Hospital
Three Arch Road
Redhill
Surrey RH1 5RH
UK

M.A. Foster
Department of Biomedical Physics
and Bioengineering
University of Aberdeen and
Grampian Health Board
Foresterhill
Aberdeen AB9 2ZD
UK

N.W. Garvie
Department of Radiology and
Nuclear Medicine
The London Hospital
Whitechapel
London E1 1BB
UK

W.E. Green
Oakwood
Orestan Lane
Effingham
Leatherhead
Surrey KT24 5SL
UK

A.L. McKenzie
Regional Medical Physics
Department
Newcastle General Hospital
Newcastle-upon-Tyne NE4 6BE
UK

M.J. Minski
Reactor Centre
Imperial College of Science
Technology and Medicine
Silwood Park
Buckhurst Road
Ascot
Berks. SL5 7TE
UK

I.D. Montoya
Affiliated Systems Corporation
1200 South Post Oak Boulevard
Suite 540
Houston
TX 77056-3104
USA

H. Moseley
Department of Clinical Physics and
Bio-engineering
West Scotland Health Boards
11 West Graham Street
Glasgow G4 9LF
UK

R.S. Osborn
Reactor Centre
Imperial College of Science
Technology and Medicine
Silwood Park, Buckhurst Road
Ascot
Berks. SL5 7TE
UK

T. Pendry
MRC Toxicology Unit
Medical Research Council
Laboratories
Woodmansterne Road
Carshalton
Surrey SM5 4EF
UK

R.G. Putney
Department of Medical Physics
The London Hospital
Whitechapel
London E1 1BB
UK

M.P. Ramanujam
Department of Botany
Centre for Post-graduate Studies
Pondicherry
India 605 008

J. Robb
The Douglass Group of
Deloitte & Touche
1200 Travis Suite 2400
Houston
TX 77002
USA

W.L. Ruff
Clinical Laboratories
Howard University Hospital
2041 Georgia Avenue NW
Washington, DC 20060
USA

E.J. Slater
Medical Physics Department
City Hospital
Hucknall Road
Nottingham NG5 1PB
UK

J. Smith
74 Cranham Close
Headless Cross
Redditch
Worcs. B97 5AZ
UK

D.M. Taylor
Kernforschungszentrum Karlsruhe
Institut für Genetik und für
Toxikologie von Spaltstoffen
Postfach 3640
D-7500 Karlsruhe 1
Federal Republic of Germany

R. Toynton
Centre for Extension Studies
Division of Continuing Education
University of Sheffield
85 Wilkinson Street
Sheffield S10 2GJ
UK

D. Whelpton
Medical Physics and
Bioengineering Department
Kings Mill Hospital
Mansfield Road
Sutton-in-Ashfield
Nottinghamshire NG17 4JL
UK

A.R. Williams
Department of Medical Biophysics
University of Manchester
Stopford Building
Oxford Road
Manchester M13 9PT
UK

A.E. Wright
The Old Smithy
Warden
Hexham
Northumberland NE48 3SB
UK

Notes on Contributors

Dr P. Bowker, CEng, MIMechE, was born in Lancaster, England, in 1946. He did his basic industrial training at AEI Ltd., and obtained his BSc in mechanical engineering (1967) and PhD in engineering metallurgy (1970) from the University of Salford. He has worked as Senior Research Associate in the Departments of Metallurgy and Engineering Materials, University of Newcastle upon Tyne, and as a Lecturer in the Department of Bio-Medical Physics and Bio-Engineering, University of Aberdeen. His present appointment is as a Lecturer in the Department of Orthopaedic Mechanics, University of Salford. He has 16 publications to his credit, including chapters in 2 books.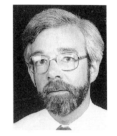

Dr (Mrs.) C. M. Chaturvedi was born in Jabalpur (MP), India in 1951. She graduated in 1969 and gained an MSc in Zoology in 1971 from Jabalpur University. After obtaining a PhD degree in Zoology (Avian Endocrinology/Reproduction Biology) in 1976 from Banaras Hindu University, (BHU) Varanasi, India, Dr Chaturvedi was appointed lecturer in the Department of Zoology, BHU in 1977, teaching graduate and post-graduate classes. Dr Chaturvedi's present appointment is as Reader in Zoology at the same university. She also joined the Department of Zoology and Physiology, Louisiana State University, Baton Rouge, USA, as a visiting scientist, for collaborative research work in 1984 and 1987. Her major research area is the neuro-endocrine regulation of seasonal reproduction and metabolic conditions in wild and domestic birds, with special reference to the thyroid and adrenal glands. She has a number of publications in the field of Reproductive Endocrinology of birds.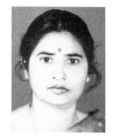

Dr G.E. Chivers was born in St Albans, England, in 1943. He was an undergraduate and research student at Birmingham University from 1962 to 1968 during which time he qualified for a BSc (Hons) in chemistry and a PhD in organic chemistry. He spent one year as a Research Fellow in chemistry at Toronto University, Canada, and one year as Research Fellow in organic chemistry at Salford University. This was followed by an appointment as Lecturer in organic chemistry at Hatfield Polytechnic. Dr Chivers is at present appointed as Senior Tutor in the Centre for Extension Studies, Loughborough University of Technology, and is responsible for the organization of post-experience short courses on occupational health and safety, risk management and industrial pollution control, and for the University Diploma in Occupational Health and Safety Management. He organizes short courses on laboratory health and safety, trains internal staff in this area and acts as a consultant on health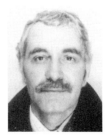

and safety in industrial and public sector laboratories. He has 4 publications on health and safety aspects in the laboratory, including chapters in 2 books.

Dr C.H. Collins MBE, DSc, FRCPath, FIBiol, was born in Luton, England in 1919 and trained as a bacteriologist with the UK Public Health Laboratory Service. He became involved in microbiological hazard investigations in the 1950s as a result of work with aerosol production from liquid cultures of tubercle bacilli and the design of microbiological safety cabinets. Dr Collins' recently retired from the Public Health Laboratory Service and now holds a Research Fellowship at King's College Hospital Medical and Dental School, London. He is also Visiting Research Fellow, Microbiological Department, Cardiothoracic Institute (University of London), Brompton Hospital, London. He is an Advisor to the World Health Organization's Special Programme on Safety measures in Microbiology and a member and Secretary to two other learned bodies in the UK, has travelled widely in Europe, India, New Zealand and the United States, studying and lecturing on microbiological hazards and tuberculosis bacteriology and has a number of important publications.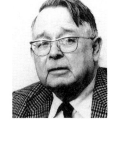

Ms Barbara Helen Czepulkowski, born in Ashton-under-Lyne, England in 1957, graduated from the University of Manchester in 1978 with a BSc (Hons) degree in genetics and cell biology. She worked as a Basic Grade Scientific Officer, Cytogenetics Department, Royal Manchester Children's Hospital for four years, following which she became a Research Assistant in the Cytogenetics Unit, St. Mary's Hospital Medical School, London, which provides a diagnostic cytogenetic service to the NW Thames Region, and also has a major research interest in the field of antenatal diagnosis, which included research on the first trimester prenatal diagnosis of chromosome defects and inborn errors of metabolism from chorionic villus biopsy. While at St Mary's Hospital Medical School, Ms Czepulkowski was also fully involved in the diagnostic work of the laboratory and the Medical School teaching programme for medical students on the paediatric course, and students in the pre-clinical year. After leaving St Mary's Hospital, she was employed by St Bartholomew's Hospital as Senior Cytogeneticist, providing a diagnostic service dealing with bone marrow studies in malignant disease. She has now moved to employment as a full-time medical writer and Editor for the publishing company 'Mediscript', based in the UK. Ms Czepulkowski has 16 publications to her credit and three chapters in books (excluding the present Handbook).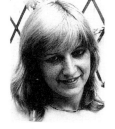

Dr B.L. Diffey, born in Bedlinog, South Wales, UK in 1948, graduated with a BSc (1st Class Hons) in mathematics and physics and an AKC in theology in 1969, and obtained a PhD in physics in 1973, all from the University of London. He became a Fellow of the Institute of Physics in 1983. He first worked as a Basic Grade and Senior Grade Physicist at the Kent and Canterbury Hospital, Canterbury and is presently appointed as a Top Grade Physicist, Northern Regional Medical Physics Department and Head of Durham Medical Physics Unit, Dryburn Hospital, Durham. Dr Diffey's special interests are concerned with the applications of ultraviolet radiation in medicine, an area in which he has made extensive contributions to the medical and scientific literature. He also provides an investigative service for patients who have skin diseases which are induced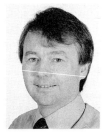

or aggravated by sunlight. More than 200 papers have been either published in the medical and scientific literature or presented at conferences and he has also written a book entitled *Ultraviolet Radiation in Medicine* published by Adam Hilger Limited (1982).

Dr D Donaldson, MBChB, MRCP, FRCPath, was born in Birmingham, England, in 1936. He graduated in medicine and surgery from the University of Brimingham in 1959, and, after various hospital appointments worked as a Lecturer in the Department of Neurology, Institute of Neurology, Hospital for Nervous Diseases, London. His present appointment is as a Consultant Chemical Pathologist at the East Surrey Hospital, Redhill, Surrey. He has 37 publications, 2 chapters in books. In 1970 he published jointly with P.T. Lascelles *Essential Diagnostic Tests* (Medical and Technical Publishing Company) and in 1990 published *Diagnostic Function Tests in Chemical Pathology* jointly with P.T. Lascelles (Kluwer Academic Publishers).

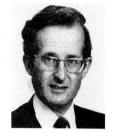

Dr Margaret Ann Hutchison (née Foster), was born in Doncaster, England, in 1940 and obtained a BSc (Hons) from Durham University in 1962, an MSc from St Andrew's University in 1968 and a PhD from Aberdeen University in 1978. She was a research student at the Gatty Marine Laboratory, University of St Andrews, Research Associate in the Department of Biological Sciences, University of Lancaster and Research Fellow in the Department of Biomedical Physics and Bioengineering, University of Aberdeen, in which department she is currently appointed as a Senior Lecturer. She is also an Honorary Senior Physicist to the Grampian Health Board, Aberdeen, and has many publications including a book *Magnetic Resonance in Medicine and Biology* published by Pergamon Press in 1984.

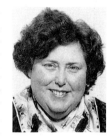

Dr N.W. Garvie, MA, MSc, DMRD, MRCP, FRCR, was born in Woking, England, in 1948, trained at Cambridge University and The London Hospital Medical College, graduating in 1972. After training as a Radiologist in Southampton, he held Senior Registrar appointments in Nuclear Medicine at the Royal Marsden Hospital, Sutton, Surrey, The Wessex Regional Department of Nuclear Medicine, Southampton and at the University Clinic, Ulm, West Germany. He is currently Consultant Radiologist at The London Hospital, London, England. His research interests include isotope bone and cardiac imaging.

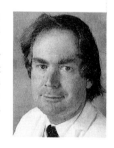

Mr W.E. Green, born in Coleshill, Warwickshire, England, in 1923, is a Fellow of the Institute of Medical Laboratory Sciences. He trained at the Royal Air Force Institute of Pathology and Tropical Medicine and at the Department of Pathology, Leicester General Hospital, England. He was appointed to the Royal Air Force Mobile Field Hospitals and General Hospitals in England, Yugoslavia, Algeria and Egypt (1942–1947), was Senior Medical Laboratory Scientific Officer and Deputy Chief Medical Laboratory Scientific Officer, Leicester General Hospital, Senior Chief Medical Laboratory Scientific Officer, Department of Pathology, Redhill General Hospital, and Principal Medical Laboratory Scientific Officer, District Pathology Service, East Surrey Health Authority. Other appointments included Lecturer in Haematology and Blood Transfusion and Secretary to the Academic Board for IMLS subjects at the Leicester

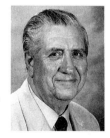

College of Technology and Commerce, Lecturer in Haematology and Blood Transfusion at the Crawley College of Further Education and Examiner in Haematology and Blood Transfusion for the Institute of Medical Laboratory Sciences. He retired from his appointment as Principal Medical Laboratory Scientific Officer in March 1987.

Dr A.L. McKenzie, who was born in Wick, Scotland, in 1949, qualified for a BSc degree from Aberdeen University and a PhD degree from St Andrews University. He worked on laser research at St Andrews University and is currently Principal Physicist in Radiotherapy, Royal South Hants Hospital, Southampton, Safety Representative to the British Medical Laser Association and Laser Safety Officer for Hospitals in the Southampton district. He has published 13 papers on Lasers and several others on Radiotherapy, Urology and Computing.

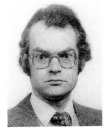

Miss M.J. Minski, BSc, CPhys, FInstP, CChem, MRSC, was born in London, England in 1937, graduated from the University of London with a BSc (1st Class Hons) in chemistry and physics in 1959, then worked for 11 years with the Medical Research Council as part of the Radiological Protection Service concerned with radiation dose assessments to man. For the last 12 years she has been first a lecturer and currently a Senior Lecturer, as well as Radiation Protection Adviser, at Imperial College, London, with research interests in the field of radioecology and trace elements in relation to disease. She has 70 publications, including two chapters in *Metal Ions in Neurology and Psychiatry*, published by A.R. Liss (1985)

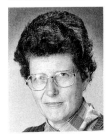

Harry Mosely is employed by the Health Board Department of Clinical Physics and Bio-Engineering in Glasgow with an honorary appointment at the University of Glasgow. He has worked in several branches of medical physics including ophthalmology in which he gained a doctorate for his thesis on fluid movement in the eye. Since then, he has specialised in non-ionising radiation. He is responsible for the provision of scientific support and for advising on safety aspects of non-ionising radiation to hospital users. He has lectured widely on medical applications and hazards and published extensively. Recently, he completed a textbook on Non-Ionising Radiation.

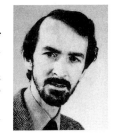

Dr I.D. Montoya, was born in Espanola, New Mexico, USA in 1950 and graduated from New Mexico State University. He trained at the Memorial General Hospital, Las Cruces, New Mexico, and is presently appointed as President of the Affiliated Systems Corporation, Houston, Texas, and Clinical Assistant Professor, University of Texas Health Science Center at Houston, Texas. Dr Montoya has published 5 papers to date.

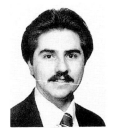

Dr R.S. Osborn, born in 1929 in Weston-Super-Mare, England was educated at Colston's Girls' School, Bristol; University College Southampton; Bristol College of Technology and Regent St Polytechnic, London. She obtained a BSc General (Lond) (Physics, Pure Mathematics, Applied Mathematics) in 1952; BSc Physics (Lond) in 1956; PhD (Crystallography) (Lond) in 1972. She did research on the physical properties of metals and alloys, and crystallography, in the aircraft industry, Bristol, 1952–1955, was Assistant Lecturer (Physics) at North West Kent College of Technology, 1956–1960, and Lecturer (Physics) at Woolwich Polytechnic, 1960–1966. Dr Osborn carried out research in crystallography, (powder and single-crystal work), at Imperial College of Science and Technology, 1966–1984, and has been a part-time assistant to the Radiation Protection Adviser, and Adviser on X-ray safety at Imperial College of Science and Technology since her early retirement in 1984.

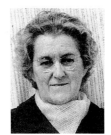

Mr T. Pendry, was born at Broadstairs, Kent, England in 1932. He is a Fellow of the Institute of Animal Technicians (FIAT). He has worked as Head Technician in a Biological Research Department (in the Pharmaceutical Industry) and as Principal Chief Animal Technician in medical research units concerned with the production and use of laboratory animals. Currently employed as Senior Scientific Officer in the Medical Research Council's Toxicology Unit in the capacity of Laboratory Manager.

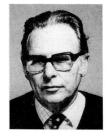

Mr R. Putney was born in London, England in 1947, where he graduated with the Master of Science degree from London University in 1974. Since then he has worked in medical physics, initially in radiotherapy and subsequently in diagnostic radiology, particularly in the field of radiation. His present post is as a Principal Grade Physicist to the London Hospital and he also provides support in the development of physics services throughout the district.

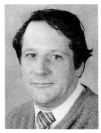

Dr M.P. Ramanujam was born on October 8, 1949 in the Union Territory of Pondicherry in India. He obtained his postgraduate degree in Botany through Presidency College, Madras in 1971 and won the 'FYSON PRIZE' for the best herbarium. Later, in 1982, he obtained a doctorate degree in Botany (Plant Pathology) from the Centre for Advanced Study in Botany, University of Madras. He is the author of several research and popular science articles. He has also received a long-term teacher research fellowship under the Faculty Improvement Programme. Actively engaged in research and popularization of science, he is also closely associated with several voluntary organizations and government agencies.

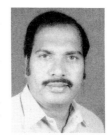

Mr J.R. Robb, born in Houston, Texas, USA in 1950, qualified as a Bachelor of Architecture from Tulane University in 1974. In 1976 he obtained a Master of Business Administration from the University of Houston. He is a Registered Architect and Member of the American Insitute of Architects. Initially, Mr Robb began his career as a medical equipment planner and he practised as a Health Care Facility Analyst and Planner for 13 years. Currently, he is a Senior Consultant with Robert Douglass Associates, Inc. assisting in planning, management, and equipping hospitals and health care facilities.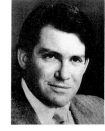

Dr W.L. Ruff, born in Columbia, South Carolina, USA, in 1938, received a BS in chemistry from Hampton Institute, Hampton, Virginia, in 1960 and, subsequently, a PhD in biochemistry from Case Western Reserve University, Cleveland, Ohio, in 1970. After graduate school, he served as a Senior Fellow in Clinical Chemistry at the University of Washington Hospital and Harborview Medical Center, Seattle, Washington. He holds a Diploma from the American Board of Clinical Chemistry and is a Fellow of the National Academy of Clinical Biochemistry. Dr Ruff is currently Associate Director of Clinical Laboratories, Howard University Hospital, Washington, DC. He is also an Associate Professor of Pathology in the Howard University College of Medicine as well as being Safety Officer and Chairman of the Howard University Hospital Clinical Laboratories Safety Committee and member of the Howard University Hospital Safety Committee. For the past four years, he has been the American Association for Clinical Chemistry's (AACC) representative on the National Fire Protection Association (NFPA) Technical Committee 56C which writes the "Safety Standard for Laboratories in Health-Related Institutions". He has been a member of the AACC Safe Laboratory Practices Committee for eight years and has presented round table discussions on laboratory safety, participated in safety workshops and published articles on safety. He is also a member of the Division of Chemical Health and Safety of the American Chemical Society.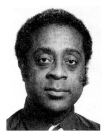

Dr E.J. Slater, CEng, MIERE, MIEE, who was born in Walsall, England in 1954, read electrical and electronic engineering at Nottingham University where he obtained a BSc degree with first class honours and subsequently a PhD for work on a blind mobility aid. He was registered as a Chartered Engineer in 1982. Currently, he is a Principal Medical Physicist in a large teaching hospital in Nottingham where he has responsibility for all aspects of electrical safety in laboratory and medical equipment. He has a number of publications in the field of medical electronics.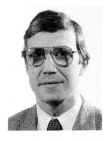

Mr J.H. Smith was born in Burton-upon-Trent in December 1941. He is a Fellow of the Institute of Medical Laboratory Sciences and worked for five years in the four major disciplines of pathology before specialising in clinical chemistry. He joined the Department of Clinical Chemistry at Birmingham General Hospital and was appointed Senior Chief MLSO in 1974. He is a part-time Lecturer and Examiner for the Fellowship Examination and his responsibilities include the position of Safety Officer, co-ordination of quality control and a special interest in analyses performed in ward areas. He has published 2 papers and a series of articles associated with reflectance meter performance.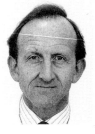

Professor D.M. Taylor, BSc (Liverpool), PhD (London), DSc (Liverpool), CChem, FRSC, MRCPath, was born in London, England in 1927. An initial training in biochemistry was followed by thirty years of research mainly in the field of radiation biochemistry, radiotoxicology and pathology. Formerly Senior Lecturer in Radiation Biochemistry and head of the Radiopharmacology Department, Institute of Cancer Research, University of London, since 1979 he has held the posts of Professor of Radiotoxicology at the University of Heidelberg and Director, Institute for Genetics and Toxicology, Kernforschungszentrum, Karlsruhe, Federal Republic of Germany. Professor Taylor has had many years of experience as a Radiation Safety Officer and as a member, or former member, of a number of local, national or international advisory committees in the field of radiation protection. He has more than 150 publications in scientific literature in the fields of biochemistry, radiation biology, cancer chemotherapy and radiotoxicology.

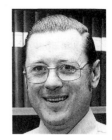

Dr R. Toynton was born in Crail, Scotland in 1952, and obtained a BSc(Hons) in Physical Geography and Geology from the University of Liverpool in 1974, followed by a PhD in groundwater pollution from the University of East Anglia, Norwich in 1979. During the period from 1979 to 1984, while Keeper of Natural Science in Scunthorpe Museum, in addition to fieldwork involved with this post, as a part-time tutor for extra-mural departments at the University of Hull and the University of Nottingham, he undertook a programme of geological expeditions with groups drawn from the general public. Since 1974, as lecturer in Earth Science with the Division of Continuing Education at the University of Sheffield, he has led a large number of such field courses in Britain and occasionally abroad. His present research is into flint formation and he has published a number of papers.

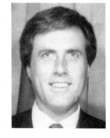

Dr D. Whelpton was born in Sheffield, England in 1938, where he obtained a BSc in physics and subsequently a PhD in medical electronics. He was employed in Sheffield and at the University Hospital of Wales, Cardiff, before moving to The Queen's Medical Centre, Nottingham. He currently serves on the UK committee for the safety of general medical electrical equipment and has a number of publications concerned with electrical safety as well as many other aspects of medical physics.

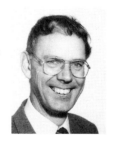

Dr A.R. Williams, born in Cardiff, Wales, UK, in 1944, obtained a BSc (Hons) degree in biochemistry, ancillary subjects being chemistry and physiology, from the University College of South Wales and Monmouthshire, Cardiff, Wales. He then held the post of Research Biochemist at the Velindre Memorial Hospital for Cancer Research, Cardiff, during which period he completed an MSc thesis. He was then appointed Research Associate at the Department of Microbiology, University College, Cardiff, and, whilst there, obtained a PhD degree with a thesis related to the biological effects of ultrasonic irradiation. His next appointment was as Lecturer in Biophysics at the Department of Anatomy, University of Manchester, followed by a year as a Visiting Scientist at the United States Food and Drug Administration, Washington, DC where his duties were to assist the Bureau of Radiological Health in their ultrasound bio-ha-

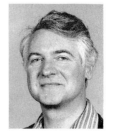

zards research programme and to help draft the performance standard for medical instrumentation emitting ultrasonic radiation. Dr Williams at present occupies the position of Senior Lecturer at the Department of Medical Biophysics, University of Manchester. In addition to this full-time post, he has been appointed Visiting Professor of Biophysics at the Department of Physiology and Biophysics, University of Southern California in Los Angeles and Visiting Professor of Physics at the Department of Physics, University of Vermont, for the duration of their periods of active collaboration. He is a founder member of the European Committee for Ultrasound Radiation Safety and is currently compiling and editing an Environmental Health Criteria Document on Ultrasound for the World Health Organization. He has also written a book on this topic which will be published by Academic Press and has a further 60 publications to his credit.

Dr A.E. Wright was born in Darlington, Co. Durham, England in 1923, and qualified in medicine at Durham University in 1948, taking the DPH in 1954 and the MD in 1957. He trained as a Microbiologist with the Public Health Laboratory Service, taking the Dip Bact at the London School of Hygiene and Tropical Medicine in 1958. He is presently Director of the Newcastle upon Tyne Regional Public Health Laboratory, Chairman of the PHLS Safety Committee and Member of the Safety Committee of the Association of Medical Microbiologists as well as Temporary Consultant to WHO on a number of technical committees on safety in laboratories. Dr Wright is the author of a number of articles and chapters on aspects of safety in the laboratory and the environment.

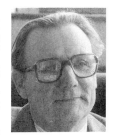

1 Organizing the Design of a Safe Laboratory

J.R. Robb

Given that the environment for scientific research plays a role integral with the realization of scientific advancement, it then becomes imperative that scientific facilities evolve as rapidly as, if not in advance of, the scientific community which they serve.

The degree to which the spatial environment suits the intended activity can have a great impact on the scope of scientific research, the efficiency with which it is performed, and the level of safety provided for both personnel and scientific data. It becomes the responsibility of the administrative authorities to manage the environment within which technical staff pursue their scientific goals.

PLANNING PHASE

Planning for the modification or construction of a scientific facility usually extends over a period of years, and requires complex compromises between service goals and financial resources. Consequently, it is essential that a Committee for Construction Planning and Coordination be formed as the initial step in a facility development programme.

It is important to realize that the planning and execution of a building programme is an evolutionary process and not a discrete task. The Committee responsible for facility development must have the longevity, or at least the mechanism for self-perpetuation, that will maintain a continuity of purpose throughout the time period required for realization of stated planning goals.

The Planning Committee should be composed of representatives from pertinent functional areas who have the qualifications and authority to make policy decisions. As Committee members, ex officio authorities and interested patrons introduce unquantifiable variables into the planning equation.

1

The Committee should include only individuals responsible for the consequences of their planning decisions, and only those individuals necessary for a fair representation of the major concerns.

This is not to state that the needs and desires of the individual user should be ignored. The Committee has a responsibility to seek out and identify these needs. When gathered at the appropriate time, and utilized as design determinants, this input becomes the data necessary to produce the only satisfactory solution to the planning equation.

The planning phase should begin with the development of a master plan for facility development. A master plan is a written document which makes specific statements regarding the scope of present and future activity, and the role of the facility within its community. These statements are usually related to 'business plans' describing service level need and the revenue streams required to support the projected activity. The plan contains explicit statements of institutional mission and the purpose behind facility development. A document of this scope should include representative opinions from all relevant areas of management and operations.

Efficient compilation of the document requires a well designed process of interview, data consolidation, management review and ratification. The following figure illustrates key issues and 'decision points' typically found in the master planning process.

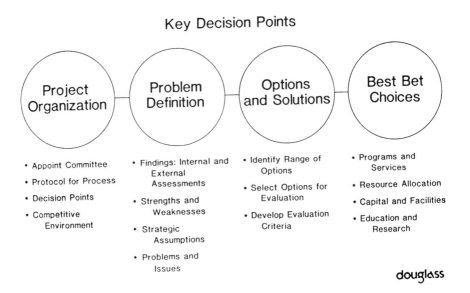

Key Decision Points

Project Organization

- Appoint Committee
- Protocol for Process
- Decision Points
- Competitive Environment

Problem Definition

- Findings: Internal and External Assessments
- Strengths and Weaknesses
- Strategic Assumptions
- Problems and Issues

Options and Solutions

- Identify Range of Options
- Select Options for Evaluation
- Develop Evaluation Criteria

Best Bet Choices

- Programs and Services
- Resource Allocation
- Capital and Facilities
- Education and Research

douglass

Figure 1.1

2

The process concludes with the formal adoption of the master plan as the elemental criteria against which all planning options are evaluated. Whether existing *a priori* or developed in process, the master plan provides the framework for future Planning Committee discussions.

Often, it is advantageous for the Planning Committee to seek the advice of an independent consultant to facilitate master plan development and subsequent planning discussions. Such individuals can provide unbiased opinions regarding the proposed scope of services, efficiency of construction methods, and industry standards for utilization of scientific facilities.

Facility utilization

Laboratory space requirements can usually be defined in terms of workload, personnel or equipment. The objective of a facility utilization review is to identify those characteristics of a specific laboratory operation which generate requirements for space. By comparing current or projected levels of service, staff or technology to planning standards, operational efficiencies and overall space requirements can be determined.

A utilization review can be approached through identification of those activities which represent 80–90% of the laboratory workload. Associated with these activities will be personnel and equipment. When possible, activities should be grouped according to procedural similarities and service requirements. Special procedures, requiring unusual amounts of facility resources, are noted separately. The procedural and service requirements for future activities should be described as completely as possible. With this data, a laboratory planner can project requirements for space which can be justified by historic and projected utilization.

Empirical data, from a broad range of existing facilities, have been used to develop statistical models which relate workload volume to square feet of space required. As utilization standards, these models quantify the amount of space required to perform various types of activities. Aggregates of space requirements, dictated by specific work programmes, can be translated into departmental area requirements. By definition, prototypical activities cannot be analysed by applying historical data. When practical, it is suggested that total space requirements be developed through aggregation of data describing relevant subtask components of the prototypical activity.

Statistical analysis provides an initial approach to the relationship between projected workload and physical space. Potential difficulties with reuse of existing space begin to become apparent. The scope of the building programme can then be tentatively established.

3

Existing facilities

For existing facilities, planning consists of achieving the spatial modifications necessary in order to meet the requirements imposed by changing technology and scientific technique.

Often, the available space is of inappropriate proportion. Inadequate floor to ceiling height can have an impact on the specific type of equipment as well as revision to mechanical services that will be required by the proposed research. Research and Development departments that are forced to operate within a series of small laboratory spaces may find the scope of their activities limited by inconvenient adjacencies, and their overall efficiency impaired.

The space available may be of inconvenient location. The hazardous nature of proposed research can create undesirable adjacencies between departmental areas. Unacceptable conflicts can be created with regard to the logistics of waste removal, materials supply, and personnel movement.

Inflexibilities inherent to the existing construction type can limit the uses of the space available. The presence of structural or mechanical elements may prevent consolidation of spaces suitable for departmental use. Relocation of departments to facilitate operational considerations may not be feasible due to the expense required for demolition and renovation.

Institutional operating budgets place constraints on the abilities of the administration to incorporate new services or technological advancements. Services provided and research performed may become dependent on short-term cost-effectiveness. Economic realities force the administration to balance the incorporation of change within the operating budgets of cost and profit centres alike.

New facilities

In the planning of a new facility, similar considerations should be given to space proportion, zoning of departmental adjacencies, flexibilities of construction type, and cost per square foot. Planning a new facility creates the additional responsibility of making decisions which will impose constraints on the decision-making process for the life of the facility.

The planning phase should begin with the development of a master plan for facility development. A master plan is a written document which makes specific statements regarding the scope of present and future activity, and the role of the facility within its community. The master plan contains explicit statements of purpose regarding facility development. It should be formally adopted as the elemental criteria by which all planning options are evaluated. Whether existing *a priori* or developed in-process, the master plan provides the framework for future Planning Committee discussions.

4

Often, it is advantageous for the Planning Committee to seek the advice of an independent consultant to facilitate these discussions. Such individuals can provide the Committee with unbiased opinions regarding the proposed scope of services, efficiency of construction methods, and industry standards for utilization of scientific facilities.

Utilization standards have been developed which quantify the amount of space required to perform various types of activities. Empirical data from existing facilities have been used to develop statistical models which relate work-load volume to square feet of space required. Aggregates of space requirements, dictated by specific work programmes, can be translated into departmental area requirements. By definition, prototypical activities cannot be analysed by applying historical data. If applicable, it is suggested that space requirements be developed through analysis of data regarding component sub-tasks.

The objective of workload analysis is to project requirements for space which can be justified with substantiating data. In addition, workload analysis begins to relate intended activity to physical space. Potential difficulties with re-use of existing space begin to become apparent. The scope of the building programme can be tentatively established.

The planning phase should have as its product an architectural space programme. This document should contain the master plan statement, statistics used in the decision-making process, and projections of space requirements based on the proposed type and level of activity to be supported. The architectural space programme documents criteria relative to the concept, form, function, and needs of the proposed facility. It acts as a useful tool throughout the design phase.

DESIGN PHASE

Although it may continue well into construction, the design phase is generally thought of as having three distinctly separate activities. They are: schematic design, design development, and construction document preparation.

Schematic design

Here the principal concern is with the organization of departmental areas as they relate to each other. Important adjacencies are identified. The flow of materials and personnel is analysed. The relationships between departmental subunits are loosely defined. Only the most general determinants of departmental location and function are discussed at the level of schematic design. The product of this activity should be schematic floor plans. These diagrams outline department areas and identify zones of related activity within the scope of the project.

Functional narratives are written descriptions of departmental operations. They should be written in non-technical language. Functional narratives provide an administrator or consultant with a general description of the mechanics surrounding specific technical procedures. Separate descriptions should be developed for proposed technical activity. The functional narrative should make specific reference to hazardous procedures and materials. The schematic floor plans and functional narratives should be discussed and formally adopted by the members of the Planning Committee. These documents may be used to develop preliminary construction budgets and estimates of project cost. The space programme, schematic floor plans, functional narratives, and estimates of project cost become a body of information often referred to as a 'Design Development Handbook'

Design development

The gathering of detailed information is now of primary concern. It is suggested that the Planning Committee form subcommittees organized around operational areas. Every functional and organizational aspect of the project should be analysed.

The physical details of the spatial environment can be more easily identified if the space is subdivided into areas referred to as 'work stations'. Work stations are spatial volumes in which specific activities occur. Every activity places service requirements on its supporting space. When a laboratory is subdivided into areas of activity it facilitates the task of determining what specific requirements will be placed upon the space by the proposed activity. Table 1.1 presents a checklist of requirements that are commonly associated with the work space. The requirements of each work station should be compared to a similar list. Special consideration should be given to areas supporting proposed prototypical activities.

Safety in the laboratory may be thought of as it relates to the safety of laboratory occupants, equipments, and data. Table 1.1 also contains attributes which relate to these aspects of laboratory safety.

Laboratory organization should take into consideration the occupational hazards involved with the handling of dangerous materials. Work areas which support the use or storage of radioactive waste should be planned in order that waste materials may be conveniently removed from the laboratory while minimizing the risk of exposure to laboratory personnel. Similar consideration should be given to the removal of biohazardous waste.

If it is necessary that the bulk storage of gases occur within the laboratory, then the designated area should be located at an exterior wall. Areas for the storage of gases should receive maximum fire protection. Light switches and fixtures should be of explosion-proof design. Anchoring devices should be provided in order that gas cylinders may be held firmly in place.

Table 1.1 Work station attribute requirements

General data	Architectural requirements	Plumbing requirements
Floor area (nsf)	Ceiling construction	Cold water
Minimum dimension (feet)	Lay-in (acoustical)	Hot water
Ceiling height (feet)	Plaster	Filtration
Occupants	Gypsum	Temperature control
Remarks	Integrated system	De-ionized water
	Metal panel	Distilled water
Special problems	Exposed	Steam
Odours	Remarks	Compressed air
Static electricity	Wall finishes	Medical air
Vibration sensitive	Plaster	Vacuum suction
Flammable or explosive	High strength plaster	Oxygen
materials	Liquid glazed coating	Nitrogen
Corrosive materials	Paint	Nitrous oxide
Volatile liquids	Wall covering	CO_2
Toxic reagents	Tile (full height)	Lab. gas
Infectious materials	Tile (wainscot)	Floor drain
Radio frequency interference	Exposed	Acid waste
Ionizing radiation	Remarks	Emergency shower
Radioactive materials	Base type	Remarks
X-rays	Straight	
Remarks	Cove	**Electrical requirements**
	Integral w/floor	Lighting level (f.c.)
Architectural requirements	Remarks	Lighting type
Special room requirements	Floor type	General
Radiation shielding	Resilient	Special
R/F shielding	Vitreous	Rheostat dimmer
Fire rated	Seamless	Emergency power
Acoustical requirements	Water resistant	Special purpose outlets
Sound trans. class	Conductive	Emergency lighting
Sound proofing	Concrete	Ground fault interrupters
Space enclosure	Carpet	Special grounding system
4-wall	Remarks	Explosion proof
4-wall w/Control		Clock system
3-wall	**Structural requirements**	Remarks
Visual requirements	Floor live load	
View out (exterior)	Suspended live load	**Communication**
View in	Special wall reinforcement	Telephone
Operable sash/vent	Floor penetration, chases	Pay telephone
Vision control	Depressed floor	Intercom
Blackout	(w/lightweight infill)	Sound system
Door type	Remarks	Nurse call intercom
Store front		T.V. antenna outlet
Solid core	**Mechanical requirements**	C.C.T.V. outlet
Hollow metal	Heat and ventilation	Data process, terminal
Vision panel	Ventilation only	Security alarm
Roll-up	Air conditioning	Doctor's register

7

Dutch
Other
Door width (inches)
  36"
  48"
  Other
Partition construction
  Metal study w/gyp. bd.
  Metal study w/gyp. lath.
  Masonry
  Solid plaster
  Demountable
  Folding
Remarks

Temperature (F.db)
Relative humidity
Room temperature control
Room humidity control
Room pressure
Total air changes/hour
Outside air changes/hour
Recirculation permitted
Exhaust
Special exhaust
Air filter effic. (pre) (%)
Air filter effic. (final) (%)
Remarks

Bed availability
Emergency call
Remarks

Fire protection
Portable extinguisher
Automatic sprinkler
Smoke detection
Fire Alarm system
Special automatic
extinguisher
Remarks

Material handling
Pneumatic tube
Automated
Remarks

Laboratory construction should provide adequate fire separations between areas of high and low hazard. Wall construction and protection for wall openings should provide reasonable protection from and containment of fire. In large spaces, where travel distance to exits is extended, it is advisable to provide 'fire and smoke partitions'. These partitions compartmentalize the laboratory, and help contain the fire. They also create areas of 'safe refuge'; through which personnel may exit to safety. Materials used for laboratory finishes should have low ratings for flame spread and smoke production.

Laboratory furnishings should include cabinets designed to store solvents and reagents. Ventilated flammable storage cabinets should be used to accommodate solvents. Impervious linings should be used in cabinets where corrosive reagents are stored.

Laboratory fixtures, intended for emergency use, should be provided in quantities sufficient for location within close proximity to all work stations. Deluge showers and emergency eyewashes must be available in order that immediate attention may be given to chemical spills. Fire extinguishers and fire blankets must be close at hand in the event of an incendiary accident. Fume hoods and biological safety cabinets should be provided in locations which are equipped with sterilizing light fixtures. When exhaust ductwork from exhaust hoods is combined into a general exhaust system, automatic dampers, with alarms, must be provided to signal the event of a mechanical failure.

Special consideration must be given to the design and installation of laboratory mechanical systems. Exterior louvres, provided for the intake and exhaust of air for mechanical ventilating systems, must be carefully placed in order to assure the safety of the air being used for ventilation. Air conditioning systems must be balanced to provide the pressurization levels required to prevent the spread of infection.

8

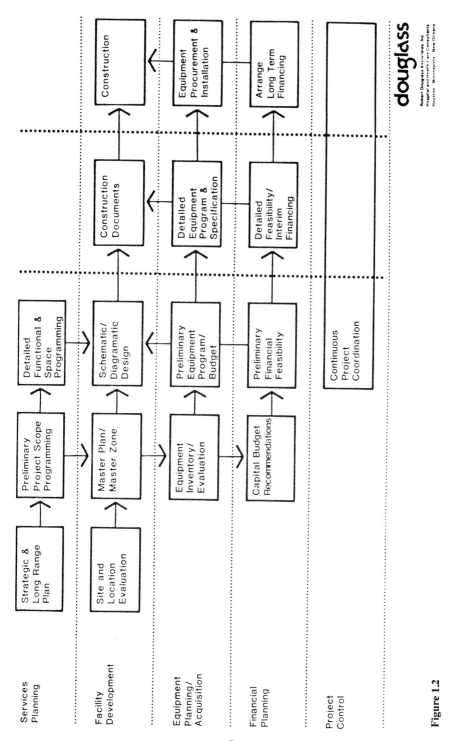

Figure 1.2

9

Emergency lighting fixtures, with independent sources of power, must be available to accomplish a safe evacuation in the event of total darkness.

Plumbing systems should include special piping and neutralization basins for the proper disposal of corrosive wastes. Lavatory station faucets should be provided with vacuum breakers. This precaution avoids the possibility of accidentally syphoning specimens into the water system via rubber tubing attached to the spigot.

Fire alarm systems should include both smoke detectors, and audible and visual alarm signals. Alarm 'pull stations' should be provided in easily accessible locations. Alarm lights and horns must be visible from all areas of the laboratory.

Protection of both personnel and equipment becomes paradoxical when considering the appropriate automatic fire-extinguishing system. Automatic sprinkling systems are relatively inexpensive to install. They can provide effective protection in an 'open plan' laboratory. However, technical equipment can be severely damaged by the water used to protect the laboratory occupants. The protection of laboratory equipment can be achieved by the provision of systems using inert gases. However, these systems require confined areas in order to be effective. This requirement precludes the amenities and efficiencies to be gained by 'open planning' of laboratory areas. A practical compromise may be reached by the development of 'equipment laboratories'. These areas may use inert gas systems for fire protection. General testing areas might use automatic sprinkling systems.

Testing equipment, particularly computerized equipment, must be protected from the electrical system which serves the laboratory. The provision of protection for computerized equipment also helps protect test data.

In the event of a sudden power failure much data can be lost. Consequently emergency power systems must be provided. Testing equipment is not usually damaged by the loss of power. However, a sudden resurgence of power can overload sensitive circuits. Whether or not power loss is anticipated, the provision of 'constant voltage transformers' is required for protection of both equipment and data from irregularities in electrical service.

Checklists, such as Table 1.1, are essential as communication devices. Questionnaires, hypothetical procedure outlines, and group discussions are other means that can also prove useful. All practical approaches should be utilized to ensure that the project has been properly researched. It is equally important to ensure that all functional groups have the opportunity to propose methods for improving their environment and performance.

Equipment planning is a separate, but no less important, aspect of the design development phase. Equipment plays a determining role in the functional and organizational reality of the scientific facility. Often, specialized equipment requires specialized spaces. The type of space required by a specific item of equipment can have a significant impact on project planning. Equipment manufacturers are good sources of equipment planning information. It is advisable to use a disinterested third party as intermediary between equipment manufacturers and the technical staff. This approach avoids confusion between products and inefficient use of technical personnel while giving fair consideration to the available equipment options. The product of the design development phase should include project meeting minutes, equipment lists, and architectural drawings. These documents compose the final chapter of the Design Development Handbook, and provide the information necessary for preparation of the construction documents.

Construction documents

Just as a photograph is a representation of an existing reality, construction documents (architectural plans and specifications) are representations of a future reality. The nature of the existing reality is interpreted from the photograph. The nature of the future reality must be interpreted from the information contained in the construction of documents. The accuracy of the physical reality depends upon the accuracy of the information, and the accuracy of its interpretation via the construction process.

CONSTRUCTION PHASE

Through construction document preparation and the subsequent construction phase, it is necessary that one or more Planning Committee members remain actively involved with the project. Revisions to code requirements, current availability of specific materials or equipment, and numerous unforeseen considerations will require direction from an administrator with the authority to make decisions for the Planning Committee and the technical staff.

The construction process will also require approval of budget expenditures and construction work at various stages of completion. The performance of continuous project administration during the period required for project completion should be seen as corollary to the function of project planning.

EVALUATION PHASE

Evaluation of the planning and construction process should result in documentation that can function as a process outline for subsequent planning efforts. It should contain a description of the planning process used, a list of programmed assumptions, and a presentation of pertinent statistics. It should make specific recommendations regarding effective approaches to future projects. As appendices, the document may include a copy of the Design Development Handbook.

CONCLUSION

The planning and construction of scientific facilities is a complex process. It attempts to define unforeseeable requirements for functional organization and occupational safety.

The process requires the conscientious participation of many individuals, with differing technical backgrounds, who interact in various capacities, over a long period of time. Large quantities of disparate information must be managed, compared, and consolidated.

The administration who undertakes a programme of facility development should be cognizant of human and technical resources required. These resources will be temporarily unavailable for normal scientific endeavours. Contingency plans should be developed to compensate for operational inefficiencies imposed by the planning process.

Before knowing the goal, an administration must create the process which will assure its achievement.

Literature consulted

Life Safety Code Handbook, 2nd edn. National Fire Protection Association, Quincy, MA, 1981
National Fire Code, Vol. 4, Chap. 56C. Safety Standards for Laboratories in Health Related Institutions. National Fire Protection Association, Quincy, Massachussets, 1981
Uniform Building Code. International Conference of Building Officials, Whittier, California, 1976

2 Electrical Safety Measures and Standards for Laboratory Facilities and Equipment in Hospitals

E.J. Slater and D. Whelpton

INTRODUCTION

Over the last 20 years or so there has been a dramatic increase in the use of electronic equipment in all walks of life, and medical electronics in particular has been the subject of much development. This growth has resulted in acceptance by the general public of electricity as an essential part of living and working. An unfortunate consequence of this familiarity is a lessening of respect for a commodity which, whilst extremely useful, is potentially lethal.

The aim of this chapter, in reviewing the particular situations found in the hospital environment, is to identify the risks resulting from electrical equipment and installations and to suggest some ways of reducing them. Because it is not possible to cover in detail all types of installation or equipment the discussion is deliberately general and applicable to a wide range of laboratories and other rooms in which electrical power is used.

The chapter naturally falls into two parts: the first considers the working environment as a whole, and the second looks in detail at the requirements for medical equipment safety. However, before either of these aspects can be considered it will be useful to take a brief look at the effect of electrical current on the body.

PHYSIOLOGICAL EFFECTS OF ELECTRICAL CURRENT

The body uses electrical signals in the form of nerve impulses to transmit information and exercise control over its components. When an external electric current is passed through the body it divides into an infinite number of routes between the point of entry and that of exit. The main physiological effect of this current is that normal neural action will be disrupted if sufficient current flows through the nerve fibres. This is particularly important when the fibres concerned are associated with the functioning of the heart or respiratory system.

It is important to appreciate that the level of physiological effect is directly related to the magnitude of the current flowing and not to the voltage driving that current. That is, with a given potential, the quality of the connection to the body is the important factor in determining the physiological effect. Normal dry skin is covered in a layer of dead skin cells and presents a relatively high resistance (> 100 kΩ) to current flow. However, this value is significantly reduced if the surface layer is rubbed away or if the skin surface is soaked with conducting fluid. Connection to the power source by moist, large area contacts (such as sweating hands) is, therefore, worse than a glancing contact via dry skin. Deliberate electrical contact to the skin for the purposes of measuring body potentials (ECG, EEG, etc) can achieve a contact resistance as low as 1 kΩ and, therefore, present a particular risk.

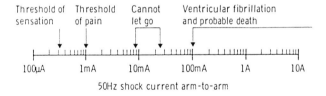

Figure 2.1 Typical physiological effects of electric current

The other major factor determining the physiological effect at a given amplitude is the frequency of the current. Most nerve pulses involved in muscle control occur at relatively low frequencies, largely below 100 Hz. Only higher level neural signals (mainly the visual and auditory systems) have significant components at higher frequencies, and even these are limited to a few kilohertz. Because of this the neural pathways of the body are specifically adapted to handle these frequencies and hence maximum disruption results from currents of about the same frequency. It is an unfortunate fact of life that the frequency of power distribution in most countries (50–60 Hz), fixed by numerous technical as well as historical factors, happens to be around the frequency at which the maximum physiological effect is obtained.

There has been much work carried out to determine the levels of current

14

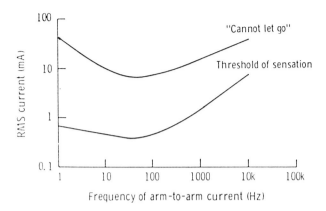

Figure 2.2 Variation of physiological effect of electric current with frequency (typical values)

at which certain identifiable effects occur. Although there are many different opinions as to the detailed values involved, there is a broad consensus on the general levels. Figure 2.1 shows diagrammatically the effects of 50–60 Hz current passing from one arm to the other in an average adult, while Figure 2.2 shows the typical variation of sensation threshold with changing frequency under similar conditions.

Another factor which plays some part in determining physiological effect is the current density where the contact is made to the body. This is because the way the current distributes itself within the body tissue will be influenced by the area of the external contacts. High current densities at the contacts will also result in localized heating effects and possibly burns. This effect, together with the insensitivity of the neural system to high frequency electrical signals is the basis of surgical diathermy. For this technique high currents at frequencies above 500 kHz are used to separate tissue, and control bleeding, by passing the current through a small area electrode at the operating site and through a large area electrode elsewhere on the body.

It is obvious that the important threshold levels are those actually measured on the vulnerable body components. When passing current directly into the muscles of the heart, for instance, the threshold for producing ventricular fibrillation at 50–60 Hz is generally below 100 μA. The importance of this value will become apparent in later discussions on permissible limits for leakage currents.

PART 1: LABORATORY FACILITIES

General aspects of laboratory safety

No matter how safe equipment may be when considered in isolation, if the basic working situation creates a shock hazard then an unsafe condition still exists. In this sense electric shock is no different from any other hazard, and the risk of it happening is increased by a number of environmental and operational factors. These factors are equally applicable to all types of laboratory.

Lighting

The provision of adequate lighting of an appropriate type is paramount to a safe working environment. Whatever the type of work being undertaken the ability to see clearly and easily what is going on has a strong influence on the safety of the situation. Workers who have to peer and crane their heads forward or reposition themselves to obtain better light increase the danger of accidental contact with dangerous parts.

The type of lighting is also important. Wherever possible the maximum use should be made of natural light. Apart from its suitability to illuminate well at low cost, the contact it provides with the outside world has a beneficial psychological effect which will itself contribute to safe working. However, even where natural light is readily available, there should be adequate provision for artificial background illumination over the whole working area. This is normally best achieved by the use of 'cold' fluorescent discharge tubes. These provide even illumination efficiently and are relatively shadow free. A minimum overall level of 150 lux should be provided in the work area.

However, except where the work being carried out is of a superficial level, additional local lighting, in the form of adjustable spot lamps, for instance, will be required to aid close work on a bench. These should raise the level of illumination to around 300 lux. As a general rule these lights should operate on low voltage supplies either locally and out of reach of the operator, or distributed from a central location. Similar power supply considerations apply to microscope lamps.

Environment

It is important to ensure than an adequate air temperature is maintained and that draught-free ventilation is provided. Once again, discomfort on the part of the worker may well lead to an unsafe situation: the propping up of a baffle to block a draught or the wearing of extra, inappropriate clothing are examples of unsafe remedies.

The subject of humidity is somewhat more difficult. Relatively few pieces of laboratory equipment are protected against high atmospheric humidity and it is certainly important that, aside from the point of view of comfort, the atmosphere should be nowhere near condensing and preferably kept to around 30–40% R.H.

Layout

A common difficulty is that a laboratory is rarely large enough or correctly shaped for its purpose, and lack of space often leads to inherent problems of safety. Although it is impossible to lay down rules for all situations, there are some important points which must be considered.

One of the biggest problems is that of providing adequate, easily accessible, storage for equipment, components, data etc, whilst providing easy access without compromising the work area.

From a safety point of view it is desirable to specify storage areas after the allocation of work areas, but it is seldom possible to treat the planning of space in such a detached fashion. In most instances all the pressures on space will be considered together and a certain amount of compromise is likely. However, there are particular standards for certain types of storage which must be considered. The storage of corrosive chemicals and inflammable or hazardous substances is obviously of prime importance not only from the inherent direct danger but also because of the hazards which they may introduce into electrical equipment. Corrosive fumes in the atmosphere may cause potentially dangerous damage to the inside of electrical equipment by weakening insulation or destroying protective connections.

Although the next section will deal with the delineation of types of activity and its influence on laboratory design, it is important to note that particular types of work require an allocation of space in order not to jeopardise safe working. For instance, it should not be necessary for a worker to carry out paperwork on one corner of a bench which has been designed for some other aspects of his work. This kind of situation can cause an electrical hazard by the introduction of extraneous equipment (pens, rulers, etc) into the work area.

Finally, on this subject, the different areas, once defined, should be clearly labelled. In some instances, as will be examined later, it may be necessary to divide the areas by doors or other barriers which should carry clear warnings and prohibitions. There is always a danger that a person unfamiliar with the workings of a particular laboratory may wander in. It is important either to provide them with sufficient warning of a hazard or to prohibit them from entry. In many cases frequent reminders to experienced personnel will not be wasted.

Types of work undertaken

Whilst the basic danger from electric shock exists in any situation where electrical equipment is being used, there are many gradations of risk spanning a wide range of work activities. For the present purpose the risks are divided into three main categories, and before looking in detail at safety precautions it is appropriate to consider the risk in each category.

Firstly, and perhaps most commonly, there is the laboratory situation where the primary work function is not electrical but where power is distributed around the laboratory and electrical equipment is routinely used for its intended purpose; that is, the equipment itself is not the subject of the investigation. This is the lowest risk category, although it probably presents the most diverse set of hazards. It is reasonable to assume that the workers in this type of laboratory have no specialized electrical knowledge. The greatest problem resulting from this is that electrical equipment may inadvertently be used for purposes, or in places, for which it was not intended. This places the onus of safe working on those responsible for the layout and design of the laboratory. This category covers the majority of hospital laboratories since virtually all modern techniques rely on the use of electrical equipment.

This category also includes situations where the primary work function is electrical but does not involve dismantling of equipment, a process which obviously creates greater risk and will, therefore, be considered separately. However, the risks may be relatively high since the work could involve deliberate contact with electrical equipment. The overall danger is reduced somewhat because the workers employed here will have some electrical knowledge and training and thus are more aware of the hazards and the ways of allaying them. The work could include routine calibration and functional checking, but not servicing or repairs. Development of electronic circuitry in a research setting where low voltage bench power supplies are used to provide power is another example of this type of work. However, in many situations work of this type is more easily categorized as the next type because of the difficulty of preventing routine calibration and checking turning into servicing.

The second category is much easier to identify. This includes laboratories intended for the testing and repairing of electrical apparatus containing exposed conductors at voltages in excess of 125 Vac or 250 Vdc, including the operation of the equipment under normal conditions but with any, or all, protective covers removed. This is the situation found in any electrical service department and calls for strict safety measures.

The third and final situation to be considered is the carrying out of electrical repair work on equipment which is fixed in a location not ordinarily provided with additional electrical safety features. This problem is encountered, for example with X-ray equipment, large automatic sampling devices etc, where the faulty item cannot be removed to the service area and repairs are carried out *in situ*.

Safety measures for hazardous situations

It is more convenient to first consider the ways of providing a safe working environment for areas which fall into the second category. In this way it is possible to see what methods are available, discuss their effectiveness, and use this knowledge later to assess the problems of the other situations. In order to achieve a safe working environment for the repair of electrical equipment it is necessary to provide the work bench area with positive protection against electrical shock risk. This approach is made in two stages. Firstly, any obvious risks inherent in the work area are removed, thereby ensuring that the remaining hazards are those associated with the actual work being carried out. Secondly, having reduced the risk to a definable level and type, all possible steps must be taken to limit the danger to the worker should he accidentally receive an electric shock. It is not possible in the type of work being considered here that there can ever be no risk: therefore, having reduced the risks to the lowest possible level, consideration must be given to making the situation as safe as possible should a shock occur.

The basic environment can be made safe by adopting some simple design rules. The aim of these rules is to prevent two possible causes of danger. The first is the danger of shock from a fault occurring elsewhere when the fault current is not safely directed to earth at the place of origin. Under these conditions the fault current may flow through the earth wiring of the work area, and, if this has a sufficiently high impedance, its potential will be raised. A person simultaneously touching this raised potential and a good earth would provide an alternative path for the fault current, thereby receiving an electric shock.

The second type of risk from the environment comes from unnecessary metalwork or conducting parts. In a situation where equipment may be operated in various states of disassembly with many electrical connections extended over the bench, then any extraneous metalwork merely creates an unnecessary risk of unintentional contacts.

So a good basic rule of work bench design is to use insulation. The bench itself should be made of insulating material (possibly laminate covered wood) with no accessible supporting metalwork. Much use is currently made of fast assembly metal framework to support bench tops and this is quite acceptable providing simple design measures are taken to prevent this material being exposed, bearing in mind the risks stated above. Similarly, all other extraneous metalwork should either be covered or replaced with insulating material. Particular attention should be paid to earthed metalwork including adjacent water pipes, radiators, electrical supply trunking and power socket boxes. One item which commonly causes problems is bench lighting. However, it is possible to obtain adjustable bench lights in which there is virtually no accessible metalwork. It is important to appreciate the reason for its existence when applying this 'metal-free' rule. It is not always possible to effect total covering of all metalwork, particularly when considering improvements to existing laboratories, when it may be necessary to exercise some judgement as to how this rule should be applied.

It is normally desirable to provide an insulating floor covering and, with modern flooring materials, this does not pose a particular problem. As an aside to the issue of electrical power shocks it is a sensible precaution to take steps to prevent the buildup of static electrical energy. Discharges from this source can be uncomfortable and unnerving: in some instances with delicate components or inflammable materials they can be dangerous. Some types of man-made fibre carpets can result in excessive static charges and the most practical solution is probably to utilize a vinyl type floor covering.

Similar comments to the above apply to the seating provided at the work bench. Whilst fulfilling an ergonomic need to prevent operator fatigue and resulting unsafe working, the seats provided should preferably be made of an insulating material which is not prone to static charge buildup.

Whilst on the subject of the safety of the working area, it should be noted that work benches provided for this type of work must not be supplied with either gas or water services. As stated earlier, work areas must be categorized by job function and any use of gas or water supplies must not take place in an area reserved for electrical repair work.

Having provided an inherently safe area for electrical work, attention must be given to the second requirement, that of protecting the worker in the event of an electrical shock. The main shock risk is the simultaneous touching of true earth and the live supply conductor; a situation for which it is relatively easy to provide protection. The shock risk that cannot be protected against is the simultaneous touching of the live supply wire and the supply return (or neutral). The shock current flowing in such a situation is no different from the normal equipment operating current and, therefore, cannot be recognized as an abnormal condition. Good working practice with adequate training is the only prevention.

The basis for protection against shock in the live-earth contact situation is the recognition that the shock current exists in addition to any normal power current. Current supplying correctly operating equipment flows conventionally from the live supply wire through the equipment and returns via the neutral return wire. Therefore, the currents in the live and neutral supply wires are essentially equal (see later for a discussion of equipment earth leakage current). If a worker touches live and earth he will cause a current to flow from the live wire which, because it goes to earth, does not return down the neutral return wire. So, the currents in the live and neutral wires are no longer equal. The difference in the two currents, which is assumed to be flowing to earth, is called 'earth leakage current' or 'residual current'.

Devices are available, known as 'earth leakage circuit breakers' (ELCB), or 'residual current circuit breakers' (RCCB), which are able to detect the current difference and, when the difference reaches a certain preset level, disconnect the supply automatically. Such a device represents the minimum level of protection required in this category of work area. It has a fast response time (10 ms) and, with a trip limit of 5 mA, will allow minimal risk and discomfort to the unfortunate person receiving the shock.

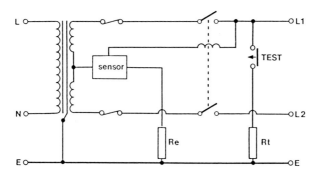

Figure 2.3 Suggested use of an isolation transformer with earth fault current detection and limit. The values of the limiting resistor *Re*, the test load *Rt* and the fault sensor are selected to give the appropriate sensitivity

Improved protection is obtained by using an isolating transformer which includes not only an ELCB but also fault current limiting so that the operator cannot receive even a transient peak shock current of a dangerous level before the ELCB operates. In Figure 2.3 the isolating transformer has a secondary winding with a centre tapping which provides the earth reference terminal so that each power line at the bench presents a potential of only half the supply voltage with reference to ground. At a given body contact resistance, this reduces the possible shock currents by a half. The resistance, *Re*, in the earth return lead is included to limit the fault current to a value which is only slightly in excess of the ELCB trip current.

One criticism of isolating transformers is that they need to be rated to operate with a nominal power transfer not exceeding about 75% of their rating in order to prevent power waveform distortion and the creation of a 'noisy' power supply. In critical applications even further derating may be necessary.

The best solution to this problem is to provide a separate isolating transformer for each workbench so that the total power throughput required is kept to a minimum. This also has the advantage of providing each worker with their own protection so that a fault on one bench does not cause power loss to any other. A sudden loss of power and, even worse, its reinstatement by someone else, is in itself dangerous. Each worker must retain control of his own bench supply, and separate supply units are the easiest way of achieving this.

The bench must also be provided with visual indication (a red light for example) that power is 'on' and also a quick, easy means of cutting off the power. An 'emergency stop' button is preferable to having to throw a circuit breaker. This button could also be the 'test' button shown in Figure 2.3, thus providing a test of the ELCB each time the bench power is switched off.

Each work station, equipped as described above, must be physically isolated from any adjacent benches, whatever their function. The particular protection provided on a bench is totally wasted if the 'protected' worker can make physical contact with either an unprotected area or even another protected area. This type of contact is referred to as 'handshaking' for obvious reasons, but it may include the passing of tools and need not even involve another person.

Such isolation can be achieved either by physical separation of the benches so that simultaneous contact of two work stations can not be made, or by the provision of barriers. In many situations, physical separation is not possible because of space limitations and the second solution is the one which has to be adopted. Such barriers must be made of insulating material and should preferably be transparent. This provides maximum distribution of light and also enables visual contact between workers, both essential for safe working. There are numerous non-flammable materials available for this purpose.

One remaining feature which offers prevention rather than cure is to provide each bench with an adequate number of power sockets. This removes the need for adaptors and long lengths of cable, both of which are common causes of electrical faults. Recommendations about the layout of the bench are not appropriate to this discussion: the particular needs of the work and the amount and shape of the space available are the prime considerations when layout is considered. However, the basic rule is to provide as much space as possible. Consider shelving above the bench to carry equipment which is in constant use as this avoids cluttering of the main bench area. As mentioned earlier, each worker should be provided with adequate storage space for tools etc., and any necessary paperwork. It cannot be stressed too much how important such considerations are for a safe working environment.

Less critical situations

The situation described above investigates safety measures for the most hazardous electrical situation found in hospital laboratories. However, the vast majority of situations will not carry risks as great as these and will fall into the 'lesser risk' category. Here it is possible to provide an adequate level of protection at a reduced capital cost. The main problem with laboratory situations whose primary work function is not electrical is that other processes, commonly involving the use of liquids, are carried on in the vicinity of electrical equipment. Some equipment is specifically designed to work in these situations and is protected against spillage. The risk is greater when miscellaneous electrical equipment is used which has no inherent protection. Often, items such as oscilloscopes, signal generators and bench top computers have a permanent home in the laboratory.

The basic rules for design are the same as discussed in the previous section. A generally insulated environment provides some protection against earth fault shocks and lessens the danger of a good earth contact should the worker touch a live supply. Also, the general guidelines concerning lighting, the adequate provision of power supply sockets, storage space and work areas still apply. Adoption of this 'safe environment' policy will provide adequate protection in most instances in this type of laboratory.

However, there are a few other precautions which should be considered highly desirable and which, at relatively low cost, will provide a much improved level of protection. In any work area where electrical power is used, some visual indication that the power is on is both desirable and easy to provide. An 'emergency off' switch should also be considered although there is unlikely to be a need for one at each work station. In principle, a single 'off' switch for each laboratory, clearly labelled and preferably sited near the exit, will suffice unless the laboratory is particularly large, when division into smaller areas may be appropriate, or equipment is present which should normally be continuously powered. This latter situation requires a separate 'off' switch with 'power on' indication and clear labelling stating the risks of turning off.

Even in the domestic environment there is an increasing trend to recommend the use of ELCBs for added protection. This is because they offer a high level of protection at a low cost and the variety and number of electrical appliances used is increasing. Much the same arguments can be put forward in the laboratory situation being considered here. The best protection will be gained by providing each work station with an ELCB. This has the added advantage of not affecting other workers should it be tripped.

Servicing and repairing in a non-electrical department

Often it is necessary to repair and service equipment which, by virtue of its size, weight or installation, cannot be moved from its normal environment. This poses serious problems for the service engineer who does not have the protection provided in the workshop and who may have to work with a number of electrically untrained staff in attendance. However, even in such circumstances it is possible to recommend procedures which will significantly reduce the risks involved.

Firstly, the person carrying out the work should be accompanied by another person whose level of electrical competence will depend on the work being carried out. In cases where there is no danger of contact with conductors at voltages in excess of 125 Vac or 250 Vdc then help may be expected from a non-technical but responsible person, possibly a member of the staff who uses the equipment. Their function is merely to be able to disconnect the mains supply in the event of an accident and to summon help. This assistance does not necessarily involve full-time attention by the accompanying person. In situations where exposure to higher voltages is possible then the accompanying person should be expected to have a level of technical competency which is greater as the risk increases. Indeed, it is likely that, in particularly hazardous situations, both the workers involved will have a similar level of electrical knowledge. In the UK, guidance on this matter has been issued by the DHSS.

Secondly, the area around the equipment being repaired should have clear notices informing other people of the dangers and prohibiting access. Here the engineer has a heavy responsibility for the safety of others who cannot be expected to appreciate all the risks.

It may be possible to make use of a portable isolation transformer and ELCB to improve the level of protection provided. Indeed, the use of such equipment in a low risk situation may reduce the requirement for an accompanying person to regular but intermittent visits.

Summary

None of the safety measures discussed here is any substitute for an adequate level of training and suitable supervision. Each department must make and enforce a set of rules and procedures for safe working. Adherence to these rules should be as much a matter of pride as is any other aspect of good workmanship.

One other part of training which must not be overlooked is that of first aid. Assuming that the above guidelines are implemented then it is unlikely that anyone will have to deal with a case of electric shock. This makes it all the more important to ensure that people will know what to do should such an unfortunate situation arise, and this may involve regular refresher courses on artificial resuscitation in particular.

It is unfortunate that no single standard exists to cover the areas discussed so far, and many of those often quoted are inappropriate in one way or another. This makes it more difficult to achieve a uniform level of safety because much has to be left to local decisions. It is to be hoped that an increased awareness of the dangers and any resulting discussions will lead to the formulation of an appropriate safety standard. This process has already taken place in relation to equipment safety in the hospital environment, as the second part of the chapter will show.

PART 2: SAFETY OF MEDICAL ELECTRICAL EQUIPMENT
Equipment hazards in hospitals

Many of the electrical hazards to be found in hospitals are comparable with those in other industries or in the domestic environment. The risk to the operators of clinical chemistry analysers, medical computers or ECG recorders is not made greater because they are operated within the hospital environment. However, the latter type of equipment introduces a different class of risk - that of risk not to the operator, but to the patient. Even in the simple case of a patient in normal health having an ECG recording made, the scale of hazard is immensely increased because it is necessary to make a good electrical connection to the patient, taking all acceptable steps to minimize the body's first stage of protection - the resistance offered by dry intact skin. Thus the skin surface is cleaned and prepared before an electrode, often with a conductive gel, is either stuck or strapped to the patient. Whilst such procedures are necessary if biopotentials of approximately 1 mV or less are to be measured and recorded, the consequences in terms of the safety standards necessary to avoid electrical hazards are considerable. The scale of the problem increases still further if the patient is anaesthetized, as he is then unable to record pain. In extreme cases the patient may have received drugs to remove muscle contractions, in which case yet another sign of the passage of electricity through the body is made much less sensitive! The ultimate in hazard is when electrical connection is made directly into the heart. In this instance the right ventricle is the most sensitive chamber, and reports have been published of currents of a few microamps producing ventricular fibrillation - uncontrolled and ineffective 'fluttering' of the heart, which would normally lead rapidly to death.

In addition to the extreme situations quoted there is much equipment which will be used with patients but without intimate electrical contact. Similarly there are devices which may be used in the patient environment, possible in conjunction with equipment connected to the patient. This category can include computers and other data collection equipment which may not be sold specifically as medical equipment.

As the range of equipment in the health care environment continues to increase, other hazards also become apparent. Throughout this century there has been a growing awareness of the hazards of ionizing radiations. In addition to equipment generating such radiations the last decade or two has seen widening applications of non-ionizing radiations in medicine covering, in particular, shortwave and microwave electromagnetic radiation, ultra-violet, visible, infrared light, including laser applications, and ultrasonic systems. Other equipment is designed to lift, position or manipulate patients, when mechanical hazards may also exist. Some equipment is designed for use in hazardous environments – either in explosive or inflammable atmospheres or in particularly moist or other difficult conditions. Despite the overall emphasis placed on electrical hazards, there is a wide range of requirements which must be met by medical electrical equipment if that equipment is to function in a way which is safe both for the operator and the patient. Whilst the electrical requirements have been of particular concern for some years, they cannot and must not be seen in total isolation.

Development of standards

As the quantity and complexity of medical equipment has grown, so too has the search for satisfactory standards. The medical equipment market is very much an international market, and the need for interrelated, if not unified, international standards is clear. However, standards normally grow from local perceived needs and different countries react in different ways to similar problems. Over the years a number of European countries have produced their own standards for differing parts of the range of medical electrical equipment. In the United States the pressures were somewhat different, and the approach, particularly of listing equipment by the Underwriters Labora-tory, was significantly different from the European solution of producing constructional guidelines which were supported to varying degrees. In the United Kingdom guidance was issued in 1963 in Hospital Technical Memo-randum 8, Safety Code for Electro-Medical Equipment. The intention of the document was defined in its opening clause as follows:

'This memorandum has been drawn up to establish adequate standards in the design and construction of electro-medical apparatus for use in hospitals, with the aim of ensuring:

(i)   Safety from electric shock to patients and to operators.
(ii)   Safety from overheating and risk of fire in both the apparatus and its surroundings.
(iii) The provision of adequate and clearly marked controls.
(iv)   That apparatus is conveniently accessible for servicing purposes'

Whilst such standards, memoranda and guidelines provided a useful frame-work against which to judge the general acceptability of equipment, it is unrealistic to expect imported equipment to be designed to meet local standards. It is clearly desirable to sweep away national standards and to replace them with an international standard sufficiently clearly thought out and expressed to be applicable on a world-wide basis.

The only forum which exists which may be considered to go a reasonable way towards reaching this ideal is the International Electrotechnical Commission. The Commission has an overall membership in excess of 40 countries, and is the leading organization for international electrotechnical standardization. It established a Technical Committee (TC 62 - Electrical Equipment in Medical Practice) with a membership of 24 countries to draw together national discussion and comment in order to produce an international standard. In 1977 the Technical Committee published the first part of its standard, IEC 601-1. This was conceived as the first part of the publication, dealing with General Requirements, and with the intention that subsequent parts of the standard would be published. In particular there would be a considerable number of 'Part 2' documents, which would deal with specific requirements for particular types of equipment, often either augmenting or replacing the requirements of particular sub-clauses of the General Standard (Part 1). There are intended to be 'Part 3' documents which will specify appropriate performance requirements for specific types of equipment.

Since its publication in 1977, IEC 601-1 has begun to be accepted as the appropriate standard for electromedical equipment. In most countries where it is in widespread use there have been a small number of particular problems - often the new standards not being as rigorous in certain details as specific aspects of the old standards, sometimes the opportunity being taken to include within the standard aspects which were merely covered previously as 'good practice'. Nonetheless, the standard has been incorporated into the national standard structure of a growing number of countries. For instance, in the United Kingdom, IEC 601-1 was adopted with 14 extremely minor textual alterations. The standard was then published as British Standard BS 5724 Part 1, and the old Memorandum HTM8 phased out.

Scope of the standards

It has already been suggested that equipment in use in hospitals covers a wide range, from that designed very specifically to perform a medical function, through normal laboratory and computer equipment to ordinary domestic equipment. A considerable proportion of this equipment may have been designed to meet a specific standard drawn up with no thought of medical application. Therefore it is important to consider which standards should apply to which equipment, and to determine what distinctions and criteria should be applied to subdivide this mass of equipment.

The normal conclusion is that IEC 601-1 deals with medical electrical equipment. This term itself was defined in the first publication of IEC 601-1 (sub-clause 2.2.15) as 'Electrical equipment specified for use in the patient

27

environment and related in such a way to the patient that the patient's safety can be influenced'.

Whilst this sub-clause is likely to be modified to make it slightly more specific the concept is clear – medical electrical equipment is that equipment relating directly to the patient, not peripheral equipment possibly accepting data from another unit which is, in itself, relating directly to the patient. This concept is strengthened by safety requirements for the input and output connections of electromedical equipment. IEC 601-1 requires that the patient should not be at risk because of foreseeable electrical hazards arising within peripheral equipment attached to the electromedical unit (Figure 2.4).

What standards should apply to equipment in use in hospitals, possibly in

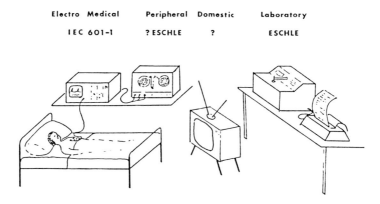

Electro Medical	Peripheral	Domestic	Laboratory
IEC 601-1	? ESCHLE	?	ESCHLE

Figure 2.4 Equipment designed to various standards will be near to the patient

the patient environment, or possibly in laboratories, but in neither case connected to the patient? For particular items of equipment specific standards (national or international) may exist. In the UK the increasing tendency is to expect such equipment to follow the guidelines of another DHSS publication - *The Electrical Safety Code for Hospital Laboratory Equipment* (ESCHLE). Thus equipment 'next' to the patient is expected to meet IEC 601-1, or the local version, BS 5724 Part 1, and other equipment in the vicinity, ESCHLE or any other British Standard which may be appropriate to that specific item of equipment. In almost all respects this places stringent requirements on the patient-related equipment, but normally only calls for accepted good practice in the other equipment.

The philosophy and requirements of IEC 601-1

The underlying philosophy of IEC 601-1 is that the patient must be safe in normal working conditions as well as under foreseeable fault conditions. However, it is considered that a fault condition will be detected and equipment withdrawn from service before a further fault arises. Thus limits are set for leakage currents for various categories of equipment under normal operating conditions and certain fault states. Because reversal of mains supply polarity is not specifically limited or prevented in many countries, interchanging the mains live and neutral connections is considered to be within normal non-fault conditions. However, circumstances which lead to an interruption of the protective earth conductor, or one of the supply conductors, are considered to be single-fault conditions (SFC), as are failures leading to mains supply voltage on the signal input or output connectors of equipment or on the applied part, as well as leakages of medical gas systems and breakdown of certain sections of insulation or failure of circuit components. In order to achieve these aims, the basic requirements of good practice in electronic construction methods are expected. In particular, specific limiting values are laid down for particular parameters.

Initially, equipment is divided in terms of Class and Type. All equipment must belong to one of four classes (sub-clauses 2.2.4–2.2.6, 14.5).

Class I is equipment in which protection against electric shock does not rely on basic insulation only, but which includes a protective earth system which will prevent accessible conductive parts becoming live in the event of failure of the basic insulation.

Class II is equipment in which protection against electric shock does not rely on basic insulation only, but in which additional precautions such as double insulation or reinforced insulation are provided, there being no provision for protective earthing.

Class III is equipment in which protection against electric shock relies on supply at safety extra-low voltage and in which no higher voltages are generated. This Class is being withdrawn.

Internally Powered Equipment must have no external connections to the power source, or electrical connection between the internal power source and an external supply must be possible only with the internal power source separated from the remainder of the equipment. Otherwise the equipment must be classified as Class I or II.

Equipment must also belong to one of three Types which are categorized by the permissible leakage current limits. The normal Type is B, whereas the more stringent classifications, BF and CF require electrical isolation of those parts connected to the patient (the applied part). Type CF is designed to be safe for application where direct contact with the heart may be anticipated.

A common misconception is that equipment which is battery-powered and has no direct electrical connection to the patient is outside the scope of IEC 601-1. Whilst the standard may not contain a great deal of relevance in such cases, if the equipment is used directly with the patient it should properly be classified as Internally Powered, Type B.

The detailed requirements of the standard specify particular qualities of insulation, mainly measured in terms of dielectric strength tests, in which test voltages and methods are specified. Climatic conditions relating to moisture preconditioning tests are also specified. All such tests are clearly potentially damaging and should be carried out only under carefully controlled conditions. They are certainly not to be reproduced in user departments. Other aspects of insulation are measured by creepage and clearance distances. These can be verified by visual inspection, where appropriate.

The other direct electrical safety measures of the standard refer to earthing and leakage currents. These parameters are in a totally different category to insulation provision – the standard assumes that a failure in the earth path will be found *before* a further fault occurs – this implies routine safety testing. Leakage currents are the major parameter to be used for assessing safety performance, thus these also must be measured routinely. Much debate has taken place about the manner in which protective earth path impedance should be measured. The compliance test within IEC 601-1 calls for measurements with a current in the range 10–25 A for a minimum of 6 seconds, and requires an impedance from the protective earth terminal to any part connected to it of not more than 0.1 Ω or, alternatively, of not more than 0.2 Ω if the measurement is made from the earth pin of the mains plug. A formula is published to enable the limits appropriate to accessories to be calculated. For routine testing the resistance values remain the same, but there is no necessity for test currents of such a high value, and there is a growing tendency to perform routine tests with a test current in the range 0.5–1 A. The claimed value of using high current testing of protective earth

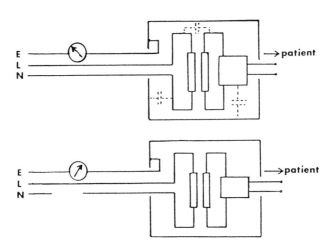

Figure 2.5 Total earth leakage current shall not exceed 0.5 mA in normal (upper), or 1.0 mA in single fault conditions (lower)

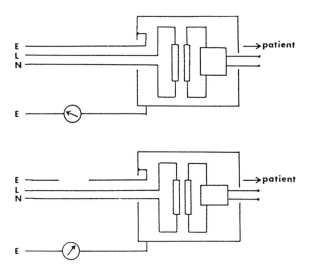

Figure 2.6 Enclosure leakage current shall not exceed 0.1 mA in normal (upper) or 0.5 mA in single-fault condition (lower)

circuits is that such currents will destroy an earth path which contains broken wire strands, but it is completed by just one or two strands. Recent work has shown that it is very unlikely that such an earth path would burn out at the current levels of the compliance tests; however these high currents are very likely to damage functionally earthed circuits if they are inadvertently included in the tests.

Type classifications are, in effect, patient leakage current categories. Three major paths for leakage current are considered. Firstly there is the current which may flow continuously in the earth conductor both in normal conditions, including reversal of mains supply conductors, and in single-fault conditions, which for this test is the condition with one supply conductor interrupted, as when a fuse ruptures or a supply connection becomes broken. This test applies only to class I equipment and imposes the same limits of 0.5 mA in normal and 1.0 mA in single fault conditions, regardless of the Type of equipment (Figure 2.5).

Enclosure leakage current is often related to the total earth leakage current. As the name implies, it is the current that will flow to earth from any part of the equipment housing. It includes currents that would capacitively couple through an insulating case to, for instance, a hand placed on the case. Enclosure leakage current is measured under normal conditions when it may not exceed 0.1 mA. (The current IEC regulations list a current of 0.01 mA for Type CF equipment. It is likely that this value will be brought into line with the 0.1 mA limit for Types B and BF). In fault conditions – protective earth conductor interrupted, or the interruption of either supply conductor

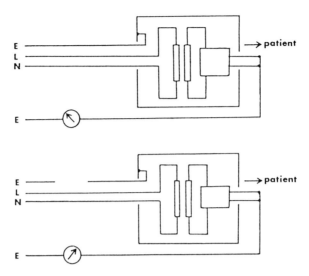

Figure 2.7 Patient leakage current shall not exceed 0.1 (normal) or 0.5 mA (SFC) for Type BF, or 0.01 (normal) and 0.05 mA (SFC) for Type CF equipment

– the enclosure leakage current limit for all Types of equipment rises to 0.5 mA (Figure 2.6). It should be noted that all these limits are around or below the lower limit normally accepted to be the most sensitive threshold of feeling. Thus, even in the case of a fault in equipment, neither the patient nor the operator is likely to feel any electric shock sensation.

Patient leakage current limits have to be set to values such that there will be no foreseeable electrical hazard to the patient. Under the normal and single-fault conditions listed above, the limits for the patient leakage current in Types B and BF equipment are the same as the enclosure leakage currents, i.e. 0.1 and 0.5 mA (Figure 2.7). The requirements for equipment which may have a direct cardiac connection are, however, ten times more stringent viz 0.01 and 0.05 mA. Further, additional fault conditions are envisaged, in particular situations where mains voltage appears on a signal input or output part of the equipment – perhaps due to failure in a peripheral device not designed to the standards of IEC 601-1 – or where mains voltage appears on the patient, perhaps again from some other source. Type B equipment must limit the current through the patient if mains voltage appears on a signal input or output part to a 'safe shock' level: 5 mA has been selected. As any patient circuitry on Type B equipment is likely to include an earth connection, it is impossible to limit the shock current if mains voltage were to appear on the patient or the applied part. Thus the standard recommends that all equipment with an applied part should be Type BF or CF with an electrically isolated input circuit. In Type BF patient leakage current in the fault condition of mains voltage on the applied part or patient is limited again to 5 mA.

However, for Type CF equipment, because it is designed to be used in direct cardiac applications, this limit becomes 0.05 mA. Limits are also imposed on the currents that may be injected into a patient in order to achieve measurements such as electrical impedance, etc. Such limits do not apply to the functional output of the equipment, and therefore do not apply to devices such as diathermy generators (electrosurgical generators) or stimulators.

Debate has taken place over recent years about the correct value for leakage current levels. For much equipment the values quoted are readily achievable with current electronic design. Thus there are arguments for making the limits even more stringent. In particular, this argument rages between the USA and Europe, and is further emphasized because of the lower supply voltage in the USA. Nonetheless, most of the published clinical work appears to indicate that the present levels are sufficiently stringent. Further, an added complication is that arising when equipment is combined in one form or another, for then the leakage currents frequently add together, taking equipment which had appeared safe and within the limits to values beyond the set levels.

Design requirements

Whilst in general terms the requirements of the standard are based on 'good practice', there is a considerable quantity of detail governing certain aspects of equipment design. These include requirements for ensuring adequate protection against the dangers of explosion, and against excessive temperatures, safety of motors and other mechanical devices as well as detailed constructional requirements for the mains part of the equipment.

It used to be considered that there was a very high risk of explosion in anaesthetic rooms and operating theatres, to the extent that all mains outlets were fitted with spark-proof switches and interlocked so that the plug could not be withdrawn whilst the socket was still alive. More recent work has identified specific zones of risk. The current standard and the draft amendments being considered envisage flammable anaesthetic mixtures with oxygen or nitrous oxide contained within specific equipment (including the anaesthetic circuit), and extending 5 cm beyond any point at which leakage may occur. Beyond that distance there is considered to be a further zone extending to 25 cm from such a point. Within this second zone there is considered to be a flammable anaesthetic mixture with air. Within the first zone only APG equipment may be used, whereas the requirements of AP equipment are sufficient in the second zone. Beyond the second zone any normal medical electrical equipment may be used. The requirements for penetration and containment of gases, and for limiting sources of ignition, are laid down for APG and AP equipment.

Overheating of equipment has two main consequences. Firstly, there is the normal hazard as a source of fire. The precautions for prevention of fire in general electromedical equipment are perfectly normal. The additional hazard is that of causing harm to patients because the equipment part to which they are connected overheats. As damage to human tissue can be caused by temperatures within 42 and 45 °C there are stringent constraints including requirements for back-up thermostats. These restraints are particularly relevant where an applied part which may be attached to an unconscious patient may overheat and cause serious tissue damage as a result.

Similarly the consequence of electrical or mechanical failure in motor-driven systems and other devices become unusually significant if the equipment is lifting or turning a patient or supporting a heavy, suspended load over a patient. Equally the consequences of mechanical failure in a ventilator, or other life-support system, can be extremely severe. The philosophy of the standard which was apparent in electrical considerations, is equally applicable to mechanical hazards. As a consequence, failure of a single protective device must not cause a greatly increased patient hazard. Further, failure of such a protective means should be detectable to the operator. Generally speaking equipment must fail safe.

Design of the mains part of the equipment

Much of the detail of the first part of IEC 601-1 is concerned with safe construction of the mains part. For all mains-operated equipment, the mains lead must be the appropriate colour code (in the UK the mains lead must have insulation coloured brown for the live, blue for the neutral and green/yellow for the protective earth conductors). The lead must be correctly rated (not less than 0.75 mm^2 Cu for mains currents up to 6 A), and be correctly terminated, either in an adequate mains terminal block, or with an adequate connector. The lead must be appropriately anchored and strain-relieved. An item of equipment may have only one mains lead. Class I equipment must be fused in each supply conductor (with the fuse connected correctly), and, if the equipment has an applied part, must have a double pole mains switch. These requirements become increasingly appropriate when it is remembered that reversal of the polarity of the supply mains is not considered to be a fault, thus both supply conductors must be fused and switched to give optimum protection (Figure 2.8)

Further clauses deal with the construction and protection of transformers. The philosophy applied is that short-circuiting of transformer windings or outputs should not create a hazard. Thus transformers must either be inherently short-circuit-proof or be so protected with secondary fusing that component failure will not leave the transformer short-circuited. Class II equipment must follow much the same construction requirements, except

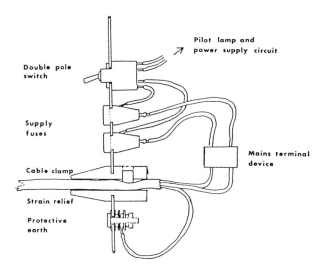

Figure 2.8 Typical layout of the mains part of equipment. (Insulating sleeves over connections have been omitted for clarity.)

that mains fusing in the live conductor only is acceptable as a minimum standard of equipment protection.

Less major design requirements which are frequently misunderstood or omitted concern the markings which equipment should carry. Normally equipment should carry adequate markings to fully identify it, in terms of manufacture and supplier name and address data, equipment type and serial number. The layout of controls should be logical, and their functions clearly marked. The ratings of equipment and protective fuses should also be clearly marked. Difficulties arise with markings of Class and Type of equipment however, as the special symbols proposed in Appendix D II (IEC 601-1) have not yet received full approval, thus equipment without Class and Type marking may be Class I Type B which is, in effect, the default category - or may belong to a more stringent category but merely be unmarked. Nonetheless, all difficulties with symbols should be dispelled by the accompanying documents which should, although frequently they do not, include specification of Class and Type.

A further aspect of marking is the use of coloured lamps and other indicators. Current emphasis is on the approach of green - safe, yellow - caution or attention required, and red - danger, urgent action required. Any other colour may also be used but not to convey the meanings of red or yellow warnings. Increasingly this colour code is being widely accepted and understood.

The philosophy and requirements of ESCHLE

The Electrical Safety Code for Hospital Laboratory Equipment (ESCHLE) has a totally different standing from that of IEC 601-1. This document was published 'to ensure the electrical safety of equipment used in hospital laboratories and similar locations where patients are not involved directly...', and has authority only in the United Kingdom. It was based on Hospital Technical Memorandum No. 8 (HTM8), one of the precursors of IEC 601-1. It has the aim of ensuring, in normal use:

(i)   safety from electric shock to operators;
(ii)   safety from overheating and risk of fire in both the equipment and its surroundings;
(iii)   the provision of adequate and clearly marked controls.

The code was envisaged as permitting manufacturers the widest possible choice in design and construction methods. It was also envisaged that where equipment complied with other appropriate safety standards, it should be considered to meet the minimum requirements for laboratory equipment.

Safety from electric shock is met through the normal equipment classification - Class I, with protective earthing, and Class II with double insulation. The requirements for protective earthing of Class I equipment are similar to those of Class I in IEC 601-1. The code envisages that type testing of Class II equipment will include a dielectric strength test. Such tests should be performed only by manufacturers or approved test houses.

The concept of single-fault condition is not directly introduced within the text of ESCHLE. Leakage current tests are described and limits set without reference even to measurements with supply conductors reversed or protective earth path interrupted although both conditions are illustrated in the explanatory figures. There is no reference to any conditions comparable to the envisaged fault conditions of IEC 601-1. Accordingly, there is only one limit quoted for permissible leakage currents for equipment other than fixed equipment. The normal limit is 0.75 mA.

In the case of fixed equipment (permanently installed equipment) a higher limit (5.0 mA) is set. However, it is suggested that the Department of Health may permit higher limits for certain non-fixed equipment, notably equipment incorporating mineral-insulated heaters or requiring specific filters for the suppression of radio-frequency interference. Thus it is clear that there is no Type category for equipment covered by this code, but rather that a universal standard be applied to all laboratory-orientated equipment in hospitals. In recent years the concept has become one of equipment interfacing with the patient meeting IEC 601-1, and all other equipment either connected to the outputs of the patient-related equipment, or used in laboratories, etc. within the hospital, meeting ESCHLE.

The constructional standards set within ESCHLE are rather more simple than in IEC 601-1, although once more the emphasis is on normal 'good practice' type of standards. Nonetheless, requirements are less stringent; for instance, whilst mains supply fusing is called for, a single fuse, or single pole circuit breaker in the line conductor is considered acceptable. Most items of equipment do not require a mains switch. However, the colour coding of panel lights and indicators is specified in a manner comparable to that within IEC 601-1.

ESCHLE has filled an important gap in the safety standards applicable to electrical equipment in hospitals, much of which is used in association with the patient or to make measurements on patient samples remote from the patient. Whilst the safety requirements for such equipment are less stringent than for equipment directly connected to the patient, the safety of all concerned is influenced by all the equipment being used, and a safety code, or better, a safety standard for such peripheral equipment is a matter of some importance.

Foreseeable developments

Most international standards are continuously evolving. The evolution tends to occur on a number of fronts. Firstly, no standard is of any relevance unless it is used. Then any standard will be reviewed, often in a fairly continuous manner. Thirdly, technical developments influence the standards and their interpretation. All these aspects arise in the case of electromedical equipment, together with a fourth aspect - there is continuous work to prepare and publish further parts of the standard, especially the Part 2 sections - Particular Requirements for specific types of equipment.

Since the publication of IEC 601-1 in 1977 it has been adopted by a number of countries. As a result, all of the major manufacturers of electromedical equipment consider it necessary that their equipment should meet those requirements, and many of the smaller manufacturing organizations have also adopted the standard as the appropriate design standard. Thus, even those countries who have not yet adopted the standard, principal amongst which is the USA, have much of their equipment manufactured to IEC 601-1. This is particularly evident where the manufacturer expects a major export market.

The existing standards are not perfect, nor are they unambiguous. Much work is in progress to produce a revised IEC 601-1. Such work is necessarily slow even on a national scale. To achieve international agreement on limits to be imposed or the precise phraseology for textual changes is a job of great magnitude. Nonetheless, changes are occurring, of which the greatest to date is the decision to eliminate Class III (equipment in which protection against electric shock relies on supply at safety extra-low voltage...). A very large number of minor changes are being considered and approved to simplify and clarify the standard. Emphasis is placed on requirements which can be tested, and those for which a test cannot be compiled tend to be removed. However, the underlying foundations are firmly laid and the associated principles are not likely to change.

Technical advances in electronics will create major changes in electromedical equipment in the next few years. One sometimes loses sight of the fact that technical advances in medicine have a similarly great effect on electromedical equipment. It is important that significant advances in either electronics or medicine are not made unusable because of unimportant and unnecessary restrictions in the safety standards. On the other hand, it is important to appreciate the reason why specific limits are set or particular requirements made in order that important safety requirements are not jeopardized.

A number of additional standards have been published recently. These are Part 2 standards, – Particular Requirements for specific items of equipment. Many more Part 2s will be published, as will Part 3s which will be Performance Specifications for particular types of equipment.

A Part 2 will contain three kinds of comment. It will confirm which sub-clauses of the General Standard (IEC 601-1) should apply to the equipment in question, it will state which clauses may not be applied and it will add further clauses as necessary. Thus a Part 2 may require all equipment of a specific function to be Type CF, by excluding the possibility of it being Type B or BF. Before Class III equipment category was abolished, each Part 2 draft was excluding Class III as equipment in which safety could not be adequately assured because of its dependence on a separate installation with no associated standards. The Part 2 will also include additional requirements which, although important for that equipment, could not be so widely relevant as to justify their inclusion in the General Standards.

Hospital-produced equipment

The standards described above are intended for commercial production. It is envisaged that a sample unit will be type tested in accordance with the compliance tests included in the standard. As a number of these tests are potentially damaging the sample unit should not be returned to the production batch. A significant amount of equipment is either produced or modified within hospital workshops in order that particular medical needs may be met. It is effectively impossible to fully test such equipment to the standards of IEC 601-1. The safety of this equipment is just as important as that of any other. Therefore, the concepts contained within the standards must be applied. Whilst equipment cannot be fully evaluated to IEC 601-1 it can, and should, be subjected to a searching acceptance test at least to the standards of the DHSS publication, HEI 95 before it is put into use. It must meet the basic constructional and labelling requirements, have adequate insulation, protective earthing, fusing and leakage currents. It must also be fully documented – an area in which much hospital produced equipment has fallen short in previous years. Many hospital departments now have their own internal guidelines for the standards appropriate to 'in house' produced equipment. A guide was recently published laying down such standards.

Implications of safety standards

The adoption of international safety standards has many implications. The major impetus for international co-operation is to remove national trade barriers, but the concept that equipment will fail safe has two detailed implications for hospital electronic servicing laboratories. Firstly, failures must be detected. A failure in a protective earth path, or other failure which may lead to increased leakage currents will not prevent the equipment functioning but does decrease the likelihood of safe failure. Thus routine safety testing is inherent in the concept.

Secondly, equipment which has developed a fault is designed still to be safe. Thus equipment being serviced is only potentially unsafe if it is operated with protective means, including enclosures, removed. Accordingly, equipment may be operated in a service laboratory in its failed state, without causing hazard. Indeed, even when the safety covers are removed, the inherent safety of the equipment design is such that it is considerably less hazardous than, for example, normal domestic electrical and electronic equipment. Nonetheless the fundamental intent of existing safety standards for electromedical equipment is to ensure that maximum feasible safety is achieved for each person associated with the equipment, be that patient, operator or service personnel.

LITERATURE CONSULTED

Brown, B.H. and Smallwood, R.H. (1981). *Medical Physics and Physiological Measurement.* (Oxford: Blackwell)

Dalziel, C.F. and Lee, W.R. (1969). Lethal electric currents. *IEEE Spectrum*, **6**, 44-50

Raftery, E.B., Green, H.L. and Yacoub, M.H. (1975). Disturbances of heart rhythm produced by 50 Hz leakage currents in human subjects. *Cardiovasc. Res.*, **9**, 263-265

Vickers, M.D. (1971). Explosion hazards. *Anaesthesia*, **26**, 155-157

Watson, A.B., Wright, J.S. and Loughman, J. (1973). Electrical thresholds for ventricular fibrillation in man. *Med. J. Aust.*, **1**, 1179-1182

Whelpton, D. and Roberts, J.R. (1982). Safety of medical electrical equipment and BS 5724. *J. Biomed. Eng.*, **4**, 185-196

BS 5724: Part 1. (1979). *Specification for safety of medical electrical equipment.* Part 1. *General requirements.* (London: British Standards Institution)

Code of practice for acceptance testing of medical electrical equipment (1981). *Hospital Equipment Information*, **95**. (London: Department of Health and Social Security)

EU7 (1979). *Engineering Data: Electronic and medical equipment. Maintenance facilities required*. (London: Department of Health and Social Security)

Electrical safety code for hospital laboratory equipment (1977). (London: Department of Health and Social Security)

IEC 601-1, (1977). *Specifications for the safety of electrical equipment used in medical practice*, Part 1: *General requirements*. (Geneva: International Electrotechnical Commission)

Management of equipment (1981). *Hospital Equipment Information*. **98**. (London: Department of Health and Social Security)

Safe design and construction of electromedical equipment. Ed. Smallwood, R.H. (1983). Topic Group Report, **37**. (London: Hospital Physicists' Association)

Safety code for electromedical apparatus (1963, revised 1969). Hospital Technical Memorandum, **8**. (London: Department of Health and Social Security)

Safety Information Bulletin (2) 14: Accompanied working (1982). (London: Department of Health and Social Security)

3 Design of Mechanical Equipment for Laboratory Staff and Patient Safety

P. Bowker

In recent years, throughout the Health Services of the western world, there has been a steady increase in the number of departments employing teams of BioEngineers and Medical Physicists. Whilst the activities of these departments range over a very wide field, they are all to some extent innovative, that is they are concerned with the development and assessment of new techniques and new pieces of equipment. This continuing process of development and improvement inevitably leads, at least in some cases, to the introduction of new pieces of diagnostic or therapeutic equipment into the clinical environment.

Whilst we cannot know precisely what new pieces of clinical equipment will be produced in the next decade, we can be certain they will be both numerous and diverse. Perhaps the two major areas of development in recent years have been in the design of electronic monitoring equipment and in the introduction of nuclear magnetic resonance imagers. These are very different kinds of products, but both, in common with all other past and future innovative pieces of equipment, have mechanical components.

This chapter then, presents the basic guidelines which need to be followed by those who design and build this new mechanical equipment for laboratory and clinical use, those people who need to regard, with paramount importance, the safety of laboratory staff and of patients.

THE DIFFERENT TYPES OF SAFETY ASPECTS

To someone required to design a piece of electrical or electronic equipment for use in a hospital environment, the need for it to be electrically safe so that

41

nobody could be electrocuted whilst using it would be obvious. Similarly, to a designer developing clinical equipment involving sources of ionizing radiation, the need to consider the safety aspect of the relevant isotopes would again be obvious.

There is, in general, a high awareness of the hazards associated with electrical installations and with the use of ionizing radiations – probably because the nature of these hazards is very specific. For example, the hazards associated with electrical equipment result from the physiological effects of electrical currents flowing into and circulating within the body or from overheating and, to a lesser extent, arcing. Furthermore, there is a uniformity of electrical components and the ways in which they are combined into circuits, which allows very specific standards to be prepared to instruct and guide designers in the preparation of sound and safe designs.

On the other hand, in the case of a piece of mechanical equipment or, indeed, of the mechanical components of a piece of electrical equipment, or of one involving isotopes, the manner and extent to which its safety aspects need to be considered may not be at all obvious. One finds in general, among both professional and lay staff, a much lower awareness of the possibility and consequences of mechanical failure than of the hazards of electricity or of radiation. This probably arises because, whereas electrical installations all present similar risks, mechanical hazards are extremely diverse, and mechanical components and assemblies infinite in nature. In this situation, the preparation of concise standards setting out requirements and guidelines for safe design is clearly impossible. The documentation required to instruct in the safe design of ALL possible mechanical components would be that needed to train a professional engineer and more.

This chapter then, can be no more than a very general introduction to the subject of safety in mechanical design. It makes no attempt to instruct on how this may be achieved, but aims to highlight the fundamental problems facing the Professional Designer and to demonstrate that the lot of the Amateur Designer is fraught with difficulties.

THE PROBLEMS OF THE PROFESSIONAL DESIGNER: WHAT ACTUALLY HAPPENS TO CLINICAL EQUIPMENT

The first point which must be made is the obvious one that any piece of equipment, large or small, simple or complex, can fail, and that in so doing may cause injury. On occasion, although fortunately infrequently, such injury can be very serious. It is the responsibility of all who produce or use mechanical equipment in a laboratory or a clinical setting to be constantly aware of this and, therefore, to exercise the greatest diligence in their work.

The responsibilities of the Professional Designer are of course particularly onerous. His task is to produce a piece of equipment which is safe and which will remain safe throughout its useful life under all the circumstances which it will encounter. What these circumstances will be, however, is not always easy to foresee. Perhaps an example may best help to illustrate the sort of contingencies for which the designer must allow.

Let us imagine that the requirement is to design, and subsequently to have built, some type of scanner which has a boom carrying a detector mounted on a rotating annulus so that the detector can be placed in any position with respect to the patient. As one possibility will be that illustrated in Figure 3.1 with the detector vertically above the patient, it is fairly obvious that the single most important design requirement is that the boom and the boom's attachments to the detector and to the annulus should be designed in such a way that, when it is in this overhead position, it will not fall on top of the patient. It is also clear that this basic requirement is met throughout the entire life of

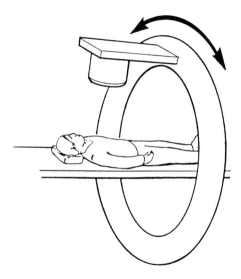

Figure 3.1 A hypothetical clinical scanner in which the safety of the patient is dependent on sound mechanical design

the scanner.

To ensure that the machine is safe beyond any doubt when it leaves the workshop is relatively straightforward. This is simply a matter of applying good analytical and practical engineering. To ensure that it is still safe a number of years later is less straightforward as things are going to happen to it whilst it is in service which will potentially make the scanner less safe. What are these things? It must be assumed that three factors will operate. The first of these is *normal wear and tear*. All moving parts are going to wear, although on a device such as this, the degree of wear is likely to be very small. There may be shock loadings applied to the structure when the rotating parts start and stop moving, and there will be stress reversals when the boom moves

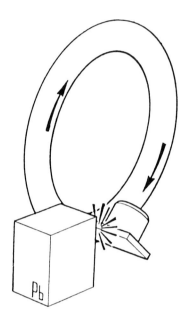

Figure 3.2 A typical example of accidental misuse discussed in the text. This incident could lead to damage which would make the structure of the scanner less safe

from the upper to the lower position. There may also be vibrations in the boom originating from the drive mechanism. There is, therefore, going to be a tendency for fatigue cracks to develop, especially if there are any preexisting defects or surface flaws, for example in the welds which may be used in the fabrication process. The stress reversals and vibrations could also cause nuts and bolts and any other sort of fastenings to work loose.

The second factor which must be considered is that of *accidental misuse* (Figure 3.2). For example, a carton of lead shielding which was delivered during the lunch break is left in the path of the boom. The operator, discussing the afternoon's work with his colleagues as he sets up the scanner for the first patient after lunch, fails to notice the carton and drives the boom into the obstruction. In the confusion which follows somebody manages to move a part of the scanner without releasing the braking mechanism, and then a small forklift truck, being used to move the carton of lead, accidentally backs

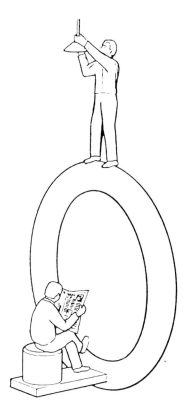

Figure 3.3 The possibilities for intentional misuse of the scanner are great. Illustrated are two situations of which the designer must take account

into some part of the scanner assembly. All these contingencies have happened before and doubtless will happen again.

And finally, the third factor which must be considered in designing for safety is *intentional misuse* (Figure 3.3). The list of possibilities here is almost endless. As a starting point it perhaps may reasonably be assumed at the very minimum, that people will sit on the detector to read the newspaper and that when the man comes to replace the light bulb he will climb on top of the frame.

These three factors, normal wear and tear, accidental misuse and intentional misuse, will subject the device to loadings and stresses which potentially will make it less safe. It is, therefore, imperative that full account is always taken of them when any structure or any mechanical component is designed and built. The Professional Engineer will do this in the preliminary phases of preparing his design before he begins his detailed calculations of how exactly each component and subassembly of the scanner should be designed.

THE PROBLEMS OF THE AMATEUR ENGINEER: IS IT SAFE?

Having dealt with these very fundamental outline design criteria which will guide the Professional Engineer when he/she is designing mechanical equipment, it is perhaps salutary to consider the shortcomings, and indeed dangers, of the design process as it has been known to be actually practised in some hospital departments. This may be a typical scenario: the term 'scientist' is used to describe anyone who is not a Professional Engineer.

The clinician and scientist who have been working together on the development of a particular clinical service, have identified a need for a new piece of equipment which they will use in the hospital as part of their routine diagnosis or treatment procedures. The scientist, very reasonably, agrees to design this piece of equipment, to make the necessary arrangements for its installation and to subsequently oversee at least the initial use of the equipment with patients.

Being a conscientious worker, he/she devotes a considerable amount of time to thinking about the problem, discussing it with his/her colleagues and reading the relevant literature. He perhaps does some calculations and makes a couple of sketches, before approaching the chief technician in the nearest mechanical workshop. The scientist describes to the technician, with great care, exactly what is required, what it does, how it works and how perhaps it may be put together. And, in the fullness of time, the device is built and the scientist, as planned, supervises its delivery to the appropriate clinical area and at the earliest opportunity, finds a patient upon whom it can be tried out.

Strictly speaking there is nothing wrong with that scenario. No laws have been broken nor any regulations contravened. Indeed there are no laws or regulations governing who can design, or build, or install clinical equipment. Nor has there been a failure to conform to the relevant 'Standard' for the design and construction of medical mechanical equipment, for, as has been pointed out, no such document exists.

Superficially then, there is nothing that should have been done that has not been done, and nothing that should not have been done that has been done. Nobody in a position of authority is going to come and ask awkward questions or quote rules and regulations, conditions or requirements. At least, not so long as the new equipment continues to work without injuring anybody. If, however, an accident does happen, the ending of the story will be rather less happy, not only for the person who is injured, but also for the amateur designer. For if we look at our scenario critically, we see that it really was rather casual. How competent were the two people who designed and constructed the equipment to do so? At what point was a fully qualified person called in to carry out a safety audit on the design? For something as important as a piece of clinical equipment, these questions can never be side-stepped.

The first point is that the scientist clearly did not appreciate the full implications of designing the device. In doing so, it very much became his/her piece of equipment and, as such, not only could the scientist claim all the credit for its success, but would also have to carry all the responsibility for its failure. And if a patient were to be injured by its failure, not only would there be a moral charge, there might also be a criminal charge, for the courts are unlikely to be persuaded that there has been no negligence if the design process has not involved a person who could clearly be seen to be professionally competent.

Once the scientist had become aware of these responsibilities, the correct course of action should have become much clearer. Unless the device had been sufficiently trivial for the non-professional to feel entirely competent to judge its safety and to be certain that no part of the design was, or ever could reasonably become, hazardous, then he/she should have consulted a competent engineer. If anything could break, bend, fatigue, rust, fall off, collapse, distort or otherwise become unintentionally modified, it should have been examined by somebody who could make sure that it did not. If it had any moving parts, it should have been designed so that these were safely constructed and safely housed. And, in particular, the sequence of events following the failure of any part of the equipment should have been fully explored. It is of vital importance, especially if the equipment is to be connected in some way to a patient, that it fails to safety. If there is any doubt whatsoever about any of these points, the design must either be entrusted to someone who is trained and is competent in this work, or, at the very least, must be fully and properly checked by them.

In a real world, it will never be possible to give absolute, 100% guarantees concerning the safety of a mechanical device. There are an infinite number of ways in which things can go wrong and in which they can be accidentally or intentionally misused, but in a finite lifetime it is only possible to think about a finite number of them. Against this background, any general pieces of advice can clearly only be rather vague. However, one point is particularly important and worthy of special mention, and that is that accidents very often occur as the result of a *combination* of unforeseen misfortunes or occurrences. This is nowhere better illustrated than in road traffic accidents. A driver may cover hundreds of thousands of miles without being involved in even the most trivial of incidents but may well come to grief when confronted, without warning, by that 'one in a million' combination of totally unexpected events, any one of which, on its own, would be insignificant.

It is, therefore, always wise to assume that two or more faults will always occur simultaneously and that their natures will be such that neither will become immediately apparent. The warning lamp will fail at exactly the instant at which the fault which it is intended to indicate occurs.

47

THE DESIGNER'S BREADTH OF RESPONSIBILITY

Having discussed the general nature of mechanical hazards and of the responsibilities encumbent on the designers of mechanical equipment, it is necessary to add three brief points regarding the breadth or extent of these responsibilities. Firstly, the title of this chapter refers specifically to the design of equipment so as to ensure the safety of laboratory staff and patients. Whilst these are perhaps the two most obvious groups of individuals for whose safety the designer carries a responsibility, it would be misleading to suggest that they are the only groups. Of course, equipment design and construction must take into account the safety of all the people who will come into contact with it, both those such as the doctors, nurses, technicians and cleaners whose daily work brings them close to it, and those such as the man who comes to change the light bulb who may see it only once in his lifetime.

Secondly, the points made so far have tended to refer to the design and use of new pieces of equipment. It is perhaps hardly necessary to add that the responsibility for the safety of such equipment continues throughout its life. It must be checked and maintained properly and regularly, and any remedial work required should be put in hand without delay. The guiding idea should be that accidents are to be prevented, not investigated. And when, eventually, the equipment becomes obsolete it should be removed and dismantled.

And thirdly, this chapter has dealt specifically with the design and manufacture of equipment from scratch. It is appropriate to add a word of caution regarding the modification of standard pieces of bought-in equipment. However seemingly small may be the changes which are made, the same standards of care as have been described for completely new developments must be applied. If anything subsequently goes wrong, it may be taken as certain that the original manufacturer will not have anything to do with it.

RESPONSIBILITIES IN LAW

In any text which may be read internationally, the author generally seeks to avoid mention of specific details which only apply in particular countries or groups of countries. However, in nearly all the circumstances in which medical equipment is designed, the designer will have certain vitally important responsibilities in law. Those responsibilities, as they apply in the United Kingdom, are very briefly referred to below. Concerned readers should consult their professional bodies for more detailed information and to determine the position in other parts of the world.

The designers, manufacturers and suppliers of medical equipment in the UK have responsibilities under two quite separate items of legislation. Firstly under the *Heath and Safety at Work Act* (1974), they must ensure, by testing if necessary, that the piece of equipment is designed and constructed to be safe and without risk to health when properly used, and that sufficient information about the safe use of the equipment is supplied to the users. Since the potential hazards associated with innovative designs are sometimes particularly difficult to foresee, the designer would therefore be well advised, in many circumstances, to formally seek a second professional opinion.

Secondly, the terms of the EEC directive on product liability, which is due to become effective in member states by 30 July 1988, make the producer of an item strictly liable for personal injury and damage to property caused by a defect in the product, that is, without the need to prove fault or negligence on the part of the producer. Whilst it appears that the designer of the product would not normally be considered to be a producer, and would not therefore fall directly within the terms of the directive, if the producer could trace the defect to a design fault, he may well seek redress in the courts through an action against the designer for professional negligence.

4 Handling of Laboratory Animals – Including Non-human Primates

T. Pendry

INTRODUCTION

Working with animals in the laboratory can be potentially dangerous to the health and safety of research workers and supporting staff.

All animals, breeding stock and experimental animals alike, can inflict physical injuries. They bite, scratch, and kick, sometimes all three at once, but correct methods of handling can do much to reduce the risks. The wearing of protective clothing and use, where appropriate, of restraining devices can also help in the reduction of this very real hazard.

An additional hazard from contact with animals is the possibility of laboratory-acquired infection from zoonoses. Most common laboratory animal species are capable of carrying, and passing on to man, a number of diseases; some, particularly those transmitted from primates, can be fatal. The handling of primates requires special precautions and care.

Allergy to animals and their waste products is an increasingly recognized threat to the health of laboratory workers, but can be substantially reduced by adequately designed buildings and protective clothing.

Finally, experimental animals subjected to certain procedures can pose a danger to the handler. Animals used to study pathogenic diseases of human origin, and those used to test known carcinogens or passage human tumour tissue, are examples.

GENERAL CONSIDERATIONS

The general rules for laboratory safety apply equally to the animal house. In fact, the problem of disposal of larger volumes of waste, decontamination of cages, room surfaces and ventilation systems, all need special consideration.

Codes of practice should include:

1.   identification of restricted areas and control of access;
2.   emergency procedures and first aid policy;
3.   smoking, eating and drinking and application of cosmetics prohibited;
4.   protective clothing to be worn;
5.   high level of personal hygiene practice;
6.   waste removal and disposal procedures.

These rules need to be drawn up in relation to the type of work and degree of hazard in each situation. Rules which are not clearly laid out, accepted as being necessary or being restrictive as to make work difficult, are less likely to be obeyed. Training and supervision are all-important, particularly with cleaners and maintenance staff who may not always have the background experience to appreciate biological or chemical hazards.

In addition to the possible dangers from contact with animals, animal waste tissues and contaminated equipment, awareness of the need for care in the use of the following is also indicated in the animal house environment.

Disinfectants, fumigants

Correct dilutions, detailed protocol and safety procedures including first aid in the event of a mishap, are advised whatever material is used. The selection of the appropriate material should be related to the organism present, and particular care should be exercised when using formaldehyde to fumigate rooms or buildings.

Anaesthesia and euthanasia

All the substances which induce anaesthesia and euthanasia are dangerous, and care in using them is vital if accidents are to be avoided. Unqualified staff should not administer anaesthetics or drugs. Detailed information should be sought regarding needs of particular species. In addition to the hazards associated with all anaesthetic substances, volatile materials can also be flammable and/or explosive under non-controlled conditions.

Glass, instruments and equipment

Accidents can occur in the animal house from broken water bottles, sharp instruments or equipment, such as autoclaves and cage washing machines.

Electrical fittings

All animal house fittings should be waterproofed, particularly in areas where hosing down is the method of cleaning.

THE HANDLING OF LABORATORY ANIMALS

The importance of this aspect of animal care cannot be over-emphasized. An animal which is not handled correctly, i.e. with regard to the safety and security of both the animal and the handler, may injure itself or the person handling it. At the very least the confidence or trust of the animal may be lost.

Correct handling is not learned by lectures or by reading, but by demonstration and careful practice. The animal should be held securely and firmly, but not tightly. An animal which has been frequently and carefully handled, quickly becomes tractable. If the animal feels insecure, it will surely struggle and/or bite and/or scratch.

A pregnant animal is handled as little as possible, but, if necessary, with great care avoiding constriction around the abdomen and giving maximum support to the hind quarters at all times.

When approaching an animal be calm, quiet and confident.

Species

Rabbit

This is arguably one of the more difficult animals to handle. Some rabbit cages tend to be restricted, denying clear access to the animal. To remove the rabbit from the cage, place one hand over the rabbit's ears grasping a large handful of the loose skin at the back of the neck. Place the other hand, palm upward, under the belly of the animal. Lift both hands together gently but firmly.

However, if you are trying to remove a large rabbit from a small cage, it may be easier to face the animal away from you and instead of putting one hand under the belly, place it between the hind legs and then lift the rabbit toward you.

To carry a rabbit, one hand is used to control the head, by placing the index finger between the ears and curling the thumb and remaining fingers around the back of the head. The other hand supports the weight of the animal under the hind quarters. The animal is held in an upright position close to the body of the handler so that it cannot kick.

To hold a rabbit in a suitable position for sexing, a large flap of scruff skin is held in one hand and the hind quarters immobilized in one of two ways depending on the size of the rabbit. A small rabbit may be immobilized by placing the other hand across the loins and upper thighs of the rabbit. The animal is then manoeuvred into a position lying tilted backwards with the weight of the animal supported on the forearm of the hand holding the scruff. If you are dealing with a large rabbit or have small hands, the hind quarters may be more efficiently immobilized by holding the hind legs between the fingers. The legs should be held just above the hocks with the index finger between the legs to avoid the joints being injured. To hold a rabbit for artificial insemination or for intramuscular injection, place the animal on a firm non-slip surface, with the head tucked into the handler's body. A hand is run down each side of the animal's body keeping the forearms close to the flanks, and one hind leg is grasped in each hand. For insemination the legs should be held raised and apart, and for an i.m. injection the leg to be injected is extended towards the person injecting for him to grasp the foot. Meanwhile, the person holding the rabbit holds the same leg high above the 'knee', to prevent the leg being drawn back.

When handling a rabbit, e.g. for sexing, remember to keep the animal's hind legs well away from everyone's face.

Guinea pig

This is a shy animal and tends to make a fuss when approached. Grasp the 'pig firmly around the thorax with the thumb under the lower jaw. If dealing with a large 'pig or if you have small hands then the thumb under the jaw is not essential as the 'pig is usually an inoffensive beast and not inclined to bite. The weight of the animal should be supported with the other hand. Pregnant guinea pigs require particular care when handled.

Hamster

Hamsters are usually lifted by loosely cupping the hands around and under the animal. To immobilize the animal for inoculation, the loose skin at the back of the neck is held between the thumb and the knuckle of the first finger. The hand is then turned over so that the hamster is lying on his back and one hind leg may be held against the animal's body by the fourth finger, or between the fourth and fifth finger.

Rat

The rat should not be picked up by the tail. This method will cause damage to the rat's spine – also it can double up and bite you. The rat should be gently but firmly grasped around the thorax, with the thumb above the forelimbs and under the rat's lower jaw. Approach the animal positively without fumbling and hesitating. The tail of the rat should also be held for manipulations.

Mouse

This is the only animal that may be held by the tail. It should be grasped at base and the weight of the animal supported on a flat surface such as a cage lid. If the hind legs are then lifted by lifting the tail the mouse may be easily sexed. For injections, etc., hold the loose scruff skin in the finger and thumb, turn the hand so that the mouse is lying on its back and secure the tail between the third and fourth fingers or the fourth and palm of the hand, depending on the size of the mouse and the hand.

Ferret

Ferrets which are handled regularly become quite tractable. Never hesitate when handling a ferret. To pick up the animal, grasp it around the neck and upper thorax making sure that the thumb is under the lower jaw, firmly, to close the animal's jaw should it attempt to bite. Support the weight of the animal with the free hand.

Chicken

Avoid quick movements when approaching birds of any type. To pick up a chicken place one hand either side of the bird's body, with the thumbs over the bird's wings and the fingers under the keel. To carry the bird, approaching it from the front, slide one hand under the bird's breast until it is between the legs, immobilize the legs between the thumb and forefinger and the third and fourth fingers. Tuck the bird's head between your upper arm and body if the bird is very frightened.

Cat

The cat is a difficult animal to handle, unless the handler is experienced and the cat is docile. The cat is blessed with five-pronged offensive, four sets of claws and one set of jaws, all of which it will put to very good effect if it feels threatened or insecure. Unless a cat is known to be exceptionally docile, it is better to be safe than sorry. Place the cat on its right side on a table, with the feet away from the handler. Hold the hind legs in the left hand, above the hocks with a finger between the legs to avoid pressure on the joints. The forelegs are held in a similar manner and the head may be immobilized by the forearm of the right arm pressing gently across the neck and shoulders of the cat. The cat's body is held firmly against the handler's body. This method will immobilize a cat sufficiently for most procedures. To pick the cat up, it may be lifted by the scruff taking care to keep the forearm in line with the spine. To carry the animal, place the head and the right hand holding the scruff, under the left arm, using the left forearm to support the animal's body holding it close to the handler's body.

When releasing the cat from restraint, release both hands at the same time, or the cat may damage itself struggling and the handler may be badly scratched.

Dog

When approaching a dog, it is particularly important to make the dog aware of your presence by talking to it. It is best with a dog to allow it to see your hands and to calm it by stroking it after first allowing it to sniff your hands well. If you are in doubt about the dog's temperament, clench the fist and offer the back of the hand to the dog to sniff. This way if it does decide to snap it will do far less damage to the back of the fist than to the fingers of an open hand. All movements should be slow and deliberate. If the dog wears a collar it may be restrained by that or, if not, grasped by the scruff, keeping the forearm in line with the spine of the dog. The other hand may be placed under the dog's brisket as an extra restraint, holding the hindquarters into the body of the handler. A particularly nervous dog may require a tape muzzle. This is effected by putting two turns of a 2-in. bandage around the muzzle and tying the ends behind the head. When using a muzzle it is useful to restrain the forelegs of the dog to prevent it pawing the muzzle. Before muzzling any animal consider if the stress would justify its use. Dogs quickly adapt to what is required of them and if well handled, eventually require the minimum of restraint.

Non-human primates

Unless it is essential to an experiment that it should not be so, monkeys should only be handled under an anaesthetic such as phencyclidine. Most modern

56

cages have a sliding crush grid which makes the drawing up of the animal to the front of the cage very simple. By grasping a hindleg through the bars, a light dose of a suitable anaesthetic may be injected intramuscularly and the monkey handled safely while asleep. Protective clothing, visors and thick elbow-length gloves, as well as the usual gown, should be worn when dealing with the non-anaesthetized monkey. The thick gloves may be replaced by surgical gloves once the animal is asleep. Though most monkeys are quarantined when imported, there is still a very real risk of transmissible disease to man. At least two of these diseases carry a very high mortality rate, so every precaution should be taken. Handling of non-anaesthetized animals involves a great deal of stress to the animal as they are either pursued until exhausted around the cage before being netted, or an excess of physical force is employed to be sure there is no risk to the handler, pinning the animal to the floor or forcing it into a narrow box, then removing it limb by limb. If animals must be handled in an unanaesthetized state, it should be done by personnel experienced in the handling of monkeys or by senior staff. On no account should it be attempted by junior or otherwise inexperienced staff. Simple procedures can usually be carried out using the crush grids, so the need to anaesthetize the animal will only arise rarely.

Health programmes Particular attention should be paid to health monitoring of all staff required to work with primates, as not only are there risks to staff from micro-organisms endogenous to simians, but human diseases can be passed to simians, increasing the potential hazards from cross-infection. A thorough pre-employment medical examination is recommended for all staff handling laboratory animals, but particularly for primate handlers.

The conditions under which codes of practice need to be drawn up will vary from country to country, but should as a minimum include:

1. Staff handling simians should be under the supervision of a veterinarily or medically qualified person, knowledgeable about the dangers of animal diseases transmissible to man. Access to medical and veterinary advice should be available at all times.
2. Everyone should always wear adequate protective clothing, and in general should handle simians only when the animals have been anaesthetized or suitably sedated.
3. Precautions should also be taken in handling blood, tissues and dead animals. Carcasses and waste materials should be safely packed and incinerated.
4. Standing orders should include instructions on the action to be taken should personnel be bitten, scratched or injured while working with simians. Wounds, whether superficial or deep, should immediately be scrubbed clean with copious supplies of soap and water, and made to bleed. A local antiseptic such as tincture of iodine or cetrimide should

be applied, and the wound covered with a sterile dressing. Immediately after the first aid treatment has been given, a doctor should be consulted about the injury.

5. It should be standard practice to ensure that those in contact with simians have been immunized against tetanus and tuberculosis.

6. When encephalitis or other disease occurs in people who have been in association with simians, the possibility of infection from the simians should be seriously considered.

Animals held on long-term experiments should still be regarded as potentially dangerous as latent infection can be reactivated under experimental stress. Specialist advice should always be sought when planning to use primates. A number of suitable sources of information are suggested in the list of literature for further consultation.

Summary

Animal areas should have clear codes of practice to identify potential hazards and suitable safeguards.

Animals should be handled by adequately trained staff with a knowledge of the needs of each species.

Proper clothing should be provided and restraining devices and/or anaesthetics should be used where appropriate.

ZOONOSES

The risk of acquiring disease from laboratory animals, both experimental and non-experimental, should be taken into account by those handling animals in the laboratory. All animals are capable of passing on to man micro-organisms which they may harbour without displaying any overt signs of disease themselves.

The diseases which can be transmitted vary from species to species, and the following examples are not intended to be a complete list, but reference is made to sources of information in specialist literature for detailed control and treatment routines.

Transmission

Diseases of animals can be transmitted to man by scratches and bites, by ingestion of parasites, via the respiratory and alimentary tracts, broken skin and mucous membranes of the urinary tract.

Bacteria, viruses, fungi, ectoparasites and endoparasites can all be potentially hazardous if the basic rules of personal hygiene are not complied with; when they are, the risks of laboratory-acquired infection will be substantially reduced. As already stated, codes of practice should include rules which will help to prevent diseases. For example, the no-eating or no-drinking rules, the wearing of protective clothing and washing of hands before leaving animal areas are simple but effective precautions.

General considerations

The source of supply of animals is of primary importance in controlling zoonotic disease.

Animals from purpose-bred colonies, in-house breeding or commercial breeders, with high standards of hygiene, disease surveillance and control programmes, offer the best protection with regard to the control of zoonotic diseases. However, even animals from known sources should always be considered a potential hazard as undetected infections can be activated by stress, the colony can be invaded by wild rodents carrying disease, or human diseases may be passed to animals and potentially passed back to man.

Dogs and cats from non-purpose-bred stocks clearly present a hazard and wild-caught animals, particularly primates, can be the most dangerous of all.

Quarantine and screening

All animals should be held in quarantine on arrival and screened before allowed contact with current stock.

The quarantine period needs to take account of the degree of hazard from a particular species of animal incubation periods and may also need to conform with certain legal requirements, for example, in the UK all mammals imported into the country must be held for 6 months under the Rabies Order.

The minimum requirements in general terms for quarantine facilities are:

1. area completely separate from main animal area with high standard of containment;
2. separate equipment;
3. separate staff where possible;
4. a high level of hygiene;
5. arrangements for safe disposal of waste;
6. no animals to leave quarantine until a full clinical and microbiological examination has been completed;
7. where known or suspect pathogens are present, isolator facilities or full protective clothing to be provided.

These are basic requirements and special consideration must be given to the quarantine of primates from unknown or suspicious sources, and should include:

1. a medical programme for all staff at risk;
2. special arrangements for sterilization of animal waste before disposal;
3. high level of supervision and training in primate handling;
4. full parasitological and microbiological screening of animals with appropriate treatment before release from quarantine.

Examples of zoonoses

Rodents

A number of salmonella infections from both mice and rats are fairly common. Among the viral diseases, lymphocytic choriomeningitis is the most hazardous, with the virus being shed from saliva and urine by carrier animals. Stock should be screened before use. Ringworm from various rodent microspore types and intestinal parasites are other not uncommon infections from rodents to man.

Rabbits

An example of an organism transmitted from rabbits is pseudotuberculosis, which can, in certain circumstances, cause serious illness in man.

Dogs

In addition to rabies, a number of other diseases can be passed from dog to man, leptospirosis and pasteurellosis among them. Fungal and parasitic diseases, particularly from non-purpose-bred dogs, are possible dangers.

Cats

The agent of cat scratch fever, nematode, *Toxacara cati* and sarcoptes mite are among the problems of handling laboratory cats.

Non-human primates

These animals, because of their evolutionary closeness to man, clearly present the greatest risk, and among the many recorded organisms which are dangerous and even fatal, are *herpesvirus simicae* (B virus), Marburg agent, hepatitis A and Yaba virus. In addition a number of human viruses transmitted from man to simian and back to man, include poliovirus and cytomegalovirus. In addition tuberculosis, shigellosis and salmonellosis are all commonly transmitted by primates. Some ecto- and endoparasites which are common to many primates can also cause disease conditions in man.

Summary

The control of zoonotic disease may be effected by obtaining animals from disease-free sources where possible. Strict quarantine procedures in high-quality buildings with clear codes of practice, should be implemented with regular health checks on staff and disease monitoring of animals before use.

An awareness of the routes of infection and an appreciation of the seriousness of the problem will all help in reducing the incidence of laboratory-acquired disease.

ANIMAL ALLERGIES

A significant number of people whose work brings them into contact with animals, develop allergic reactions during their working lives. Some become highly sensitized and must avoid all contact with animals. One estimate is that between 15 and 20% of exposed persons develop allergic symptoms, e.g. conjunctivitis, rhinitis, dermatitis and asthma. In some rare cases anaphylaxis occurs.

Some people develop reactions against a single animal species, some to more than one. Allergies to rats, mice, guinea pigs and rabbits are the most commonly occurring. However, all animals should be regarded as a potential hazard in relation to the development of allergies.

Hair, fur, feathers, dander, dried faeces and urine from most animals can cause a reaction in a sensitized person. Direct contact, for example, from urine on scratches can cause a severe dermatitis, the allergen almost certainly being a urinary protein. Wearing gloves and long-sleeved clothing can help to reduce this type of contact.

Respiratory reactions, however, are more difficult to control, as high levels of airborne allergens will be present in most animal houses. Some control can be achieved by high air-flow levels to remove allergens. Reasonable stocking levels, the use of solid-sided cages and the monitoring of the environment for the presence of animal debris, will all help to reduce exposure.

Control of animal allergy

Employers of staff in contact with animals should be aware of the problem and do all they can to prevent the condition from developing. The provision of high standards of accommodation and adequate protective clothing, suitable training, medical and welfare arrangements, will do much to keep this industrial disease under control.

Accommodation

Good animal house design, particularly of the ventilation system, can provide an environment in which allergy to animals is less likely to develop.

An adequate ventilation system will provide sufficient air movement to supply oxygen and remove the products of respiration, odours, excess of body heat, and dilute dust and other particles, thereby reducing the risk of allergy.

A well-designed ventilation system should provide 15–20 complete changes of fresh air every hour and be capable of distributing air evenly within each animal room. The siting of inlet and outlet grilles must be considered with this in mind.

Another aspect of animal house design which contributes to the reduction of allergic conditions is the control of humidity, as dry conditions increase the incidence of dust and other particles of matter. For most species relative humidity of $55 \pm 15\%$ at $19 \pm 2\,°C$ is optimum.

The provision of adequate staff and service areas, to allow separation of activities, helps to reduce contact with allergies. Provision of common rooms, showers and changing rooms ensures staff change into protective clothing and maintain high standards of personal cleanliness. Service areas to house waste awaiting disposal, equipment being cleaned, and food and bedding stores, separate from animal holding areas, all help to reduce particulate matter in the environment.

Stocking densities

This is a difficult matter on which to be precise as cage size, group size, age of animal and method of husbandry all have an influence. However, some generally accepted levels which many laboratories find acceptable can be taken as a guide.

Number of animals/m^2 of animal room:

175 mice
40 rats
30 hamsters

18 guinea pigs
4 rabbits.

Some variations, depending on experimental needs, different countries' regulations, and of course the age, size and species of animal will affect the level of stocking.

The number of animals should be related to the animal house and air extraction design.

Protective equipment

Gloves, long-sleeved clothing, respiratory protection and eye wear, all offer a degree of protection, but may be inadequate when the degree of challenge is high or the worker particularly sensitive. In such cases, the provision of a personal protective hood (Figure 4.1) can offer a high degree of protection

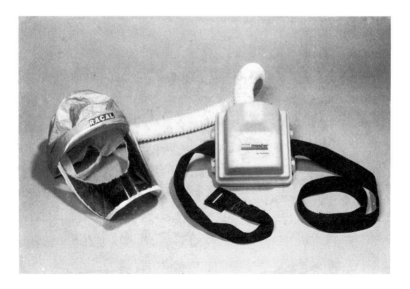

Figure 4.1 Personal filter hood

if properly used. Care must be taken when removing the caps, and the filters need periodic attention. In use, the device is very comfortable and in addition to protecting from respiratory allergens, also offers eye protection.

Any protective equipment, however, should be regarded as a supplement to good environmental control and not as an alternative.

One way of controlling the environment to protect staff in areas which are not ideal as far as ventilation rate is concerned is the use of positive pressure

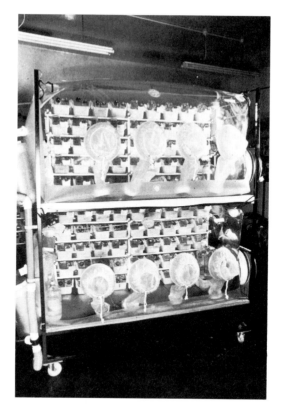

Figure 4.2 Positive-pressure isolators

isolators (Figure 4.2). These provide total containment of the animal and have proved highly effective, not only in the use for which they were designed, i.e. maintaining gnotobiotic animals, but as a cheap effective way of upgrading animal facilities to provide an allergen-free environment.

Summary

The problem of animal allergy should be fully appreciated by those working in animal areas. Provision should be made for medical and welfare guidance and information and suitable protective clothing provided.

The design of animal working areas and the modification of stocking levels and necessary working practices is critically important.

HANDLING EXPERIMENTAL ANIMALS

Animals undergoing experimental procedures can present additional dangers to staff handling them, the degree of danger being related to material introduced into the animal. The normal precautions already outlined to safeguard staff from physical dangers and transmission of disease need to be supplemented with more stringent controls taking into account the particular hazard of each experiment.

Awareness of the possible hazards before the experiment begins, and the drawing up of a protocol detailing the means of reducing them, prevent serious mishaps.

Microbiological research

The degrees of hazard are difficult to assess accurately. Attempts have been made to group biological agents used in research into groups - some of them overlapping. It is outside the scope of this section to deal with this complex subject in specific detail, as high-risk pathogens that are known to cause severe, even fatal, diseases in man can only be handled in high-grade containment areas with specialist equipment and staff.

The authorization to handle these organisms will be the subject of controls in all countries and reference will always have to be made to medical and environmental control authorities in each case. Some examples of high-risk organisms are:

Lassa fever virus
Smallpox virus
Marburg virus
Simian herpes (B) virus

These and other organisms will need the highest possible containment and special endorsement.

Other groups of organisms which offer special hazards to laboratory workers and need special accommodation and conditions include:

Brucella
Salmonella paratyphi A
Yersinia pestis
Mycobacterium tuberculosis

This is not intended to be a complete list, and reference should always be made to current regulations in each country.

The high-grade facilities needed to house high-risk experimental animals will also need a code of practice for the prevention of infection. These codes will need to be related directly to the level of hazard; however some basic rules apply when handling animals capable of passing on diseases to man.

All staff must have training in the handling of the species of animal to be used, and all contact with the animal, its waste and any equipment used, must be under supervision of the person responsible for the experiment.

Codes of practice must include:

1. animal rooms must be adequately ventilated, easy to clean and access limited to authorized staff;
2. adequate means of sterilization of waste and equipment;
3. hands must be washed and disinfected after handling animals;
4. suitable protective clothing must be worn at all times;
5. eating, drinking, smoking and application of cosmetics are strictly forbidden;
6. all waste to be incinerated and transported without spillage.

These general rules should be incorporated into a local code of practice and should be reinforced by constant updating, checking and supervision.

All areas where pathogens are used should be clearly marked with appropriate biohazard warning signs.

In many cases it will be considered wise to ensure that extract air is filtered by HEPA filters to safeguard the external environment.

The level of containment within the experimental facility again will depend on the level of hazard. A number of devices are available. Negative-pressure flexible-film isolators have proved to be useful in the containment of certain organisms where the reduction of aerosols is an important consideration.

Full air-filtered suits or respirators may also be used to separate the animal from the staff.

The approach should be maximum protection for the staff, with the minimum degree of inconvenience taking the needs of the animal into account.

All manipulations, inoculations, necropsy, tissue and body fluid sampling should be carried out in an appropriate microbiological cabinet or in isolators.

Human tumour material

The xenografting of human tumours into immunologically compromised animals has increased over recent years, and some concern has been expressed as to the potential biohazard in two areas in particular. Firstly, the immune deficiency of the animals may make them more susceptible to various human organisms which will from time to time be associated with the implanted tumours. In addition there is the possibility that oncogenic materi-

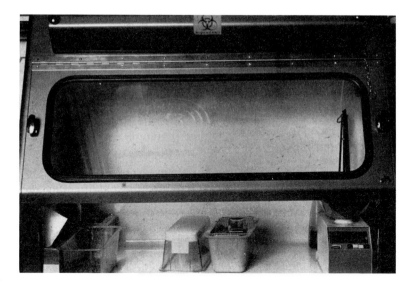

Figure 4.3 Filter top box in safety cabinet

al, perhaps of viral origin, will be activated in the animal and present a hazard to man.

These may be low-risk hazards but as the likelihood is to some extent unknown, it is reasonable to take precautions without undue inconvenience.

Filter top cages used in conjunction with a safety cabinet, as shown in Figure 4.3, offer a reasonable degree of protection.

Where the material is known or suspected of being infected the negative pressure isolator system offers a suitable alternative.

Carcinogens

The introduction of chemical carcinogens into animals creates problems not encountered with their manipulation in the laboratory. Carcinogens may be converted into a number of different metabolites. These metabolites, which may be more or less carcinogenic than the parent compound, are often found in the excreta of treated animals. Therefore not only must the compound be handled safely but the animal and its waste must be treated with care.

The assessment of the hazards of chemical compounds and the excretory products of animals receiving the compounds is difficult because there are large numbers of suspect agents, the metabolites are difficult to predict or assess, and there are differences among species with regard to the metabolism of chemical carcinogens.

The risks to staff will be clear when known or suspect carcinogens are administered to animals. The route of administration is an important factor. Carcinogens incorporated into powdered diet, thereby generating dust which comes into direct contact with staff, or is deposited in cages, on walls, and floors, are a serious hazard which should be controlled. Drinking water used as a route of administration can also present hazards from aerosols, droplets and spillage.

Other routes of administration by intubation, skin painting and various parenteral routes are more controllable and therefore safer, but all present some hazards and should be carried out in suitable containment. Volatile compounds, or those administered as gases by inhalation are of high risk and should only be carried out in suitable areas under controlled conditions with efficient exhaust systems to prevent personnel from inhaling the carcinogen. It is essential that staff wear appropriate protective equipment and clothing.

Animal house design

The considerations which apply to the design of laboratories where carcinogens are used in substantial amounts, apply even more so to animal areas. In general terms walls, floors, and ceiling surfaces must be defect-free, and finished to withstand frequent washing.

They must be well ventilated and under negative pressure and sited so as to avoid risk to adjacent areas.

Washing facilities and showers must be provided.

Strict codes of practice which prohibit eating, drinking and smoking in the area, together with rules regarding the treatment of waste, should be im-

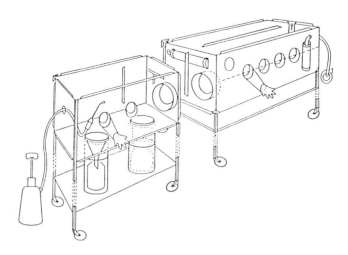

Figure 4.4 Negative-pressure isolator with cleaning module

plemented. However, to meet these requirements, particularly in regard to decontamination of cages and ventilation systems, is extremely difficult. The problems include the volume of waste, generation of aerosols and dusts, relatively large areas of space needing decontamination and the particular problem of holding animals in cages, not primarily designed for carcinogen work. One successful way of overcoming these problems has been the introduction within a carcinogen suite of negative-pressure isolators. There are a number of advantages in using this system. These are:

1. Total separation of personnel from the animal and test substance.
2. A high level of filtration, both into and out of the isolator.
3. All aerosols and dusts generated inside isolator are confined and controlled.
4. Decontamination during and at end of experiment is possible without contact.
5. A closed-circuit system for the removal of waste, dead animals, and samples by use of attachable modules.
6. The removal and disposal of filters if possible from within isolators with no operator contact.
7. Can be adapted for use with volatile carcinogens.
8. All cleaning of surfaces can be done without contact. Cages and equipment cleaned in washing machines by transfer without staff contact.
9. A more positive control over health status of animals under test, with less risk of intercurrent infection.

The isolator can be linked to a cleaning module as shown in Figure 4.4.

Within the module, waste material is transferred into double bags ready for incineration. Liquid waste can be neutralized before being disposed of in an appropriate manner depending on the material. This is clearly a very safe way of handling waste as the contaminant is contained, and no direct or aerosol contact is made.

Summary

All animals under experiment need to be handled with regard to the procedure, the degree of risk assessed, and appropriate measures taken.

CONCLUSION

The handling of animals in the laboratory can be a potential danger to those who use them, or care for them. The animals themselves, their waste products, and the organisms or compounds tested in animal systems are potential hazards. Training in handling techniques, well-designed animal areas, and adequate protective clothing and equipment together with clear codes of practice can do much to reduce the danger.

LITERATURE FOR FURTHER CONSULTATION

Animals (Scientific Procedures) Act 1986

Code of Practice for Housing and Care of Animals used in Scientific Procedures. (1988) London: HMSO

Clough, G. and Gamble, M.R. (1979). *Laboratory Animal Houses. A Guide to Design and Planning of Animal Facilities*. LAC Manual Series No. 4. (London: Medical Research Council)

Control of Substances Hazardous to Health (1988) London: HMSO

Handling Chemical Carcinogens in the Laboratory (1979). IARC Publications No.33. (Lyon, France: International Agency for Research on Cancer)

Hazards in the Chemical Laboratory. 2nd edn (1977). (London: The Chemical Society)

Laboratory Animal Handbooks. No. 1: Hare, R. and O'Donoghue, P.N. (1968) *Design and Function of Laboratory Animal Houses*; No. 5: Semer, J. and Wood, M. (1981) *Safety in the Animal House*; No. 7: McSheehy, T. (1976) *Control of Animal House Environment*. (London: Laboratory Animals Ltd)

National Cancer Institute (1979). *Chemical Carcinogen Hazards in Animal Research Facilities*. (Rockville, Maryland, USA: Office of Biohazard Safety)

National Cancer Institute (1979). *Biological Hazards in the Non-human primate Laboratory*. (Rockville, Maryland, USA: Office of Biohazard Safety)

Newman Taylor, A. (1982). *Eur. J. Resp. Dis.*, **63**, Suppl. 123, 60-64

Newman Taylor, A., Longbottom, J.L. and Pepys, (1977). Respiratory allergy to urine proteins of rats and mice. *Lancet*, **2**, 847

Sainsbury, D. (1967). *Animal Health and Housing* (London: Tindall and Cassell)

What You Should Know About Allergy to Laboratory Animals of U.K. Health & Safety Commission. HMSO London

World Health Organization (1979). *Safety Measures in Microbiology. Minimum Standards of Laboratory Safety*. Weekly Epidemiological Record, **44**, 340

5 Health Care of Laboratory Personnel

A.E. Wright

Laboratory personnel, particularly those working in departments of microbiology, may be exposed to the risk of infection in the course of their daily work. That infections do occur from time to time is well documented. Sometimes it is the individual worker who becomes ill and in this case, if the infecting agent is common in the community, proof that the infection occurred in the laboratory may be difficult to obtain. Occasionally, many staff may be infected at the same time and if the organism is known to be absent from the community then the source, the laboratory, is apparent. Such an incident indeed took place in Michigan, USA, in 1938/39 when 45 clinical cases of brucellosis occurred in association with a laboratory. The infecting organism *Brucella melitensis* had not been isolated in that territory in recent years and all milk consumed by those infected was known to have been pasteurized. Rarely, infection of a laboratory employee leads to spread of disease in the community, as happened with smallpox in London in 1973. Such clear-cut examples of hazards in the laboratory do not, fortunately, occur very often but now that infectious diseases have decreased in importance in the western world such outbreaks can have profound repercussions. There is foremost the personal tragedy of deaths such as occurred in the London smallpox outbreak, or there may be chronic ill-health which follows infection with brucellosis. In addition there is inevitably an over-reaction in the community which may result in the imposition of stricter regulations over a wide field of laboratory work. In some instances such regulations may lead to safer working conditions and should be accepted and implemented by those concerned. In other instances regulations 'across the board' can lead to restrictions of activities in fields where hazards are more imaginary than real and thus curtail research and routine work to the detriment of patient care. At the lowest level such restrictions are seen by workers to be unnecessary and are therefore ignored, bringing all safety regulations into disrepute.

For all these reasons it is essential that management and worker should co-operate to reduce hazards in the laboratory. One aspect of the reduction of hazard is to look after the health of the laboratory worker. It is the objective of this chapter to outline the steps which should be taken in this direction. In the UK an Act of Parliament *The Health and Safety at Work etc. Act 1974* has clearly defined responsibilities in this field. A Health and Safety Commission is responsible for policy decisions which are translated into action by inspectors of the Health and Safety Executive. Such inspectors have the power to visit and advise on safety in all occupations including laboratories. In this they have support in law. In addition, and probably more important than the legal aspects of health and safety at work, management, usually in the form of the director of the laboratory, has a moral responsibility to look after the health of his staff. On the other hand, each individual worker has a legal and moral responsibility for safety, for his actions may imperil his fellow workers or members of the community in which he lives.

Further to the Health and Safety at Work Act of 1974 new regulations in this field came into force in the UK in 1989. These are the "Control of Substances Hazardous to Health Regulations" requiring an employer not to expose employees to any substance hazardous to health unless an assessment has been made of the risks and steps taken to mitigate against these. Employees must be informed of the risks and the precautions that must be taken. Clearly, these Regulations include chemicals and micro-organisms, methods of handling, and in particular, ventilation systems and biological safety cabinets.

As in all respects of Health and Safety, the keeping of records is of primary importance.

The employer, although responsible, is able to delegate implementation of these Regulations to the Laboratory Director who will be assisted by the Laboratory Safety Officer and the Laboratory Safety Committee.

As these Regulations apply to the whole hospital as well as to laboratories the Health Authorities may appoint a Coordinator and Control of Hazardous Substances Team.

FITNESS FOR EMPLOYMENT

The health care of laboratory personnel should commence when the candidate first presents himself or herself for a job. No interview is complete without

(a)   the candidate's medical questionnaire;
(b)   an explanation of the work and possible hazards involved.

72

REFERENCE C.A.M.R.

PUBLIC HEALTH LABORATORY SERVICE

CONFIDENTIAL

1.	NAME IN BLOCK LETTERS	a. Surname ....
		b. Other names (in full) .... Age last birthday ....

2. Situation or class of appointment for which you are a candidate

3. What is your height (without shoes)?

.... ft .... ins or .... m.

and your present weight .... lbs.
in indoor clothes
or............................... kg.

			YES or NO	(IF APPROPRIATE GIVE FURTHER DETAILS).
4.	a.	Is your eyesight satisfactory for all normal purposes (with glasses if necessary)?		
	b.	Is your hearing in each ear good for all purposes including telephoning?		
	c.	Are you free from any defect of speech?		
	d.	Are you free from any other physical defect or disability?		
	e.	Are you now and generally in good health?		

			YES or NO	(IF ANY REPLY IS 'YES' GIVE PARTICULARS)
5.	a.	Are you at present under medical treatment or observation?		
	b.	Are you taking any medicines, tablets or drugs of any kind?		
	c.	Have you ever had treatment in hospital, undergone any operation, or had any serious accident?		
				DATE
	d.	Have you ever had treatment by radium or radio-therapy?		

Figure 5.1 This figure is included by kind permission of the Director of the Public Health Laboratory Service UK, Dr J.E.M. Whitehead

Figure 5.1 *Contd*

	YES or NO	(IF ANY REPLY IS 'YES' GIVE PARTICULARS INCLUDING LENGTH OF ILLNESS WITH TREATMENT AND APPROXIMATE DATES)	DATE(S)
6. Have you ever had:			
a. fits, fainting attacks, blackouts or epilepsy ?			
b. mental ill-health, nervous breakdown or nervous debility ?			
c. heart trouble, including rheumatic fever or high blood pressure ?			
d. asthma, bronchitis, tuberculosis or other chest disease ?			
e. gastric or duodenal ulcer or other digestive or bowel disorder ?			
f. kidney disease or bladder trouble (including stone or gravel) ?			
g. arthritis, rheumatism, or gout ?			
h. any back or joint trouble including prolapsed disc ?			
i. any blood disease ?			
j. any skin disease ?			
k. diabetes ?			
l. eye disease ?			
m. ear disease (including running from the ears) ?			
n. rupture ?			
o. varicose veins ?			
p. any other illness or disease ?			
7. a. Do you suffer from hay fever ?			
b. Are you allergic to anything ? (eg. eggs)			

Figure 5.1 *Contd*

	YES or NO	(IF ANY REPLY IS 'YES' GIVE PARTICULARS AND APPROXIMATE DATE)	DATE(S)
8. Have you ever left employment on ground of ill health or unsatisfactory attendance ?			
Have you been medically rejected for service in HM Forces ?			
Has any insurance company declined to accept a proposal to insure your life ?			

9. Have you required a doctor during the last 3 years ?   (Please answer YES or NO) _____

If the answer is YES please give the following particulars for each occasion:

Nature of ailment (use a separate line for each illness)	Dates of beginning and end of illness (as near as you can give them)	Number of weeks unable to attend school or to follow usual occupation

10. a.   What is the name and address of your doctor ?

    b.   May we approach him if necessary ?

I declare that all the foregoing statements are true and complete to the best of my knowledge and belief.

I understand that I may be required to undergo a medical examination.

Signature of Candidate _____ Date _____

75

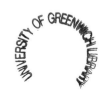

The medical questionnaire

Some authorities require a full medical examination report before appointment. There are occasionally indications for this to be done but such routine examinations are not always a necessity for civilian appointment. It is often just as rewarding to ask the candidate to answer a series of questions on his health and to indicate that untrue statements may lead to the loss of the job. It is rare for the candidate to lie. A typical form is shown in Figure 5.1. The important questions include age, height and weight, and these should be compared with tables showing the normal distribution. A marked difference, over 10% from the normal, should lead to examination by a medically qualified practitioner. It is essential to establish previous medical history with particular emphasis on mental outlook, a history of allergies or skin diseases and previous accidents or operations. The introspective individual may allow imaginary hazards to prey upon his mind, the allergic may not be able to work with animals, and the individual who has had a severe accident may be physically incapable of certain duties. Drugs should be declared. The candidate on immunosuppressive drugs is unsuitable for work in a laboratory. The vaccination history is important. Those who have never received any form of immunization may be in this situation because of the attitude adopted by their parents, but it does not mean that they are themselves opposed to such policies. The question should be asked either on the form or at interview.

A radiograph of the chest may be indicated but certainly a question should be asked about vaccination against tuberculosis. If the individual has had BCG it is as well to examine the site to establish without doubt that this has been done.

Variations from the normal should be investigated sympathetically. Some 8% of men are red/blue colour-blind but for women the incidence is less than 1%. This should not necessarily exclude a good candidate from employment in a laboratory. The intelligent individual soon learns to compensate for this minor defect and many good technical workers recognize the tubercle bacillus through a microscope as much by its shape and size as by its colour. Even epilepsy has not debarred all laboratory workers in the past. Providing the condition is well controlled, or the individual has rare attacks with adequate premonitory signs, he or she can perform laboratory duties successfully.

An explanation of the work and possible hazards involved

This is an important element of the interview. The candidate's reaction to the need to receive a series of vaccinations should be judged. The requirement for the worker to be vaccinated should be clearly stated and the candidate should not be appointed if objections or doubts are raised. The attitude adopted to the prospect of being involved in experimental work with animals should also be explored. Both these questions can save a considerable amount of trouble at a later date.

ON EMPLOYMENT

The employee's medical questionnaire should be filed and a medical record card completed bearing important details from the questionnaire. This card should be designed to display the complete immunization history. For the small laboratory this procedure is adequate, but it requires a conscientious and dedicated approach to health care for these cards must all be checked at intervals year after year to ensure that the employee is offered booster vaccine doses at the proper intervals. A much more efficient method applicable to larger laboratories is to place the individual's medical history on a computer with safeguards to ensure that only those authorized can recall the information. Using modern data-handling equipment it is possible to have available each month a list of those individuals who require booster doses of vaccine during that calendar month. This leads to greater efficiency in recall and it also spreads the load for the doctor who is called upon to give a few injections each month throughout the year instead of dealing with larger numbers at infrequent intervals. This has the added advantage of making the employee feel that he is being treated as an individual instead of one of a herd. The shrewd doctor will take advantage of this situation as it gives him time to make enquiries concerning health and personal problems and thus to anticipate and often deal with difficulties before they assume major proportions.

The medical record card should display the employee's name and address, his or her next of kin and the name of his medical practitioner. When this is completed, and before any arrangements are made for immunization, a letter should go to the medical practitioner telling him that the individual has started work in a microbiological laboratory. This will be filed with the patient's records and should alert the doctor if his patient develops an unexplained fever. The letter should also explain that the employee will shortly be offered immunization against a variety of infectious diseases unless the doctor writes to register any objection or would prefer to administer the prophylaxis himself. It is rare for any such objection to be raised if this procedure is followed, but problems can arise if the employee is immunized without prior notice to the doctor.

Two further steps should be taken at this stage. The employee should be issued with a personal card to be carried at all times. This card should show the name and address of the holder and the name and telephone number of his doctor. In addition, the card should state where he or she works and the telephone number of one or more senior members of the medical staff of the laboratory. This card should be produced to the attending physician if the laboratory scientist is taken ill. Such a card will alert the physician to the possibility of a laboratory infection and enable him to discuss the case with laboratory staff who will know if indeed any such hazards exist.

The second step is the collection of a specimen of blood to provide serum for a double purpose. The serum can be screened for the presence of antibody to a variety of infectious diseases and will be discussed under these headings. The specimen can then be stored for retrieval at a later date, to provide a 'baseline' specimen if the employee falls ill.

Finally the new recruit should where possible be given an *induction course*.

The amount of time which can be allocated to an *induction course* for newly appointed personnel will vary with the size of the laboratory. The small diagnostic laboratory taking on one or two new workers at any one time may be unable to allocate any formal teaching at this stage. It is useful to attach the new staff to the laboratory safety officer for a brief period so the importance of observing safety precautions is instilled from the first day. Safety is largely an attitude of mind and the new recruit should be clearly shown that such precautions are taken seriously in the laboratory. In larger laboratories one or more days may be set aside for an induction course and this, although emphasizing safety, may be used with advantage to allow the recruit to find his way about in what may be a complex and unfamiliar world. Such a course should include lectures or demonstrations on:

(a) laboratory hazards with an introduction to the literature on the subject;
(b) legal aspects of safety at work;
(c) the use of protective equipment such as safety cabinets and clothing, e.g. respirators and Martindale suits;
(d) how to write a protocol for a work programme so that potential hazards can be highlighted and obviated;
(e) how to handle animals safely;
(f) specialist fields such as chemicals and gases, if these are relevant;
(g) the safe transit of specimens as laid down by the Health Services Advisory Committee.

Finally, consideration should be given to offering a protective vaccination against the following diseases.

Tuberculosis

Laboratory-acquired tuberculosis was first shown to be a problem in the UK by Reid, who demonstrated in the early 1950s that laboratory workers were from 2 to 5 times more likely to contract tuberculosis than a control group. It had been known for many years that this disease was a hazard to those who handled clinical material but this work was the first to use a control group.

Similar figures were shown in France and Canada and again in the UK 20 years later. In retrospect it is disturbing that such a hazard should have persisted into the 1970s for the dangers to young nurses of contact with cases of open tuberculosis had been recognized for a generation. The role of BCG vaccination in prevention had also been well documented. The incidence of tuberculosis in the general population, although falling steadily over the years, remains appreciable. In England and Wales in 1987, 4000 cases occurred in a population of approximately 50 million. Such cases are well investigated, it being usual to send at least three specimens of sputum to the microbiological laboratory for culture for *M. tuberculosis* and subsequently to send specimens at monthly intervals to determine the effect of treatment and to confirm that the organism remains sensitive to antituberculous drugs. The development of antibiotic resistance may also require further laboratory investigations. Routine procedures of this type ensure a steady flow of potentially infectious material into the laboratory. The following precautions should be taken:

(a) Technical procedures should be used which are known to be least hazardous. Work should be done in safety cabinets in a room designated for this purpose. Facilities such as disposable caps, gowns and handwashing facilities should be available.

(b) Staff should be tuberculin tested and their BCG status should be known. It is not sufficient to ask if vaccination has been done (few countries in Western Europe make such vaccinations compulsory); the vaccination site should be inspected. If evidence of successful vaccination is present this should be recorded together with the results of the tuberculin test. There is good evidence that the administration of BCG gives long-lasting immunity to those living in the UK even if their skin sensitivity has waned. If no typical scar is present it should be assumed that no vaccination has been done and BCG should be given. Unvaccinated staff with little induration with the Mantoux test (less than 5 mm diameter) or Heaf test grade II or less should also be vaccinated. Skin reactions greater than those described raise the question of active tuberculosis and further investigations including a chest radiograph will be necessary. It is possible that routine BCG vaccination of schoolchildren will soon be stopped in the UK. Special groups may continue to be vaccinated and it is reasonable to argue that scientists working with Mycobacteria should be one of these.

Routine chest radiographs are of doubtful value, but the recommendation that they should be done is found in all the codes of practice for the care of the health of laboratory staff. Thus laboratory workers should be encouraged to have repeat chest radiographs at 2-3-year intervals, especially if they work with the agent.

Newly joined staff who have spent their early life overseas should be assessed carefully. BCG has not proved as effective in India as in the West. It is not known if this finding is due to the BCG used or to the individual's exposure to related mycobacteria prior to vaccination. Until this finding is explained consideration should be given to revaccination even in the presence of evidence of a successful 'take' if this has been given in the tropics.

Enteric disease

Although vaccines have long been available against typhoid fever and para-typhoid A and B, only the monovalent typhoid vaccine is now used in the UK. This vaccine contains 1000 million *Salmonella typhi* per ml, a much lower dose of organisms than in the polyvalent preparation which used to cause appreciable side-effects. The monovalent vaccine is less troublesome, but whether this is due to the reduction in the numbers of organisms injected or to the absence of the paratyphoid element is not clear. Side-effects do still occur and are more likely the more frequently the vaccine is injected and the older the recipient is. At one time those who had received many booster doses of this vaccine were advised against further injections when they had reached the age of 35. Of course such a recommendation would not apply if exposure to infection was likely.

Typhoid disease has always merited a prominent place in the list of laboratory infections and the danger has been highlighted in recent years in the USA. In America *Salmonella typhi* is used as a quality control organism and distribution to laboratories there resulted in a number of laboratory infections. In the UK this organism has not been distributed in this way although there is no reason why it should not be so used. Cases of typhoid in the UK, however, rarely exceed 150 each year but even so one death in a laboratory worker was recorded in the 1970s. The vaccine confers some 70–90% protection for a period not exceeding 3 years and booster doses are recommended at that interval after a basic course of two injections at 1-month interval. Medical opinion implies that all laboratory workers should be protected and certainly all those who handle specimens, especially faeces, urine and blood, should be inoculated. The administration of the vaccine to all other members of staff, including office workers and cleaners, can be a difficult decision in countries where the disease is rare. The infection is not airborne and in theory only those handling specimens and cultures should be at risk, but at least five cases have occurred in the USA in laboratory workers who were described as 'merely present in the laboratory'. Vaccination should only be offered after due consideration of the potential hazard.

Live oral typhoid vaccines using the Ty21a *S. typhi* strain are not showing as much promise as was hoped and it may be that a genetically engineered vaccine will be used in the future.

Tetanus

A few cases of tetanus infection have occurred in laboratory workers, but this is not a disease which normally presents a hazard in the diagnostic laboratory. In the research laboratory where the toxin itself may be produced and manipulated the situation may be different. Nevertheless, on general medical grounds no opportunity to vaccinate against tetanus should be missed. The disease, now rare in the West, is still capable of causing death, and in the UK occurs in the young athlete and the middle-aged and elderly gardener. The laboratory workers may at some time or other fall into one of these groups and should, therefore, be offered vaccination. Many European countries recommend tetanus vaccination and in some it is compulsory.

The basic course consists of three injections of absorbed tetanus toxoid with an interval of 6–8 weeks between the first and second doses and 6 months between the second and third. Booster doses should be given at 5 and 10 years. Many children receive their basic course at an early age combined with diphtheria and sometimes with whooping cough. In these instances the laboratory worker will only require a booster dose. Too many booster doses may cause local or even general reactions.

Rubella

All women of childbearing age should be vaccinated against rubella, and most countries in Western Europe have a vaccination policy recommending this at ages 12–15 years. The baseline serum collected from newly appointed laboratory workers should, therefore, be examined for evidence of immunity and if such evidence is lacking the live attenuated rubella vaccine should be offered. No reliance should be placed on a history of a rubella-like illness in the past as other virus infections are known to cause similar illnesses. The vaccine is contraindicated during the first 3 months of pregnancy and con-ception should be avoided for 3 months following vaccination. Immunity should be checked 8 weeks after vaccination.

The introduction of measles, mumps, rubella vaccine (MMR) for all children in the UK from 1988 should eventually reduce the risk of rubella infection in pregnant women.

Hepatitis

Hepatitis has been known to occur in laboratory workers for about a century, but it is possible that some of these early cases may have been due to any one of the several different viruses now known to cause this disease. There is, nevertheless, clear evidence of cases occurring following contact with blood

81

and serum, and these were most certainly due to hepatitis B. Blood is not easy to aerosolize and in any case we have no evidence that hepatitis can be spread by the airborne route. It is, however, very easy to splash blood as a result of many manipulations commonly done in the laboratory. Opening containers, especially those with a plug-type closure rather than a screw-capped container, is a case in point. Such splashes will contaminate equipment and bench surfaces and thus the clothing and skin. The virus seems able to penetrate into the blood stream via minute cuts and abrasions, but more dangerous are cuts from sharp instruments such as scalpels and penetrating wounds from needles, the so-called needle-stick injury. Such minor accidents are not infrequent in laboratories. The virus of hepatitis B is thought to be carried by persistent human carriers forming a vast global reservoir estimated as exceeding 150 million persons. The geographical variation in incidence is wide, ranging from 1 in 800 blood donors in the UK to some 10% of the population in certain parts of Asia and Africa. It follows from this that all blood handled in a laboratory is potentially dangerous and should be treated with a degree of care. Gloves should be worn and protection taken against splashes to the eyes. This may be done by wearing goggles but many prefer to use a safety cabinet which has the added advantage of allowing work to be done behind a glass screen. Needles should be replaced by cannulas, and glass pipettes by plastic disposables. Cuts and scratches should be encouraged to bleed, treated with a disinfectant and covered with a dressing. Technical procedures should be carefully reviewed at intervals to ensure that personnel are handling material with care. Guidelines should be written out and displayed so that no worker has any doubt concerning his responsibility.

In addition to the general guidance already given the laboratory director should make certain that testing of specimens for hepatitis markers is only done by experienced staff. If the skin is punctured or contamination of mucous membranes is known to have taken place hepatitis B immunoglobulin may be administered. This should only be given if the specimen is known to be positive and the individual is tested to see if he is susceptible. Such a step will not be necessary if all those involved in the testing of such specimens are offered inactivated hepatitis B virus vaccine which has been available since 1982. This vaccine is an inactivated, alum-adsorbed suspension of surface antigen particles. These are purified from human plasma by a combination of physical and chemical procedures followed by a triple process of inactivation each of which are known to inactivate HB and other viruses. The vaccine has now been administered to many persons in various parts of the world and although its safety has been questioned there is no real evidence to raise any doubts. Such questions on the safety of the vaccine arise from the well-known fact that the vaccine is derived from human plasma and that some of the donors may have been homosexuals and that cases of AIDS are known to have occurred in the cities where blood was collected to make the vaccine.

In spite of the fact that AIDS may take years to develop there is no evidence to implicate the vaccine in its spread.

The vaccine course consists of three intramuscular doses, the second dose being given after 1 month and the third 6 months after the first. Such a course produces antibody in over 90% of those vaccinated and persists for some years; the exact period is yet to be determined.

Since 1986 a new genetically engineered vaccine has become available produced by *Saccharomyces cerevisiae* into which a plasmid has been inserted containing Hepatitis B surface antigen gene. The immune response to the recombinant HB vaccine is satisfactory when given as a three-dose course. (This vaccine is now replacing the plasma-derived vaccine.)

A small proportion of vaccines, less than 10%, give a poor response so that when attempting to protect the individual laboratory worker, tests for anti-body response may be indicated. (If there is less than 50 i.u./litre of anti HBsAg in the serum of the vacinee a fourth dose should be given.)

Although the hazards of handling blood are stressed it should be noted that neither in the USA nor in the UK are laboratory workers considered to be a high risk population. Immigrants and refugees from areas of high endemicity, those who work with the mentally retarded, homosexuals and drug abusers are all more likely to become infected than those who work in laboratories. In fact, the application of good basic microbiological techniques appears to have caused a fall in the incidence of this disease in those who work in laboratories in the UK. Nevertheless, health service staff who develop infection with hepatitis B often fail to identify an accident or incident, and the annual incidence of infection in laboratory scientific staff was quoted as 37 per 100 000 compared with four among nurses in 1980–84. The comparable figures for 1985–88 are 10 and 2. Clearly there is a case for extreme care in handling blood and vaccination should be offered, but in spite of the fact that 5% of the 6,696 cases of hepatitis B in England & Wales and Northern Ireland in the years 1980–84 occurred in health care workers, the uptake of vaccination remains poor.

Poliomyelitis

Vaccination against poliomyelitis is recommended in most countries in Western Europe and is compulsory in some. Laboratory workers should be offered and encouraged to be vaccinated, especially if working with faeces as in a routine bacteriology and virology department. Some specialist laboratories handle faeces from abroad, including the tropics, and here vaccination is most important.

The vaccine is available as an oral attenuated strain of each of the three types of poliovirus and produces by multiplication a local gut immunity and a serum antibody response. The basic course is three doses at intervals of 6-8 weeks and 4-6 months between the second and third respectively. Contraindications include pregnancy, gastrointestinal upset and hypersensitivity to antibiotics used in the preparation of the vaccine. A killed vaccine is also available if the live vaccine is contraindicated.

Live vaccine should only be given to laboratory workers if their families are to be vaccinated at the same time as there is a remote chance of enhanced virulence if the vaccine strain is passaged through young siblings. In this situation it is often wiser to use the killed vaccine.

Reinforcing doses are only required if there is no clear history of such a dose being given on leaving school.

Diphtheria

Diphtheria is a rare disease in Western Europe due to the immunization schemes which exist either as recommendations or in compulsory form in different countries. Most children have some basic immunity due to childhood vaccination but few receive booster doses in later life.

Only staff to be exposed to a case of diphtheria or swabs and cultures need to be vaccinated. This can be done using diphtheria vaccine depending upon the results of a Schick test. Such a procedure is cumbersome and takes time, and for this reason it will probably be replaced by the use of diphtheria vaccine for adults (adsorbed) which is now available. The preparation may be used for the immunization of persons aged over 10 years. Primarily designed for boosting immunity in adults such as laboratory staff it may be given without Schick testing. Neither the immune nor the hypersensitive are likely to experience reactions other than mild side-effects.

Other vaccinations

These should be confined to those who work with agents in highly specialized laboratories. Vaccines are available against *rabies*, *anthrax* and *botulism* as examples.

Rabies immunization is usually done using a three-dose regimen on days 0, 7 and 25, of human diploid cell rabies vaccine produced by the Merieux Institute. The usual dose is 1.0 ml by intramuscular injections and this gives adequate titres of antibody. Because of the cost of this vaccine the practice of giving three doses of 0.1 ml by intradermal injection has become commonplace but the efficacy of this procedure has been questioned. Doubts arose because of a case of human rabies in a Peace Corps Volunteer working in Kenya, and subsequent investigation revealed that the intradermal route did not always result in good protection. If the intradermal route is chosen serological testing should be done 2–3 weeks after immunization and if a titre of less than 1 in 16 recorded, additional doses given until that titre is reached or exceeded.

Anthrax injections in laboratory workers have been reported at intervals since 1914, and Pike has recorded 45 deaths from this disease. The hazard lies in inhalation and is, therefore, largely confined to research institutions where aerosols may be created, particularly by those who have an interest in biological warfare. A vaccine is available prepared from a growth of the Sterne strain of anthrax and rendered sterile by filtration and the use of thiomersal as a preservative. The alum-precipitated anthrax antigen is given as a course of four intramuscular injections each of 0.5 ml. The first three doses are given at intervals of 3 weeks and the last dose 6 months later. Reinforcing doses are given annually. Local erythema and swelling may occur and less often regional lymphadenopathy and pyrexia. In the UK this vaccine is prepared for the Department of Health and Social Security, Russell Square, London by the Public Health Laboratory Service.

Botulism has not been reported as a laboratory infection but the vaccine is given when work with the toxin of *Clostridium botulinum* is done. A pentavalent toxoid aluminium phosphate-adsorbed vaccine is available from the Centers for Disease Control (CDC), Atlanta, Georgia, USA. It contains toxoids from formalin-inactivated partially purified types A, B, C, D and E containing thiomersal as a preservative. The vaccine is given deep subcutaneously in a dose of 0.5 ml in three doses at intervals of 2 and 12 weeks with a booster dose at 12 months. Subsequent booster doses are required every 2 years but are only given if antibody levels judged by antitoxin levels in the serum are not satisfactory. At the time of writing *Botulinum* toxoid is not a licensed product in the USA and is only available under strict conditions laid down by CDC. Moderate local reactions do occur and are an indication to reduce subsequent doses.

THE ANIMAL HOUSE

The general recommendations concerning staff health working in laboratories also apply in the specialised area of the animal house. Conditions may be warm and dusty and the physical effort greater than in the main laboratory. Pulmonary diseases, especially of an allergic nature, preclude employment there. Vaccinations against tuberculosis, rabies and tetanus are essential, but other modes of protection of the animal attendant are equally important. These include the training of the worker so that he or she has some knowledge and understanding of animals, and that safe methods of handling and the means to do this are clear. Protective clothing, clean clothing and facilities for changing and showering are all important.

Animals are a reservoir of disease agents some of which can be transmitted to man, and in some surveys have been shown to be the cause of over 10%

of laboratory infections. Although the skin is often breached due to bites and scratches accidents with syringes and needles often occur in association with animals due to careless handling. Animals too are responsible for aerosols either from their fur or via urine and faeces allowed to dry in bedding. Such aerosols may be inhaled by handlers causing respiratory distress due to allergy. Material from animals can also get on to the hands and clothes of workers, and thus be transmitted to the eyes.

The organisms being injected into the animals are also a hazard at this stage. Air in syringes should not be expelled into the room but into a small pledget of cotton wool soaked in disinfectant. It is also just as important to disinfect the skin of the animal after the injection as before. This is because the agent injected is frequently present at the site of infection and often is released into the atmosphere in the form of an aerosol. After injection the agent may be excreted via the urine, the faeces and open lesions, and from the respiratory tract in coughs and sneezes. Changing the bedding, just as in a hospital ward, increases the number of bacteria detectable in the air.

Care should be exercised with animals newly introduced into the animal house. The stress of travel and of new surroundings and handlers may play a part in an increased susceptibility to disease. Animals may themselves be suffering from diseases such as tuberculosis but may be exposed to such a disease from a human handler. This situation is a particular hazard in monkey colonies. These animals may also be a source of *Shigella* and *Salmonella* infections as well as parasites such as *Strongyloides*, *Entamoeba* and *Giardia*. Adequate quarantine facilities will deal with these infections and the outbreak of Marburg disease which occurred in Marburg, Frankfurt and Belgrade in 1967 is a salutory reminder of what can occur if quarantine regulations are ignored. Infection with B virus should not occur if only seronegative animals are used and screening for this highly dangerous disease should be done during the quarantine period.

Smaller animals are known to carry *Salmonella*, *Yersinia*, *Leptospirosis* and lymphocytic choriomeningitis, and outbreaks of disease in man have all been traced back to the animal house. Skin infections appearing in animal handlers may be the first intimation of widespread infection of animals, with *Trichophyton* and *Microsporon* fungi. *Toxoplasma* and *Toxocara* may be caught from dogs and cats.

We do not know the risk from tumour viruses, and indeed it may not exist at all because of species specificity. Nevertheless, we cannot ignore the possibility of transmission to man and hence materials derived from such tumours should be handled with care.

SPECIAL SITUATIONS

HIV infections in health care workers

There is considerable apprehension among health care workers with regard to the dangers of handling blood from patients who are antibody positive to the human immunodeficiency virus. Guidelines for handling this material are available and concentrate on good basic techniques. No vaccine is available. Exposure to possible infection in health care workers due to splashing, cuts or needlestick injury must have occurred on thousands of occasions, but evidence of transmission of infection based on seroconversion appears to be confined to 19 cases, all of whom appear to have had substantial exposure to infection. There have also been a number of large surveys in which those exposed to infection as a result of a recorded incident have been followed up without any seroconversion taking place. Thus it is clear that handling HIV positive material is hazardous, but the risk is small and probably less than that from handling hepatitis B positive material. Such hazards should be clearly explained to all laboratory workers.

Pregnancy

The effects of rubella in pregnant women are well documented, and similarly the dangers of Cytomegalovirus infection are understood. Other viruses are suspect as causes of malformation in babies if the mother is infected in the early stages of pregnancy. Many such infections may not be teratogenic, but a number, such as mumps, are associated with abortion. Women who are hoping to become pregnant, and those who are pregnant, should not be allowed to work in a virus department. The chance of infection occurring elsewhere in the laboratory and causing harm is very low, so it is usual to move such female employees to a different task. This change in occupation can often be provided in the media preparation department or possibly handling environmental specimens such as food and water. The baseline serum collected on joining should have been tested for the presence of rubella and CMV antibodies and vaccination offered against the former. Cytomegalovirus, although clearly a cause of congenital infection, sometimes with severe abnormality in the offspring, is much less common. Vaccination is rarely done for female laboratory staff unless work with the virus is part of the research programme.

Absence due to illness

Staff should be instructed to send a message to the laboratory when they are unable to work due to illness. This should always be done on the morning of the first day of absence. If no message is received a colleague should visit to make certain that the absentee is not suffering from some illness associated with his work. Such a step is of paramount importance if the employee is known to live alone.

Disaster services

Although it is unlikely that accidents can be foreseen and plans made to cope with the incident, an attempt should be made. The advantage of thinking ahead in this context is that the exploration of an imagined incident in the form of discussion with those likely to be involved will stimulate ideas. These ideas should be committed to paper in an incident or disaster file, and should be available to all in authority at all times. The file should commence with a statement of the action to be taken by the staff involved in order (a) to mitigate the effects of the accident on him or her and (b) to prevent others being involved. This section of the file should be circulated to all staff, and in large establishments where research is done staff should sign to signify that they have read the contents. The subsequent immediate action to be taken will depend upon the agent involved and the degree of contamination which has taken place. This may be decided by the most senior member of the staff present at the time, or may concern the physician if he is called.

Subsequent entries in the file may be administrative in the sense that it may simply consist of a list of names and telephone numbers of those who must be informed. Such lists are extremely useful in an emergency.

Finally, the outline procedure should be laid down for an inquiry to be held. This should always be done however trivial the accident may seem, for it establishes two principles:

1. no grade of staff is immune from an injury;
2. All procedures leading up to the accident are liable to investigation and modification to prevent a repetition

Such a routine approach to all incidents establishes the fact that inquiries are not designed for disciplinary reasons but as a process in preventive health. Should disciplinary action be indicated this should follow a separate investigation by the employer, and the physician should avoid taking part unless required to give medical evidence. It is most important that the preliminary internal enquiry should be established as a routine so that all staff are not afraid to report incidents or to co-operate in the investigation.

There is in addition a legal requirement for all such incidents to be reported to the Health and Safety Executive

CONCLUSIONS

The occupational health physician concerned with the health care of laboratory personnel has an important task to perform. On the one hand he must be aware of, and instruct others on, the hazards associated with work in the laboratory, but on the other hand he must do this without overstating his case. His difficulty lies in the fact that there is ample evidence, collected over many years, of examples of illness and death attributed to handling micro-organisms. Nevertheless, this evidence is mainly anecdotal. There are very few studies in which the incidence of illness in laboratory workers is compared with a control group in another occupation. Furthermore, in the few studies in which comparisons have been made with controls, no attempt has ever been made to do serological studies to detect subclinical infections. Thus, as in many other fields of medicine where our assessment of a degree of hazard from many procedures is limited, so in the laboratory we cannot judge the risk of infection. It is, however, probable that even were we able to measure the risk, and to compare it with the risk of working elsewhere, decisions with regard to isolated incidents would still be made on an emotional rather than a scientific basis. It is doubtful if there is justification for large epidemiological studies to establish the degree of hazard unless designed to establish the efficacy of a projected and very expensive preventive measure. In fact it could be extremely difficult to collect the required statistics. For instance in England and Wales the notification of respiratory tuberculosis has now fallen to the order of 4000 cases per year (1987) in a population of some 50 million. To detect a small but statistically significant increase in the incidence of this disease in a few thousand laboratory workers would require them to be followed up for very many years. Such an investigation is not feasible nor indeed required. We know how tuberculosis is transmitted and we know the steps which should be taken to prevent the transmission. The physician should, therefore, be aware of the mode of transmission of diseases and should familiarize himself with the microbiological techniques used in the laboratory. This knowledge will enable him to give sound advice and apply the other preventive measures such as vaccination mentioned in this chapter.

LITERATURE CONSULTED

Advisory Committee on Dangerous Pathogens (1986). LAV/HTLV III - the causative agent of AIDS and related conditions: Revised Guidelines

Blaser, M.J., Hickman, F.W., Farmer, J.J. III, Brenner, D.J., Balows, A. and Feldmen, R.A. (1980). *Salmonella typhi*: the laboratory as a reservoir of infection. *J. Infect. Dis.*, **142**(6), 934-938

Centers for Disease Control (1983). Field Evaluations of Pre-exposure use of Human Diphoid Cell Rabies Vaccine. *Morb. Mortal. Weekly Rep.*, **32**, 601-603

Crombie, D.L. (1983). Immunization procedures in Europe. *Health Trends*, **15**, 86-90

DHSS (1970). Precautions against tuberculosis infection in the diagnostic laboraotry H M 70/60. (London: Department of Health and Social Security)

DHSS (1978). Code of Practice for the Prevention of Infection in Clinical Laboratories and Post Mortem Rooms. (London: Department of Health and Social Security)

Fascaldo, A.A., Erlick, B.J. and Hindman, B. (1980). *Laboratory Safety: Theory & Practice*. (London: Academic Press)

Harrington, J.M. and Shannon, H.S. (1976). Incidence of tuberculosis, hepatitis, brucellosis and shigellosis in British medical laboratory workers. *Br. Med. J.*, 1, 759-762

Health and Safety at Work (etc) Act (1974). (London: HMSO; reprinted 1978)

Health Services Advisory Committee (1986). Safety in Health service laboratories: the labelling, transport and reception of specimens. ISBN: 0 11 883893 8 (London: HMSO)

Huddleson, I.F. and Munger, M. (1940). A study of an epidemic of brucellosis due to *Brucella melitensis*. *Am. J. Publ. Health*, 30, 944-954

Kinnersley, P. (1990). Attitudes of general practitioners towards their vaccination against hepatitis B. *Br. Med. J.*, 300, 238

Lach, V.H., Harper, G.J. and Wright, A.E. (1983). An assessment of some hazards associated with the collection of venous blood. *J. Hosp. Infect.*, 4, 57-63

Levine, M.M., Ferreccio, C., Black, R.E. and Germanier, R. (1987). Large-scale field trial of Ty21A Live Oral Typhoid Vaccine in enteric coated capsule formulation. *Lancet*, 1, 1049-1052

McEvoy, M., Porter, K., Mortimer, P., Simmons, H. and Shanson, D. (1987). Prospective study of clinical laboratory and ancillary staff with accidental exposures to blood or body fluids from patients infected with HIV. *Br. Med. J.*, 294, 1596-1597

Merger, C. (1957). Hazards associated with the handling of pathogenic bacteria. *Canad. J. Med. Technol.*, 18, 122-125

MMWR (1982). Recommendations of the Immunisation Practices Advisory Committee: inactivated hepatitis B virus vaccine. *Morb. Mortal. Weekly Rep.* (CDC, Atlanta), 24, 317-328

MMWR (1983). Current Trends: the safety of hepatitis B vaccine. *Morb. Mortal. Weekly Rep.* (CDC, Atlanta), 32, 134-136

MMWR (1987). Recommendations of the Immunisation Practices Advisory Committee: Update on Hepatitis B Prevention. *Morb. Mortal. Weekly Rep.* (CDC, Atlanta), 36, 353-360

Pike, R.M. (1979). Laboratory-associated infections: incidence, fatalities, causes and prevention. *Ann. Rev. Microbiol.*, 33, 41-66

Polakoff, S. (1986). Acute viral hepatitis B: laboratory reports 1980-84. *Br. Med. J.*, 293, 37-38

Reid, D.D. (1957). The incidence of tuberculosis among workers in medical laboratories. *Br. Med. J.*, 2, 10

Report (1974). Report of the Committee of Inquiry into the Smallpox outbreak in London in March and April 1973. Cmnd 5626 (London: HMSO)

Report (1980). Report of the Investigation in the Cause of the 1978 Birmingham Smallpox Occurrence. No. 668. (London: HMSO)

Seamer, J. and Wood, M. (eds.)(1981). *Safety in the Animal House. Laboratory Animals Handbooks*, No. 5, 2nd edn. (London: Laboratory Animals Ltd)

Smith, C.E.G. Lessons from Marburg Disease Scientific Basis of Medicine Annual Reviews 1971

6 Responsibilities of the Director of Laboratory Medicine for Health and Safety Issues in the Laboratory

I.D. Montoya

By nature, the position of Director of Laboratory Medicine is problematic. The position requires management of the laboratory's policy with regard to occupational health and safety in an effective and expeditious manner. Often, however, the means required to administer this policy are either unavailable or limited. To begin with, the Director may have the title of Director, Administrator, Manager or Chief of the Laboratories. Each of these titles connotates a different degree of scientific, financial and administrative responsibility. Regardless of the title assigned to the Director of the Laboratory, the overall responsibility for the health and safety programme belongs to this individual.

Often the Laboratory Director reports to an administrator who has little or no scientific training. The administrator may have difficulty in viewing the health and safety programme of the Laboratory as anything but an academic exercise on the part of the laboratory staff that requires minimal training and no resources. It is thus imperative that the Laboratory Director design a health and safety programme that is understandable to the administrator as well as the laboratory staff to ensure that it receives support from both parties. This programme should be structured in such a manner that the outcome is measureable (i.e. number of accidents, lost work time due to accidents). It is also important that the Laboratory Director alert his/her administrator about potential risks encountered should the laboratory not have a sound health and safety programme, and the threat this poses to the laboratory employee as well as the institution itself.

The following activities are recommended to help the Laboratory Director in meeting his/her responsibilities.

NEEDS ASSESSMENT

A needs assessment must take place before a health and safety programme is designed, or an existing one modified in any fashion. The following parameters should first be identified:

-       scope of the health and safety programme required;
-       strengths of the existing programme;
-       weakness of the existing programme;
-       resources required to achieve desired status; and
-       workplan to develop and implement needed components.

This assessment will allow the Director to plan, prioritize and secure the needed elements of the programme, and effectively utilize the available resources.

Typically, the needs assessment is structured in a questionnaire or checklist format. This instrument is developed based on the needs of the particular laboratory and the requirements imposed upon it by the Government, funding sources, accreditation/licensing agencies and local regulations. It is important to include the requirements of other areas within the institution that interface with the laboratory. Such areas may include housekeeping, maintenance and public relations programmes who often provide tours of the laboratory. The content of the needs assessment should address both technical and educational requirements.

It is recommended that a needs assessment be conducted annually in every laboratory to ensure that the health and safety programme is meeting current guidelines.

PROGRAMME DESIGN

Designing a health and safety programme is facilitated by utilizing the information obtained in the needs assessment. The information available from the needs assessment identifies the areas of strength and weakness. Many times the strengths can be used to overcome the weaknesses.

Since most laboratories respond to various types of agencies, it is not inconceivable that a laboratory may meet the requirements of one agency but not another. It is even possible to obtain conflicting information from

92

different agencies. In designing a health and safety programme, it is most effective to begin by preparing a master list of health and safety requirements from the standards utilized by the agencies reviewing the laboratory. In cases of duplication, the most stringent requirements should be selected.

Having compiled a master list, a Laboratory Director must consider the educational/training programme needed to implement these requirements.

IDENTIFICATION OF RESOURCES

Implementation of a new, or changes to an existing, health and safety programme can be hampered without sufficient resources; therefore, it is necessary to seek these resources wherever possible. When seeking resources for implementation, one should investigate sources both internal and external to the institution. For instance, other departments within the institution may have the necessary audio-visual material to assist in training programmes. Some institutions have departments whose sole function is staff training and development. If provided with the necessary training curriculum they will prepare, present and evaluate the programme for the Laboratory Director. Other departments may have existing policies and procedures developed that can be useful as models. Outside resources may include other laboratories who have developed the mechanics for implementing and maintaining their health and safety programme. Community based organizations such as the Red Cross or the Heart and Lung Association may provide valuable resources for a health and safety programme in the form of pamphlets, programmes and statistics. Educational institutions may also provide resources in the form of students seeking projects, e.g. art students may design the necessary artwork for drawings or training material. Often, these resources are available at either no charge, or at a nominal fee.

Some laboratories seek an outside consultant to assist them with this endeavour. If a Laboratory Director is pressed for time or lacks experience in health and safety programmes, hiring a consultant may be in the best interest of the laboratory.

STAFF EDUCATION

Many excellent health and safety programmes can be found in bookcases in the Laboratory Director's office, however, laboratory staff have generally not been familiarized with these. This is unfortunate because a health and safety programme is only effective when the laboratory staff have knowledge and access to the programme materials. This is especially true when staff must respond to accidents and/or emergencies.

The educational/training component of the health and safety programme should include instruction for present employees as well as an orientation for new employees. Periodic reviews during staff meetings is advised, as well as simulations of various hypothetical emergencies (i.e. fires, explosions, floods).

Continuing education should be viewed as an opportunity to enhance the skills of the laboratory staff, as a means of contributing to the welfare of the staff. To do this effectively, the Director must ensure that the training presentations are well planned and utilize adult learning techniques. If the staff perceives these training sessions as repetitious or trivial, then the effectiveness of the programme is minimized. It is a good idea to administer evaluations of the training sessions for use in upgrading future presentations. Some laboratories administer safety examinations to their employees and the results are kept as a part of the employees personnel file.

POLICY AND PROCEDURE MANUALS

Health and Safety policy and procedure manuals should be updated on a regular basis. In addition, a copy should be readily available at each workstation or section within the laboratory. It is the responsibility of the Laboratory Director to ensure that these manuals are up to date and available in the laboratory.

The contents of a comprehensive policy and procedure manual will include the following:

Goals and Objectives;
Staff Training;
Staff Protection Measures;
Hazards in Laboratory
Operations;
Toxic and Hazardous Substances;
Solvents, Fire Hazards and Explosions;
Biohazards;
Radioactivity;
Cryogenic and Compressed Gases;
General and Electrical Systems;
Environmental Systems;
Laboratory Housekeeping; and
Emergency Procedures.

When preparing policy and procedure statements, it is wise to follow the **RUMBA** concept. This acronym dictates that all procedural policies should be:

Realistic,
Understandable,
Measurable,
Behavioral, and
Achievable.

Statements such as 'We will provide a high quality safety programme' is neither understandable nor measurable. The term 'high quality' does not mean the same thing to all staff. If **RUMBA** is kept foremost in mind, the content of policy and procedure manuals will meet the needs of the laboratory staff.

Figure 6.1 illustrates a page from a policy and procedure manual that depicts **RUMBA** in a procedure that is difficult to address.

INVENTORY SYSTEMS

Traditionally, the maintenance of inventory levels has been viewed as an administrative/financial function rather than a component of the health and safety programme. However, this function is necessary to the success of both programmes. Laboratory Directors may forget to evaluate the effect different levels of laboratory supplies may have in the event of an emergency. When determining the 'safe' level of inventory required, a Laboratory Director would be wise to consider laboratory supplies stored off-site, stored elsewhere in the installation and stored in the laboratory itself.

The inventory review should address the qualities of supplies as well as the inventory system as a whole. The review should include issues such as storage conditions (i.e. temperature, humidity, location, air circulation), transportation of inventory items and record keeping of all transactions.

MONITORING THE HEALTH AND SAFETY PROGRAMME

Once the health and safety programme has been implemented, the Laboratory Director must monitor the programme during its' maintenance mode. The monitoring activity is best accomplished by compiling relevant statistical data. This information combined with other operational statistics together create the database for the Laboratory's Management Information System (MIS).

Health and safety reports are useful for indicating the effectiveness of procedural policy. The report should contain statistics regarding:

1. Number of accidents by type of accident;
2. Number of injuries resulting from accidents;

AFFILIATED SYSTEMS CORPORATION

SOURCE MANUAL: Phlebotomy Policies and Procedures

PROCEDURE: Preventing Shock

Shock usually accompanies severe injury or emotional upset. It may also follow infection, pain, disturbance or circulation from bleeding, stroke, heart attack, heat exhaustion, food or chemical poisoning, extensive burns, etc.

Signs of Shock include: Cold and clammy skin with beads of perspiration on the forehead and palms of hands. Pale face. Complaint by the victim of a chilled feeling, or even shaking chills. Frequently, nausea or vomiting. Shallow breathing.

DO: 1. Correct cause of shock if possible (e.g., control bleeding).

2. Keep victim lying down.

3. Keep his/her airway open. If s/he vomits, turn his/her head to the side so that his/her neck is arched.

4. Elevate victim's legs if there are no broken bones. Keep his/her head lower than trunk of the body if possible.

5. Cover the victim to keep warm.

6. Call the Emergency Room Physician.

DON'T: Do not give fluids to unconscious or semi-conscious persons.

Do not give fluids if abdominal injury is suspected.

NOTE: All Laboratory Staff must complete training in this procedure and demonstrate competence in the procedure annually.

Figure 6.1

3.   Number of employees requiring physician visit due to work related accidents;
4.   Number of employees requiring hospitalization;
5.   Number of training sessions held;
6.   Number of employees attending each session;
7.   Number of simulated accidents/emergencies;
8.   Number of employees participating in simulated accidents/emergencies;
9.   Number of laboratory audits to secure compliance with health and safety policies and procedures;
10.   Average cost per accident (lost time, reagents, etc.);
11.   Average cost per injury;
12.   Total number of lost days due to laboratory accidents; and
13.   Cost of unexpected repairs due to accidents (equipment, facilities, inventory).

The data collected from the health and safety report will be useful in the day to day operation as well as serving as the data baseline for next years needs assessment.

INSURANCE

Depending on the nature of the health care system of a given country, some laboratories are covered by insurance and others are not. Those that are self-insured will have particular interest in the statistics describing their health and safety programme. These numbers will assist the institutions risk manager in the containment of cost. For those facilities that maintain insurance coverage with an independent company, these figures are equally important. In certain cases, if an institution can demonstrate a sound health and safety programme and the statistics reflect a low accident rate then the institution becomes eligible for lower insurance rates. It is up to the Laboratory Director to secure this information pertaining to coverage in the laboratory and the cost of such coverage.

NEWS MEDIA

One of the most difficult areas a Laboratory Director has to deal with, in a health and safety programme, is the news media when an accident/emergency occurs. A wise Director will know in advance what the institution policies regarding news media are.
    During an accident/emergency, the Director must make many decisions in a short period of time. If news media personnel are present, they may

hamper the expediency with which an emergency is handled, and may endanger their own safety. It is the Laboratory Director who must ensure the safety of these personnel.

In some cases, providing news media personnel with information about the accident/emergency situation is the responsibility of the Laboratory Director. It is essential that the media be provided with facts and not speculations. The resulting story could be unnecessarily detrimental to the institution, and it may take many years to shed a bad reputation caused by one episode. If properly informed, both sides of the story, including the laboratory's safety precautions, will be revealed. Positive working relationships with the news media will help in ensuring fair and accurate coverage of any accident in the laboratory.

QUALITY ASSURANCE PROGRAMME

Quality Assurance Programmes have received much attention in the past few years. However, many definitions exist among various institutions. Quality control, risk management, chart audits and peer review are all terms used interchangeably, and incorrectly, with Quality Assurance. Simply stated, Quality Assurance is an interdisciplinary review process that assures internal against select criteria are being provided in a timely and cost-effective manner.

It is evident that the laboratories health and safety programme is a major component of the Quality Assurance Programme. Data collected from the health and safety programme should be available to the Quality Assurance Programme for further review, and comparison to programmes of other departments. Many times the activities of the Quality Assurance Committee are closely related to the activities of the laboratory's health and safety programme. Examples might be a relationship between findings of the infection control department and the laboratory's findings in a clinical setting. For those in a public health setting, a correlation between environmental findings and the laboratory's health and safety programme may be relevant.

In any case, it is best to use the data readily available from the health and safety programme than collect the data from another source for the Quality Assurance Programme.

NEW FACILITY PLANNING

Planning a new laboratory can be an exciting and rewarding experience. It is the sole responsibility of the Laboratory Director to orchestrate the smooth series of events that must occur. Planning for health and safety needs in the laboratory must take place early in the planning process. This allows time to secure information on the most current requirements and give the architect time to plan for these health and safety features.

The architect will rely entirely upon the Laboratory Director to provide the direction necessary for health and safety features appropriate to the laboratories procedural policy. The Laboratory Director must monitor the plans, drawings and construction to ensure the health and safety features are not compromised.

LITERATURE CONSULTED

Faulkner, W. and Meites, S. (1982). *Selected Methods for the Small Clinical Chemistry Laboratory*, Vol. 9. (Washington DC: American Association for Clinical Chemistry)

Flury, P.A. and Deluca, K. (1978). *Environmental Health and Safety in the Hospital Laboratory*. (Springfield, IL: Charles C. Thomas)

Green, M.E. and Turk, A. (1978). *Safety in Working with Chemicals*. (New York, NY: MacMillan)

Hartree, E. and Booth, V. (1977). *Safety in Biological Laboratories*, Spec., Publ. 5. (London: Biochemistry Society)

Henry, R.J., Olitsky, I., Lee, N.D., Walker, B. and Beattie, J. (1976). *Safety in the Clinical Laboratory*. (Van Nuys, CA: Bio-Science Enterprises)

Manufacturing Chemists Association (1978). *A Guide for Safety in Chemical Laboratories*, 2nd Edn. (New York, NY: Van Nostrand, Reinhold Press)

Muir, G.D. (1977). *Hazards in the Chemical Laboratory*, 2nd Edn.. (Letchworth, Herts., UK: Chemical Society)

Pecsok, R.L., Chapman, K. and Ponder, W.H. (1975). *Chemical Technology Handbook*. (Washington, DC: American Chemical Society)

Report Corporate Capabilities (1987). (Houston, TX: Affiliated Systems Corporation)

Report Safety in Health-Related Institutions (1980). Publ. 56C. (Boston, MA: National Fire Protection Association)

Report Safety in Laboratories Using Chemicals (1981). Publ. 45. (Boston, MA: National Fire Protection Association)

Report Strategic Documents for Planning Systems in the Memorial Care Systems. (Strategic Plans Resource File) (1984). (Houston, TX: Affiliated Systems Corporation)

Steere, N.V. (1971). *Handbook of Lab Safety*, 2nd Edn. (Cleveland, OH: Chemical Rubber Co. Press)

7 Health and Safety Hazards and Precautions in Chemical Laboratories

G. E. Chivers

INTRODUCTION

This chapter will discuss the hazards involved in using chemicals in laboratories rather than restricting discussion to laboratories formally designated as chemistry laboratories.

While attention will be concentrated on chemical hazards in laboratories making extensive use of chemicals, this is not to imply that chemicals cause the majority of accidents in such environments. A survey by Harrington of accidents in medical laboratories in the United Kingdom showed that cuts from glassware contributed to over 40% of recorded accidents. Cuts from knives and other equipment were responsible for a further 32% of accidents, while gassings caused only 1% of accidents and explosions 0.8%. On the other hand, a separate survey by Dewhurst ranging across all types of laboratories showed that gassings and other poisonings were the cause of death for 27% of laboratory accident fatalities, while explosions caused a further 12% of such fatalities.

Consideration of occupational health hazards also gives good grounds for concentration on chemical hazards in laboratories. The evidence for occupationally induced cancer amongst laboratory workers is admittedly weak, despite the wide range of known or potential human carcinogens to be found in laboratories. However, it has been shown that the contraction of dermatitis or an allergy has frequently been the reason for laboratory workers leaving their jobs. The Dewhurst surveys in the UK found that of all laboratory accidents resulting in the necessity for a change of employment, dermatitis and allergy development were the problems identified in 55% of cases. Many accidents, including laboratory explosions have often resulted from a solvent spillage generating flammable vapour in the vicinity of a faulty electrical system which was producing sparks. Explosions have been caused by mechanical blockages in equipment giving rise to pressure build-up and the explosion has flung a chemical into the face of a laboratory worker. Such events will be regarded as 'chemical' accidents rather than electrically or mechanically caused accidents.

CHEMICAL HAZARDS IN LABORATORIES

Before considering precautions against hazards to health and safety arising from chemicals, it will be helpful to review the types of hazards presented by chemicals in laboratories and exemplify these by reference to actual accidents.

Chemical hazards in the laboratory may be divided into three very broad categories:

1. hazards to human health where a chemical can come into contact with the human body (toxic and corrosive hazards);
2. fires arising from or involving chemicals;
3. explosions caused by or involving chemicals.

These categories are not mutually exclusive, and many laboratory accidents involve a combination of hazards. Thus a solvent fire may result in a subsequent gas cylinder explosion.

Toxic and corrosive hazards of chemicals

To harm the human body a hazardous chemical must come in contact with it. Depending on the chemical and the nature of the contact, the harmful effect may be localized on the outside surface of the body (for example, dermatitis of the hands or eye damage), or it may be systemic and deep within the body (for example, carbon monoxide poisoning of the blood).

The localized surface attack on the body may be classified as a corrosion phenomenon, while systemic attack on the internal operation of the body may be classified as a toxicity phenomenon. Again, these are not mutually exclusive phenomena and there are numerous chemicals such as phenol which if splashed onto the body will both burn the skin and penetrate it to cause toxic effects towards vital organs.

Corrosive chemical hazards

Accidents caused by contact of the body with corrosive chemicals are still distressingly common in laboratories. The Harrington survey of medical laboratories mentioned earlier showed that splashes, spills and leaks of chemicals gave rise to some 6% of medical laboratory accidents. The Dewhurst survey of all types of laboratories reported that of 67 accidents in laboratories which caused the loss of one or both eyes, chemical reagents in the eye caused 13 of these sad cases.

Chemical attack on the skin or eyes often involves strong acids. The unwise addition of water to concentrated sulphuric acid has frequently led to the contents of test tubes and flasks being violently ejected into the face of laboratory workers. The shaking of flasks or separating funnels containing acids at eye level to observe effects has been the frequent cause of splashes of corrosive chemicals into the eye.

Acids form a major group of chemicals which can attack and burn the skin and eye. Other broad categories of corrosive chemicals are alkalis and bases, chlorides of the non-metals, desiccant compounds generally, the halogens and oxidizing agents particularly.

Acids vary greatly in their effects depending on their type and strength. Mineral acids are generally more hazardous than organic acids, although even these in concentrated form can cause deep-seated burns, especially on prolonged contact.

Hydrofluoric acid is unique in being a relatively weak acid compared with other mineral acids, but a strong biological poison. This combination of properties makes concentrated hydrofluoric acid an especially insidious and dangerous hazard. Because it is not a strong acid, contact with the skin produces no initial sensation of burning. Thus it may stay trapped inside a leaky rubber glove for hours in contact with the hand. Subsequently, and perhaps outside the workplace, extensive blistering of the skin will take place resulting in intense pain without any apparent cause. Despite this property, hydrofluoric acid and hydrogen fluoride gas have been used without sufficient safeguards and the chemical has been squirted into the eyes and ears of laboratory workers. Phenol is another acidic material which causes skin burns after a delay period because of no immediate stinging sensation. The skin will often go white and become anaesthetized and insensible to touch. The true extent of the burn is only evident many hours afterwards. The severity of the burn depends on the time during which the phenol is in contact with the skin, and again trapping some inside a glove is a common way for this to occur.

The strong alkalis and bases such as sodium hydroxide, potassium hydroxide and calcium oxide generate considerable heat in contact with water and are all able to attack the skin, and especially the eyes. Strong alkaline solutions do less damage to the skin than strong acid solutions if rapidly washed off, but have caused severe eye damage. Strong ammonia solutions

103

deserve special mention in this context, and the blinding effect of this reagent is well known to criminals.

Chlorides of the non-metals are less often recognized as dangerous chemicals. This is unfortunate as they are widely used and are a frequent source of laboratory accidents. Phosphorus trichloride, boron trichloride, aluminium trichloride and silicon tetrachloride, and the corresponding bromides all react violently with water and are extremely dangerous to the eyes.

Desiccant materials also need careful treatment for the same reason. The eye consists substantially of water behind a relatively thin membrane, and powerful desiccants in the eye will abstract water, generating large amounts of heat.

The halogens are another class of hazardous chemicals with respect to skin and eye damage (in addition to toxicity effects). Fluorine gas is so reactive towards organic materials that it will burn in contact with them. The consequences of jetting fluorine gas into the face or hands therefore need no elaboration. Chlorine is less reactive but still very harmful, while bromine has been a particularly prevalent cause of eye damage. This is undoubtedly because, in neat form or in strong aqueous solution, it has been used as a test reagent in qualitative analysis. Laboratory workers have held test tubes and flasks close to the eyes to observe effects, and the liquid bromine or the heavy bromine vapour has made contact with the eyeball, by splashing or just evaporation.

Oxidizing agents in general are harmful to the skin and eyes (as well as being potential ingredients of explosive mixtures). Thus peroxides, chlorates, some nitrates and other oxidizing agents in concentrated form should not be allowed to make contact with the body.

Less corrosive chemicals can still be very harmful to the skin if there is significant contact, and especially if contact is repeated. Some chemicals are potent skin irritants and even one slight contact can cause problems. 1-chloro-2,4-dinitrobenzene is an example of a chemical with this effect which has been produced as an intermediate in student practical classes and given rise to severe and distressing rashes to hands. A wide range of chemicals can give rise to dermatitis, and the sensitivity of individuals towards a particular chemical agent can vary widely. Solvents are often implicated in incidents of dermatitis, and if common solvents cause severe reactions in individuals it may be impractical to continue with laboratory work. As with many insidious occupational diseases, often insufficient care is taken to avoid skin contact with chemicals before symptoms become apparent, by which time the damage has been done.

Toxic effects of chemicals

For chemicals to exert effects on the body other than at the surface they must penetrate within it. There are three routes for chemicals to enter the body; they can be taken into the mouth and swallowed, they can contact the skin and pass through it, or they can be breathed in as gases, vapours or fine dust particles. Once they are in the body they may cause toxic effects at one place near the point of entry (such as the stomach or the lungs) or they may be dispersed to other sites in the body, possibly changing chemical composition en route, and cause toxic effects at sites remote from the point of entry. When considering toxic effects of chemicals we tend to think of substances which cause acute poisoning effects, such as cyanide or carbon monoxide. However, toxic chemicals can produce long-term effects, perhaps because of steady accumulation in the body as with lead or mercury, or perhaps because there is a long time delay before onset of the disease, as with many chemically induced cancers. Some laboratory chemicals will cause toxic effects on first exposure to very small quantities, while others will only produce symptoms of ill-health after prolonged exposure to large quantities of the chemical. Allergic reactions (including dermatitis and asthmatic lung complaints) caused by chemicals are a frequent reason for laboratory workers leaving laboratory employment. The survey by Dewhurst found that amongst 129 cases of this type formalin alone was responsible for 32 serious allergic responses, organic chemicals for 13, inorganic chemicals for 14, and polymer chemicals including monomers and catalysts for 12.

Further areas of concern in terms of long-term health hazards caused by chemicals in laboratories include reproductive problems and behavioural changes. A number of common organic chemicals have been shown to cause reproductive hazards for test animals in terms of miscarriages, still-births or birth abnormalities. This discovery has led to calls for young women who may become pregnant to be excluded from laboratory work with chemicals. However, it should be pointed out that some of these chemicals have been shown to cause sperm abnormalities also, so a case could similarly be made for the exclusion of men who might wish to become fathers. Recent research has shown that common solvents at low concentrations in air can affect the behaviour and performance of tasks in test animals. Such effects amongst laboratory workers would be worrying in their own right and could constitute a safety risk if workers were to lose concentration or co-ordination when carrying out potentially hazardous tasks. Dewhurst has reported a statistically significant correlation between the degree of solvent exposure and the extent to which laboratory workers reported feelings of tiredness, sickness and nausea, and headache. Few laboratories in his survey took special precautions to ensure removal of organic solvents from the laboratory atmosphere, and in over 16% of laboratories organic column chromatography was still being carried out in the open laboratory rather than in fume cupboards. Half of the respondents reported that the laboratory atmosphere contained fumes which irritated the eyes from time to time. Furthermore, it is clear that the solvents and chemicals commonly used in laboratories include suspected human carcinogens.

Chloroform was used as least once a week by more than 24% of respondents, carbon tetrachloride at least once a week by some 16% and benzene at least once a week by 10%.

Acute toxicity problems, while less common, are by no means rare in laboratories. In the Dewhurst survey gassing and poisoning were responsible for 27% of reported laboratory accident fatalities, while suicide by poisoning accounted for a further 18% of laboratory deaths. While many of these poisonings result from breathing in toxic fumes, poisoning by ingestion of chemicals is still reported. In this context it is interesting to find in the survey that eating of food was allowed in 27% of laboratories, making of tea and coffee in 24%, while for 17% a vending machine or trolley service for drinks was provided adjacent to the laboratory. Fortunately, the survey also showed that mouth pipetting, previously a common means of accidentally ingesting chemicals, is a declining practice.

A wide range of acutely toxic gases and vapours is commonly encountered in laboratories and poisoning by the breathing in of such substances is far from rare. The maintenance of fume cupboards is often neglected despite the fact that they provide the main line of defence against the effects of toxic fumes on laboratory workers. Hydrogen sulphide, chlorine, sulphur dioxide, hydrogen cyanide and ammonia are acutely toxic gases commonly employed in laboratory work or generated in the course of it.

Chronic illness may arise amongst laboratory workers from repeated exposure to low concentrations of chemicals in the atmosphere. The classical example is undoubtedly mercury poisoning, where spillages of mercury have not been properly cleaned up and a significant concentration of mercury vapour is maintained in the laboratory atmosphere at all times. Such occupational illness may be difficult to identify because the symptoms are not very specific.

Aerosols of chemicals are an increasingly common source of chronic diseases amongst laboratory workers, especially where they routinely carry out thin-layer or paper chromatography. Many aerosol sprays for development contain harmful chemicals in relatively high concentrations. In fine droplet form these chemicals can be readily carried down into the worker's lungs during normal breathing, unless sufficient precautions are taken.

A range of laboratory chemicals can produce both acute and long-term effects. Alkyl sulphates are a class of compounds of this type which have caused a good deal of recent concern. Dimethyl sulphate (DMS) is a very versatile laboratory reagent, and its use has increased in recent years. DMS has long been known as an extremely hazardous poison, causing severe inflammation of the eyes, nose and respiratory passages. This poisoning effect is caused by hydrolysis of DMS in the body to form sulphuric acid and methyl alcohol, both potent poisons in their own right. Recently, DMS and other alkyl sulphates have been reported as cancer agents causing cancer of the larynx in both test animals and exposed workers. Exposure of a range of rodents to levels between 0.5 ppm and 2 ppm led to tumours developing in the nose, lung and thorax of the animals. These results show the dangers of focusing only on the acute effects of harmful chemicals and assuming that if exposure is kept below levels at which obvious distress symptoms appear no ill-health problems will arise in time.

When considering toxicological aspects of the exposure of laboratory workers to chemicals special consideration should be given to the question of possible interaction of chemicals. In many laboratories, especially chemistry laboratories, it is common for a wide range of chemicals to be used during one working day. Workers are quite likely to be exposed to a number of harmful chemicals either simultaneously or in rapid sequence. As a minimum the additive effect of these chemicals in toxicological terms should be considered in trying to set standards for maximum exposure. In addition, some chemicals and substances produce synergistic effects in animals and man, such that the combined effect is much greater than would have been anticipated by adding together the known effects of each separate chemical. Research into the possible synergistic effects of chemicals in combination is now proceeding rapidly as it has been recognized that effects of this type greatly reduce the meaningfulness of any standards set for maximum exposure to chemicals in the workplace. Furthermore, there is a need to consider the interaction of chemical exposure of workers with cigarette smoking and alcohol consumption. Smoking should be prohibited in laboratories on both health and safety grounds. In addition to the potential for ingesting toxic chemicals from the outside of the cigarette or fingers, and the obvious fire hazards, cigarettes can also convert chemicals in the atmosphere to more harmful forms. Well-known examples are the conversion of organochlorine vapours such as chloroform in laboratory air to highly toxic phosgene when smoked through the high-temperature zone of a cigarette, and the conversion of polytetrafluoroethylene dust on cigarettes to toxic organofluorine compounds. Studies on possible synergistic effects of smoking and working with chemicals with carcinogenic properties are in their infancy.

The consumption of alcohol during the working day is another serious consideration; even small quantities of alcohol are known to reduce mental and physical performance.

Again, the combined effects of drinking alcohol and breathing in solvent vapours in the laboratory are only just beginning to receive attention. The same comments apply to the consumption of other drugs for pleasure and laboratory working.

The fact that laboratory workers are inadvertently exposed to chemicals with pleasurable and narcotic effects can give rise to problems. Laboratory staff have become addicted to a wide range of solvents over the years. Laboratories working with well-established drugs of abuse and addiction require special security precautions to avoid abuse and theft by laboratory workers and others.

Finally, in this review of toxic hazards in laboratories the problem of suicide by deliberate ingestion of poisons should not be overlooked. The survey by Dewhurst showed that 18% of reported laboratory fatalities were suicide cases. There is no evidence that laboratory workers are more prone to suicidal tendencies than other workers. The sheer availability of well-known poisons unfortunately puts temptation in the way of laboratory staff who may be suffering a period of depression for either work-related or domestic reasons. Poisons of the cyanide category should be stored in a special cabinet under lock and key with restricted access. Staff should be encouraged to report to the management signs of severe depression amongst work colleagues with access to poisons, in the best interests of all concerned.

Fires involving chemicals in laboratories

It is well known that burns or scalds from fires, flames, hot surfaces and hot liquids are relatively common in laboratories. The Harrington survey revealed that burns constituted 7.2% of all injury accidents reported from medical laboratories. Dewhurst reported that 11% of fatal accidents revealed in his survey resulted from laboratory fires. Furthermore, over 20% of laboratories reported fires which required use of a fire extinguisher breaking out at least once during a year, while 2% reported fires requiring the fire brigade. Major fires could involve substantial loss of life of laboratory and non-laboratory workers, while property damage could be extensive.

The most common cause of serious fires in laboratories where chemicals are involved concerns the ignition of flammable solvents. Comments have already been made about the relatively careless use of solvents in laboratories in the context of toxic hazards. Despite the increase in use of non-flammable solvents, highly flammable solvents with low flash points are still widely used in laboratories (Table 7.1).

Table 7.1 Closed cup flash points of some common laboratory solvents (°C)

Acetone	−18	Methanol	10
Cyclohexane	−17	Toluene	4
Diethyl ether	−21	Xylene	24
Ethanol	12		

Commonly, organic liquids with flash points of less than 32 °C are designated as highly flammable and therefore dangerous. On this basis all of the above solvents are dangerous. Most of these solvents are relatively dense compared with air when they are cool, so that if they are allowed to evaporate into the laboratory atmosphere during an experimental procedure, or following a spillage, they will tend to drift to floor level (or into below-floor recesses), and spread over large areas of the laboratory in relatively concentrated form. Contact with an ignition source will then lead to a fire or explosion, and probably a flash-back to the original source of the solvent vapour. Ignition of solvents in liquid form is also common, either because of incorrect use of a naked flame in heating beakers or flasks containing solvents, or because solvent interacted with a hot surface or a non-protected electrical heater.

A great deal can be done to reduce the incidence of solvent fires and their development into major conflagrations. Some of these precautions are obvious, such as the use of smaller quantities of flammable solvents, storage where possible in non-breakable and non-spill containers, special care when heating or distilling such solvents and minimizing sources of ignition.

A less obvious hazard which has caused serious accidents is the storage of vessels containing flammable solvents in domestic-type refrigerators. Such refrigerators usually have electrical contacts inside for the thermostat and lighting, which can be a source of sparks. If the level of flammable solvent vapour inside the refrigerator exceeds the lower explosive limit any spark can ignite the vapour and cause an explosion or fire. In the worst cases the explosion has been triggered by a laboratory worker opening the refrigerator door, causing a spark from the lighting system. Fatalities and serious injuries have resulted from the door being blown out into the body of the worker.

Another less obvious source of solvent fires arises from the use of rotary reduced-pressure evaporators, where not all the flammable solvent vapour evaporated off from the sample is recondensed into the solvent receiver. In such cases the vapour is carried down the water pump into the sink and away to drain.

Another less obvious cause of solvent explosions and fires is the distillation to low volume of ethers containing organic peroxides. A number of common ether solvents generate peroxides on standing in air and sunlight. If such ethers are distilled to very low volume or near dryness, the peroxides will decompose violently giving rise to an explosion and almost inevitably to a major fire from ignition of the solvent vapour and liquid. A recent example of this type of accident involved the purification by distillation of some 2 litres of tetrahydrofuran which had been used in an instrument. There was a sudden explosion, followed by a fire which caused extensive damage. Analysis of subsequent bottles of the same batch of tetrahydrofuran awaiting recovery by distillation showed that some contained dangerously high levels of organic peroxides. These can be destroyed by addition of a reducing agent prior to distillation. Testing of ethers for peroxides, protection from sunlight and avoidance of distillation to very low volume (or the production of 'hot spots' in the distillation vessel) are all necessary precautions.

Solvent fires in waste bins are not uncommon. Here solvent-soaked rags or paper have been deposited and a still glowing match or cigarette stub has followed. Solvent-contaminated materials should be kept in separate metal bins with lids and clearly marked as such, including the appropriate hazard warning symbol.

Laboratory fires, whether started by solvents or not, are potentially much more dangerous if large volumes of solvent are habitually left in the laboratory when not in use. An important aspect of safe laboratory practice is to ensure that solvents are used in minimum quantities and returned to purpose-designed stores when not required.

Having emphasized the importance of highly flammable solvents as a cause of laboratory fires it should be stressed that many other substances can provide a fuel for laboratory fires. These range from hot oil in oil baths which become overheated, to flammable gases from cylinders (or public supply), and even to certain metals in finely divided form. Some very reactive chemicals are spontaneously flammable, such as certain metal hydrides and metal alkyls, phosphorus or phosphine. Others such as sodium and potassium are flammable in the presence of moisture, while strong oxidizing agents can begin to burn if in contact with organic materials. This type of reaction has led to numerous fires in chemical waste bins and at waste tipping sites.

Some years ago a serious fire in a hospital laboratory was reported. The fire started when a member of staff extinguished a cigarette end on the laboratory floor with her foot. Subsequent investigation showed that this wood block floor had been subject to a large spillage of perchloric acid some years previously, and the chemical had presumably dried to a dangerous state.

Explosions involving chemicals in laboratories

Many laboratory explosions which might initially be considered as of chemical origin prove on investigation to be essentially mechanical in nature. High pressures or near-vacuum conditions are a feature of many laboratory experiments today, and faulty equipment under such conditions can give rise to explosions or implosions.

Mechanical explosions of equipment often result from the blockage of tubes or vent ports which are supposed to allow release of gases or vapours as they expand under heating. A violent explosion caused facial injuries to a research student when a U-tube was withdrawn from a coolant liquid nitrogen bath. The student had unwisely closed the Rotaflow taps at the top of each arm of the U-tube, and then allowed the U-tube to warm up to atmospheric pressure. The pressure increase from cold trapped nitrogen gas as it warmed and expanded must have exerted several atmospheres pressure on the U-tube. In addition it was considered likely that liquefied oxygen had collected in the U-tube, always a danger when liquid nitrogen is used as a coolant. The rapid evaporation of the liquid gas in the U-tube had placed intolerable strains on the glass of the U-tube. The chemical present in the U-tube was not considered to have played any significant part in the explosion.

The survey by Dewhurst reported 13 cases where the loss of one or both eyes of a laboratory worker had resulted from such mechanical explosions, as against 26 eye losses from chemical explosions. Another source of stress in laboratory equipment arises from the need for very high or very low temperatures in experiments. Rapid temperature changes in glass, for example, can eventually lead to sudden shattering.

Chemicals are often involved in pressure explosions, either directly or indirectly. A recent example involved a laboratory worker being sprayed with 0.88 specific gravity ammonia following a pressure explosion. The worker merely opened the cap of a Winchester bottle of this compound and the contents erupted violently. About half of the ammonia in the bottle splashed out onto the worker and he had to be taken to hospital. Such reagent bottles should always be opened in a fume cupboard and suitable eye protection should be worn. Breathing apparatus should be available in case of emergencies.

Chemical explosions are still distressingly common and are a cause of serious injury to numerous laboratory workers. The survey by Harrington reported 0.8% of laboratory injury accidents being caused by chemical explosions. A number of chemicals are recognized explosives in that they will detonate at room temperature under mechanical shock (impact or friction) or on gentle warming. Examples include certain polynitro-aromatic or -aliphatic compounds, nitroamines, organic nitrates, peroxides and azides, metal salts of nitrophenols, acetylides and azides of heavy metals. Other chemicals are known to explode on strong heating and there are often reports of the discovery of chemicals which exploded when distilled for the first time. The attempt merely to establish the melting point of some new solid chemicals has led to the destruction of the melting point equipment in violent explosions. Such unpredictable explosions are unfortunate and it is certainly essential to treat all newly synthesized or little-known chemicals with care, working with minimum quantities to establish basic properties. However, in reviewing the safety literature for this chapter it was distressing to find how often the same chemicals were implicated in explosions. Perchloric acid and a variety of organic and inorganic perchlorates and chlorates were the culprits in many of these explosions. While some organic perchlorates seem to be hazardous in their own right, perchloric acid is a hazard because it has been deliberately used to digest biological material, and provides the classic

111

example of the dangers of heating (or grinding) strong oxidizing agents with organic materials.

An equally high number of explosions are reported involving chromic acid. Unfortunately, despite the range of proprietary glass cleaning agents on the market, many laboratory workers still insist on using chromic acid for this purpose. Heating strong nitric acid solutions with organic materials has also given rise to explosions. In this context it should be noted that nitration of organic compounds is, nevertheless, routinely carried out using strong nitric acid or nitric/sulphuric acid mixtures. Other strong oxidizing agents which can cause explosions include inorganic nitrates, peroxides, permanganates, chlorates, perchlorates, chromates and chromic oxide as well as liquid oxygen and air. Apart from most organic compounds, readily oxidizable elements which can give rise to violent oxidations with the above reagents include sulphur, phosphorus, boron, silicon, carbon and most metals in powder form. Some metals are susceptible to oxidation to dangerous oxides and peroxides with air. Potassium has the potential to be surface oxidized to explosive peroxide even when stored under oil. There have been numerous reports of violent explosions when 'old' samples of potassium metals were cut with a knife, and a trace of peroxide was subjected to frictional forces.

Chemicals which react violently with water are another source of laboratory explosions. The alkali metals come to mind particularly in this connection, but at least the hazards of sodium and potassium in contact with water are well recognized. Many other chemicals react with water explosively, or generate considerable pressure in closed containers if moisture is allowed to enter. Amongst inorganic chemicals, the halides of the non-metals are particularly common sources of violent explosions, often caused by ignorance of their reactivity. Acyl halides and other compounds which hydrolyse to give gaseous products such as hydrogen chloride are liable to generate pressure in glass containers which may explode if sufficient moisture is present.

Less well recognized is the ability of alkali metals and other finely divided metals to react violently with halogenated organic solvents. Numerous explosions have been reported where such mixtures have been tried, for example, involving aluminium powder and carbon tetrachloride. Chlorinated organic solvents are by no means as stable as is widely expected. One particularly hazardous practice which has caused explosions is the mixing together of acetone and chloroform, either deliberately or accidentally, in disposing of waste solvents. The reaction of these solvents is catalysed by bases and is strongly exothermic leading to the formation of 'chloretone' (1,1,1-trichloro-3-hydroxy-3-methyl ketone). One reported accident involved the disposal of waste solvents used for chromatography. In this case chloroform was added to a residue bottle containing other solvents including acetone. Vigorous reaction took place and a few seconds later the bottle exploded with considerable violence, and two people were injured by flying glass.

Hazards of gases under pressure and in liquefied form

The hazards of gases contained under pressure in gas cylinders, or in low-temperature liquid form, require special consideration. A whole range of laboratory accidents from gassings and skin burns on the one hand to major fires and explosions on the other have resulted from unsafe use of gases in these forms.

Firstly the energy contained in pressurized or liquefied gases purely because of their condensed form must always be considered. The sudden release of pressure from the contents of a full gas cylinder, usually as a result of knocking the cylinder over and cracking open the cylinder head valve, can result in the cylinder shooting off in jet-propelled fashion. Large cylinders have been known to smash through the walls of laboratories and kill or seriously injure workers in adjacent laboratories. Small gas cylinders are known to have flown through the air to ceiling level after being dropped from waist height and damaged in this way.

Many laboratory gas cylinders contain toxic or flammable gases, and sudden release of these, either directly from a cylinder, or from equipment connected to a cylinder, will immediately generate a high-risk situation. Many toxic gases are also corrosive, such as chlorine and sulphur dioxide, and accidents have frequently arisen because the cylinder valve has become corroded and jammed when the cylinder has not been used for some time. In trying to force the valve open it has been suddenly released and become jammed in the fully open position so that toxic gas poured into the laboratory.

Oxygen gas in cylinders is dangerous because it can cause spontaneous fires if released from cylinders with grease or organic debris around the cylinder head. Another danger is the failure to identify gas cylinders correctly, resulting in the connection of highly reactive oxygen gas to equipment in mistake for inert nitrogen or helium gas.

Of the flammable gases hydrogen and acetylene deserve special mention. Hydrogen in cylinders or under pressure generally is especially dangerous because it forms explosive gas mixtures in almost any ratio with air. Thus, even small leaks from equipment can give rise to serious explosions in the presence of an ignition source.

Acetylene is a relatively unstable gas. It has been known to decompose under relatively non-extreme conditions of mechanical shock or heating. In addition, acetylene is violently reactive with numerous chemicals and materials, including materials commonly used for laboratory equipment. One particular danger is the use of copper tubing to carry acetylene gas, when explosive copper acetylide may be formed.

Flammable gases in cylinders, including acetylene are frequently employed as fuel for high-temperature burners both inside and outside laboratories. An important laboratory use of high-temperature flames is in glass blowing. In addition to the hazard of explosions when flammable gases leak from burners while not in use, and burning of users when they are operating, such systems are also subject to hazards from 'flashback' and explosions within the equipment. As the name implies 'flashback' involves the progressive travel of the burner flame front back down the burner from the orifice, into the connecting tubing and ultimately back to the gas supply cylinder itself. The ignition of cylinder gas following flashback has given rise to many serious fires and explosions. Explosions within burners occur when the air or oxygen supply is allowed to mix with the fuel gas supply while the equipment is out of use. Lighting up the burner before mixed gases are purged from the system can give rise to explosions at the burner or in the supply system. Non-return valves should be placed in the fuel gas line to stop oxygen (or air) forcing its way down the fuel line if unequal pressures arise.

Further hazards arise with gas cylinders when they are accidentally allowed to become warm from direct sunlight or placed close to heaters, or when they are allowed to become part of stray electrical circuits. Cylinders are a special hazard if they are present during laboratory fires as they are pressurized by the temperatures involved and weakened by the heat so that they can explode very violently.

Explosion hazards from liquefied gases which are trapped by accident in sealed containers at low temperatures and then allowed to warm up have already been mentioned. Water vapour condensing to ice on the necks of containers of liquid air or nitrogen and blocking the only route of gas to escape has been a common cause of explosion. Liquid oxygen is extremely dangerous because violent reactions with organic materials are possible. While this material is rarely used as a coolant, workers frequently overlook the ability of liquid nitrogen or liquid air to preferentially condense oxygen from the atmosphere. Any liquid air container open to the atmosphere should be emptied from time to time rather than just topped up so that this oxygen enrichment is eliminated.

GENERAL CONSIDERATIONS WHEN PLANNING TO AVOID CHEMICAL ACCIDENTS IN LABORATORIES

There are three broad aspects to the prevention of chemical accidents of the types described above in (or associated with) laboratories. Firstly, it is important to plan the layout of laboratories, their facilities and equipment with chemical hazards in mind. Many laboratories are laid out in ways which are inherently hazardous, or contain facilities and equipment which have built-in hazards. Having provided a suitable 'hardware' environment it is essential to institute safety 'software' systems which give full consideration to chemical hazards. Safety 'software' in this context covers laboratory safety rules, permit to work systems, chemical hazard data sheets, chemical ordering and disposal systems which take account of hazards, the development of safe systems of work, safety audits and inspections, safety training and other related matters. Thirdly, there are special precautions which can be adopted to deal with the known or suspected hazards of specific chemicals that may have to be used in laboratory work. Before going on to summarize these precautions, however, there are some very general points which can be made about chemical hazards and safeguards. Many laboratory accidents involving chemicals occur because the workers involved did not appreciate the hazards of the chemicals they were using. In some cases the hazard was not known about at all, while in other cases it was underestimated. New or little-known chemicals obviously present a special category of risk. Early experiments should involve the preparation and testing of only small amounts with full precautions until the hazards, if any, are better established. In many countries it is becoming a requirement that new chemicals to be brought on to the commercial market in any significant quantities must be subjected to a battery of tests, including preliminary toxicity tests, and that these tests should be reported to an appropriate government agency. Obviously, this requirement should greatly reduce the number of cases where the hazard of a new proprietary material has only been realized after a workplace accident has taken place.

However, it must be stressed that the majority of chemical accidents involve commonly used substances with well-established hazard potential. Some recently reported laboratory fires, for example, involved flammable solvents such as toluene or diethyl ether which have been causing laboratory fires for well over 100 years. Similarly, cyanide has been poisoning laboratory workers for a long time and is still doing so. Greater effort is therefore needed to make laboratory staff aware of known hazards by labelling of containers with hazard symbols and precautionary information, the employment of hazard data sheets for individual chemicals drawn from stores, and adequate health and safety training. If necessary, pressure should be applied to suppliers of chemicals to provide adequate hazard information. The extent to which certain laboratory chemicals are hazardous should be brought home to laboratory workers by use of accident case studies in training, and the development and distribution of hazard/accident bulletins. Staff should be encouraged to report minor accidents and near-misses, and laboratory managers should be encouraged to ensure that serious incidents are brought to the attention of the scientific and safety media, for the benefit of others.

The inherently hazardous nature of chemical laboratory working does not allow a lenient attitude towards deliberate risk-taking and the flouting of safety rules and regulations. Laboratory workers have traditionally often developed their own programmes and systems of work with minimum consultation with others. If these working practices are seen to be hazardous it is essential that management intervenes on behalf of all employees. Very often the hazard is created by one careless laboratory worker and another more careful worker suffers the accident injury.

A further point is that the term 'laboratory worker' should not be taken to mean only those who work most of the time in laboratories. A whole range of workers have access to laboratories, work in them from time to time, or provide a service to them. Thus, in addition to scientists and engineers, technicians and students, laboratories may be places of work for administrators, porters, storemen, cleaners, waste disposal workers, maintenance workers and others. Maintenance staff are worthy of particular mention in that they may be put at considerable risk by hidden hazards in laboratories. Conversely, incorrect or inadequate maintenance of plant and equipment by such staff may create subsequent hazards to laboratory workers. Examples of the former problem include plumbers being overcome by toxic fumes while attempting to clear blocked drains in laboratories, and ventilating engineers being injured in explosions while checking fume cupboard ventilation in hospital laboratories because of a build-up of perchloric acid (from digester fumes) in ducting. Inadequate or incorrect maintenance work can lead to fume cupboards blowing air out into the laboratory instead of withdrawing it, or electrical equipment sparking near sources of flammable vapours and gases.

All staff who have any involvement with laboratory working and can be exposed to chemical hazards require adequate training. They need to know the range and limitations of their work (for example, what the cleaners are supposed to clean), what involvement with chemicals there could be, what hazards can be involved, and what precautions they should take. For non-scientific staff the whole area of instruction, provision of information, safety labelling of all containers (including waste containers) and adequate supervision becomes doubly important.

LABORATORY PREMISES, SERVICES AND EQUIPMENT IN RELATION TO CHEMICAL HAZARDS

This aspect of hazard precautions has been placed first because it is often the most neglected. Poor design and layout of laboratories and services are often the basic underlying reasons for high accident levels. Thus, chemical accidents arising from apparent poor housekeeping and cluttered bench tops may be due to insufficient separate storage space for chemicals, or long distances between storage areas and laboratories so that staff resist returning chemicals to the stores after use. The same general point applies to equipment, including safety equipment. For example, badly designed and poorly sited fume cupboards will never be efficient despite the best efforts of laboratory-based users, and the potential for toxic hazards in both the short and long term will be enhanced.

Aspects of basic laboratory installation which are of particular concern in the context of chemical hazards include:

116

1.   space requirements, positioning of benches and means of escape;
2.   surface finishes;
3.   laboratory furniture and chemical stores;
4.   heating, ventilation and lighting;
5.   bench services;
6.   fume cupboards;
7.   hazard laboratories;
8.   instrument rooms.

Equipment considerations include:

1.   glass and plastic ware;
2.   heating and cooling equipment;
3.   mixing and stirring equipment;
4.   vacuum and pressure equipment;
5.   laboratory instrumentation and services;
6.   gas cylinders;
7.   waste disposal facilities;
8.   safety and first aid equipment.

Space requirements

No absolute rules can be made about space requirements for laboratory work because of the great variety of work undertaken. Although laboratory work is becoming less labour-intensive with the move towards automation and instrumentation, the machinery itself tends to decrease the free-floor and bench space. Underprovision of storage facilities is a false economy as valuable laboratory space is then devoted to storing portable and seldom-used equipment and chemicals, increasing the potential for accidents.

The positioning of doors and their design is of critical importance. Means of escape for laboratory workers in case of accidents or emergencies must be convenient and well marked. The relationship between the positions of doors and benches must be carefully considered to ensure that workers will not be trapped if fire breaks out suddenly. Where special fire escapes are necessary these should be checked regularly for ease of opening and safe construction. Laboratory doors should be constructed so that they are fire-resistant, but not so heavy or stiff that they are difficult to open. Visibility through doors is important to ensure that collisions with people or apparatus are minimized.

Surface finishes

Again, the requirements of specific laboratories will vary depending on the type of work carried out. Floor coverings should be comfortable and slip-resistant, durable and resistant to spills of water or common chemicals (especially solvents and acids). Flooring consisting of small units joined together, such as tiles or wood blocks, is particularly unsuitable. Any spilled liquid chemicals will run down into joints and decontamination is then impossible without taking the flooring up. Linoleum sheeting is being replaced by impervious PVC sheeting with welded joints and coved edges. This material is suitable for laboratories not subject to heavy solvent contamination, wheeled traffic or standing of heavy semi-portable equipment. For heavier duty, resin screeds, or ceramic tiles set in resin cement, may be necessary.

The long-standing tradition of making bench tops from very expensive hardwood is now dying both on grounds of cost and lack of durability or ease of cleaning. Press-bonded melamine-faced laminated boards are coming into common use for general laboratory benches while epoxy resin surface boards are employed for bench tops which are likely to be heavily contaminated, such as fume cupboards.

Laboratory furniture and chemical stores

Laboratory cupboards are now most commonly provided as modules to fit under the continuous runs of impervious benching favoured on health and safety grounds. Wooden furniture is of proven durability in most laboratory atmospheres, and should be designed for ease of access with well-fitted doors and drawers. High wall-mounted or free-standing cupboards should be discouraged as these require workers to stretch above head height to lift equipment or chemicals from shelves.

The integration of water, gas and electrical services and their controls with laboratory furniture needs careful consideration from the safety viewpoint, particularly with regard to convenient access, protection from knocks, and ease of maintenance.

Reference has already been made to the dangers of collecting large quantities of chemicals on the bench. To enable workers to reduce their holdings of chemicals in the laboratory to a minimum it is essential to provide a separate chemical store. This should be separate from the laboratory, preferably a purpose-designed free-standing structure at ground level, but fairly close to the working areas. Full discussion of the design of chemical stores is beyond this review, but certain basic principles should always be borne in mind. The separate store should be lockable to prevent unauthorized entrance. It should be designed to allow good natural ventilation so that any spillage or leak of chemicals does not allow a build-up of toxic or

118

flammable vapours. The structure should be windowless but with a light roof and large explosion vents to ensure that any explosion blows upwards through the ceiling and not out through the walls. The entrance door should be raised to allow a bund wall to be constructed which will contain completely leakage from the largest full container in the store. Gently sloping ramps should then be provided to allow easier raising of heavy containers over the bund wall. Internally, the main features should include separately bunded areas for different types of chemicals which are incompatible and dangerous when mixed. These areas should be clearly labelled, as should every container in the store. Waste chemicals and empty containers are best kept in a separate similar storage facility to await collection. Internal lighting must meet a high standard of safety with regard to operation in a potential flammable atmosphere. 'No smoking' signs should be posted outside and inside the store, and large toxic and fire explosion hazard warning signs with symbols should be affixed to the outside walls. Chemicals should not be dispensed inside the store itself, but in an adjacent open area, again bunded to contain any spillage. The store should be provided with its own equipment in case of emergencies, including a spillage clean-up kit, fire-fighting equipment and protective clothing. Mechanical aids to lifting and carrying should be employed, from trolleys with clamps for large drums, to hand-held glass bottle carriers. Adjacent to the laboratory itself there may need to be a separate storage area for large numbers of small containers. Again, good ventilation is essential, as is a degree of basic segregation of chemicals. A common hazard of such stores is the provision of large amounts of high racking which is hazardous in its own right and encourages the storage of very large quantities of chemicals adjacent to the laboratory. Racking should be sufficiently strong for the purpose, well secured and with a corrosion-resistant, non-skid surface and edge protection to prevent bottles being pushed off accidentally and to contain leaks and spills. Heavy containers should be placed at low level and smaller containers above, with the precaution that containers of particularly hazardous chemicals should be placed where they are least likely to be dropped and broken. Water-reactive chemicals should be stored above floor level in case of water flooding. Where dispensing of chemicals into smaller containers is to be carried out there should be provision of benching with spill trays adjacent to the store. Toxic chemicals which give off hazardous vapours or dusts on pouring should be dispensed within a fume cupboard.

Laboratory heating, ventilation and lighting

In modern chemical laboratories general heating and ventilation is provided by a ducted air system which should give 10–12 air changes per hour. This is not difficult in principle, but where fume cupboards with high extraction rates are employed there can be problems. Unless some special provision is made the extraction rate of air from the laboratory into the fume cupboards will lead to cooling of the laboratory as make-up is drawn in from air gaps in doors and windows, etc. If these are sealed, the performance of high-rate fume cupboards will drop off. In such cases provision of a ducted supply of unheated make-up air to the fume cupboard can overcome the problem.

Many laboratories consist of buildings adapted from other purposes and present considerable problems with respect to heating and ventilation. There is a tendency to introduce portable heaters into older underheated laboratories and these can be extremely dangerous. No heating system should be employed which involves naked flames, glowing electrical wires or very hot surfaces. In older laboratories the best approach may be to utilize existing hot-water radiators and introduce a heating and ventilation system via ducted air as a back-up.

Lighting is a particularly important service in chemical laboratories where hazardous procedures may be undertaken. Best use should be made of natural daylight which gives best colour rendering, by placing benches for common low-risk work near windows. It is particularly important to ensure that fume cupboards for hazardous work are well-lit by lamps with intrinsically safe electrical wiring on a system separate from the general laboratory lighting.

Bench services

Benches and other working areas may require a considerable number of piped services to provide the facilities necessary for modern chemical laboratory work. Pieces of equipment and instruments may each demand general service connections. The use of a colour code for supply lines of electricity, water, gas and so on has much to commend it.

The most widely required service is electricity, usually at mains voltage, although high voltages may be required for some equipment. The electrical supply to fixed equipment should be placed in conduit, or armoured cable to avoid damage. Where flexible leads are necessary on portable or semi-portable equipment the leads themselves and all connections require regular examination for damage. In addition to the normal checks for mechanical and electrical integrity special attention should be given to evidence of atmospheric corrosion. This could cause damage to the earth continuity of socket outlets for example. Faulty switches, insulation damage or any other fault which might give rise to sparking or arcing when the equipment is switched on must be replaced to avoid ignition of flammable materials. The adoption of temporary electrical wiring should be strongly discouraged. If significant amounts of flammable liquid are normally present, a flameproof installation may be required. Electrical wiring must not be placed where water or chemical spills are likely to make contact, and certainly not close to sinks. In hazard areas it may be advisable to provide mushroom-headed panic buttons so that the whole electrical supply can be very rapidly switched off. Certainly, the switch-off control or controls for the laboratory must be plainly visible and clearly marked, with one near each exit door so that the electricity can be readily switched off during any emergency evacuation. The same requirement applies to other laboratory services, and it is sensible to group these master switches close to each other.

Chemical laboratories require substantial supplies of water and sinks for cooling water, washing-up and for use in experiments. Water used for cooling generates hazards if connected to equipment with low-quality flexible tubing improperly secured. Changes in water pressure can then cause the tubing to be blown off the equipment, or old, perished tubing may split and leak. If this happens outside normal working hours the incident may go undetected for some considerable time and cause extensive flooding. Loss of coolant water may give rise to a hazard. Many water-cooled instruments now contain thermostat devices to detect excessive temperature increases and switch off the heating system. Distillation and reflux apparatus is usually water-cooled, and loss of coolant water can give rise to a dangerous build-up of flammable or toxic vapours. Special monitoring devices can be fitted to such equipment, either to detect excessive temperature increase, or preferably the initial loss (or excessive reduction in flow rate) of cooling water. Suitable, well-fitted tubing secured by purpose-designed clamps must be used, rather than twisted wire or string.

The sinks and drainage system should be made of corrosion-resistant materials with precautions against blockage by discharge of gross solids, and traps to prevent back-diffusion of any volatile vapours. Abuse of sinks is one of the commonest sources of hazard in laboratories, and every effort should be made to prevent the discharge to drain of reactive chemicals, solids (including paper and glass), or water-immiscible liquids. Pouring quantities of flammable liquids down drains is a very hazardous practice. Apart from causing hazardous chemical interactions or fires, reactive and corrosive chemicals and solvents discharged to drain will probably damage the drain itself. This may ultimately lead to a need to carry out expensive and potentially hazardous repairs to the drains. Even the relatively routine unblocking and cleaning of chemical laboratory sinks, traps and drains can be hazardous. Release of toxic fumes is likely and precautions must be taken to counter this hazard. Explosions have occurred, especially where maintenance staff have been smoking. A potential source of explosions arises where hospital laboratories have discharged waste sodium azide to drains containing runs of copper tubing. Explosive copper azide can be formed and set off by the mechanical shock or friction involved in dismantling sink traps or runs of drains.

As already indicated, the use of pressurized gases in laboratories gives rise to many hazards. Discussion of control of these hazards is a very important part of laboratory safety precautions.

Fume cupboard design and siting within laboratories has often been extremely poor leading to short- and long-term health and safety hazards to laboratory workers. Recent concern about laboratory hazards has led to extensive research and rethinking about fume cupboard performance and design. Attention must be given to the purpose of a fume cupboard, its design and location, fans and ducting, exit gas discharge point, maintenance and correct use.

Hazard laboratories

Some chemical laboratory work is so dangerous that there is a case for it to be carried out in a separate small 'hazard laboratory'. In this way the hazard is isolated and the risks to people and plant not involved in the experiment are minimized. Examples would include the opening and use of containers of highly toxic substances, where one or two workers could wear appropriate breathing apparatus for a short period as a precaution. Potentially explosive reactions or those with a high fire risk could be carried out in such hazard laboratories. It would also be best if experiments which must be continued overnight when nobody is present, were located in a separate hazard laboratory. Ideally, this laboratory should be a separate building from the main laboratory complex and purpose-designed with fire-resistant materials and roof explosion vents.

Instrument rooms

The concept of protecting sensitive and valuable instruments by reserving a room separate from the main laboratory is not new. Balance rooms have been provided adjacent to chemical laboratories for many years, away from the risk of damage from being knocked into or attacked by corrosive fumes and liquids.

There are certainly strong arguments for keeping modern analytical equipment in a clean, safe environment in view of its sensitivity, cost and importance in providing a service to laboratory work. Having provided a separate instrument room it is important to ensure that the room itself and the individual instruments are not put at risk by chemicals carried in from the main laboratory. Good-quality fire doors should be fitted and these should be kept closed as far as possible, so that instruments are protected from fumes and fire smoke as far as practicable.

SAFETY ASPECTS OF CHEMICAL LABORATORY EQUIPMENT APPARATUS AND CHEMICAL CONTAINERS

The most obvious feature of any chemical laboratory is the prevalence of containers and apparatus designed to hold chemicals. Traditionally glass has been used almost exclusively for containers and apparatus because it is very resistant to chemical attack and transparent, allowing a clear sight of chemical contents. Unfortunately, glass is extremely brittle and readily broke. the broken pieces being jagged and sharp. As discussed earlier cuts from glassware are the most common source of laboratory accidents. Glassware is broken by dropping it onto the bench, onto other glassware or hard apparatus, into sinks or onto the floor. If the glassware contains a chemical its breakage will give rise to a chemical spill and possibly an injury accident. Explosions of chemicals in glass apparatus give rise to fragments of glass being fired out into the laboratory, unless special precautions have been taken.

The chemical resistance of glass and its transparency have allowed it to retain its predominant place as the material of choice for most chemical apparatus, despite its obvious limitations. However, chemical containers are now made from a range of materials other than glass and these can offer significant advantages in safety terms. Large containers of solvents are made of metal so that they do not break under mechanical shock unless this is severe enough to split seams of drums and cans. There is increasing pressure from safety experts for smaller containers of solvents and other appropriate chemicals to be made of metal so that the dropping of small sealed containers does not give rise to breakage and spillage hazards. In the same way, bulk supplies of corrosive chemicals such as acids are most frequently provided in corrosion-resistant plastic containers with low risk of breakage.

Whatever materials are used to contain chemicals, regular checks should be undertaken to ensure that containers and apparatus are in good condition. Stressing and scratching of glassware should be avoided as much as possible since invisible stresses may build up and breakage occur later, and unexpectedly, under low-stress conditions. Stresses in glass apparatus are often induced by incorrect clamping and lack of proper support for the weight. Obviously, cracked glass apparatus should not be used under any circumstances.

Heating and cooling equipment

Heating equipment for experimental work in chemical laboratories includes furnaces and ovens, drying plant, electric isomantles and heating tapes and electric hot plates, as well as gas burners, which have already been discussed. Any electrical equipment which is likely to come in contact with flammable liquids, gases or solids in finely divided form should be electrically flameproof to avoid fires and explosions. However, it must be realized by laboratory workers that many flammable materials do not require the presence of a naked flame or a spark to ignite. Many fires have been caused by placing containers of low flash point solvents in ovens at temperatures where they will ignite. A common example is the drying of wet flasks by washing out with acetone or methanol, draining off most of the solvent-water mixture and placing the flask in a drying oven. The remaining solvent has then evaporated and ignited. Every effort should be made to avoid hot flammable solvents boiling over and running down onto electrical heating equipment. Oil baths require careful control to ensure that the temperature does not approach the flashpoint of the oil vapour.

Cooling equipment includes refrigerators and vessels to contain coolants, from ice-water, through organic solvent-carbon dioxide mixtures to liquefied gases. The hazards and precautions required with such cooling systems have already been discussed in outline. Any apparatus or vessels which are going to be subjected to shock cooling should be carefully checked beforehand for any indications of faults. Possible failure should always be planned for in terms of protection against flying glass and chemical spurts or spills.

Mixing and stirring equipment

Many laboratory accidents with chemicals involve either excessive or insufficient mixing and stirring; often, one chemical needs to be added very slowly to another, with good mixing at each addition to achieve smooth reaction and avoid localized overheating. The taps of addition vessels must be checked and greased to ensure that they will not fail during the addition, either by falling out or jamming open. Appropriate stirrers are available for all types of tasks and selection between, for example, mechanical rotating blade devices, driven by electric or compressed air motors, and magnetic stirrers should take full account of potential hazards. Magnetic stirrers are frequently selected on the grounds of convenience, but the magnetic stirrer bar is not up to the task of stirring the liquid effectively, either because of its large volume, viscous nature or the shape of the reaction vessel. Mechanical stirrers often have an extensive spark source at the commutator and are therefore unsuitable for direct stirring of reactions involving highly flammable liquids or flammable effluent gases. Spark-free ac-only motors, or still better compressed air motors, should be used in such cases.

Vacuum and pressure equipment

Vacuum pumps are expensive and easily damaged pieces of equipment and laboratory staff need proper training in their safe use. The hazards of glass apparatus under vacuum are poorly understood. Implosions can create as much accident potential as many explosions in terms of flying glass and spurting chemicals. Vacuum lines should be placed behind fixed shatter-proof screens, and any equipment in the line, such as gauges or valves, should be verified as able to withstand the vacuum applied. Accidents often arise from deliberate sudden release of the vacuum within equipment, and workers should be trained to equalize pressures slowly when experiments are completed. Pressure vessels, whether to maintain air pressure above atmospheric, or to create pressures of reactive gases, are inherently dangerous items of equipment. High-pressure hydrogenation, for example, requires a purpose-designed autoclave. High-pressure equipment should be fitted with bursting discs or other pressure-relief devices to avoid explosions in the event of over-pressurizing (for example, by runaway exothermic reactions). Regular inspection and planned preventive maintenance of all such equipment by qualified engineers is essential, and is required by law in many countries.

Chemical waste disposal facilities

Many limitations on the discharge of chemical wastes to drain and subsequently to sewer have already been indicated. In addition to these, there are limitations because of the potential for chemicals to cause hazards and damage in the sewerage systems or at the sewage works itself. Thus, toxic inorganic chemicals such as heavy metals or cyanide, or toxic organic compounds such as organochlorines, can interfere with biological treatment at sewage works, or make sewage sludge too toxic to go on to land.

Legislation in many countries prevents the burying of chemical wastes by laboratory staff on a casual basis, or the burning of wastes in open bonfires. Increasingly, waste chemicals are therefore having to be collected from laboratories for proper disposal by legally authorized methods. Such collection services are often expensive for the relatively small quantities of chemicals involved. Good laboratory management should ensure that chemicals are not over-ordered because the cost of disposal of excess chemicals can far exceed the initial purchase costs. Chemical waste disposal services are often not prepared to collect unlabelled chemicals whose nature and hazards cannot be determined. Indeed, in some countries it may be illegal for them to attempt to dispose of unknown wastes. Thus, proper labelling of all chemical containers is essential, including experimental and analysis samples. Staff leaving the laboratory on change of employment should be required to clear out all their chemical stocks and label every container clearly with details of the contents and hazards (if any). Failure to enforce this requirement can lead to laborious and costly detective and analysis work later.

Inventories of chemical stocks should be taken periodically and an investigation made of all likely 'hiding places' for chemicals. Failure to do this can lead to very hazardous situations, such as the discovery of large containers of picric acid which have dried out and are potentially explosive.

Suitable containers for waste solvents should be provided and clearly marked so that incompatible solvents are not mixed together. As a minimum, waste solvents should be segregated into organochlorines, water immiscibles and water miscibles. Apart from creating hazards, the mixing together of chlorinated and non-chlorinated solvents is costly since the mixture will be regarded as 'chlorinated' by the waste disposal services, and charged at the much higher collection and disposal rate necessary for these difficult chemicals. All waste containers should be of sound construction, clearly labelled and safely stored for collection. Where purification and recycling of chemicals, especially high-value solvents, is practised it is essential that all staff understand the importance of not contaminating recovered material with other wastes. Hazards and costs of chemical waste disposal can often be reduced or eliminated by treatment of the waste in the laboratory to remove the hazards. Thus, dilute cyanide solutions can be detoxified by hypochlorite treatment, or solutions of oxidizing agents reduced. Staff involved in chemical waste disposal must be appropriately trained, and provided with necessary carrying equipment and protective clothing.

Safety and first aid equipment

Reference has already been made to a range of equipment which provides an increased element of safety in laboratory working, such as fume cupboards, safety screens and flashback arrestors. Here discussion will be restricted to air pollution monitoring equipment, protective clothing, emergency showers and eyewash stations, fire-fighting equipment, breathing apparatus, chemical spillage clean-up kits and first aid equipment.

A wide range of air sampling and analysis devices are now available for use in connection with analysing the atmosphere in the workplace. As scientists, engineers and technicians, laboratory staff have no excuse for not monitoring the atmosphere in their own laboratories and their own breathing zones. The Dewhurst survey indicated that the atmosphere in many laboratories causes discomfort to workers. It may also be endangering their health in the long term. Equipment ranges from simple chemical tube indicators through which air samples are pumped, to instruments which are specific to particular (usually inorganic) chemicals and to activated carbon sampling systems, which when connected to a gas chromatograph can identify a whole range of organic vapours and quantify their levels in the laboratory atmosphere. There is a strong movement towards personal monitoring of individual workers in addition to general environmental monitoring, and even to the development of chemical badges to be worn and analysed like radiation badges.

Protective clothing includes eye and face protection, laboratory coats and chemically impervious overalls and aprons, gloves and boots. Eye protection should be comfortable for the individual wearer and offer both good protection and good visibility. It should be readily available in a clean condition. Goggles are to be preferred to safety spectacles where corrosive materials can spray into the face. Face-masks should be used with or in preference to goggles where any significant quantities of corrosive materials are involved.

Laboratory coats should be kept buttoned up in chemical laboratories, and there is a strong case for rear-fastening coats where chemical splashes are at all likely. If significant quantities of corrosive materials are to be poured, protective overalls of chemically resistant materials such as PVC should be employed. Gloves should be worn against both corrosion and dermatitis hazards but should not be regarded as a panacea against careless work. Nearly all types of glove material can be penetrated by one chemical or another, and it is essential to minimize contact and check that the gloves are suitable as protection against the chemical or chemicals involved. Gloves should also be checked for holes or tears and replaced if there are any doubts. Ordinary shoes and sandals offer scant protection against chemical spills onto the feet, or accidentally walking through or standing on spilt chemicals. Thus, where significant quantities of hazardous chemicals are carried or dispensed chemically resistant boots should be worn. These should also offer protection against weights, such as the edges of drums, falling onto the toes.

Emergency showers are now often regarded as essential safety equipment in chemical laboratories. There have been many examples of accidents involving chemical splashes and leading to severe chemical burns which would have caused little or no injury if emergency showers had been available. Standard laboratory taps and sinks are not designed to quickly wash down a person soaked with corrosive chemicals. Showers must be checked periodically to ensure that they are in good working order and their location and controls clearly marked.

Chemical splashes into the eye should be treated by flooding with large quantities of water for at least several minutes, using a gently running tap or a purpose-designed eyewash bottle. Care must be taken not to use a powerful water jet. The water to be used for eye washing, whether from the tap or an eyewash bottle, must be essentially sterile to avoid injecting disease organisms into the eye. Thus tap water should be from mains supply, and eyewash bottles must be changed periodically before they exceed their shelf-life.

Effective and swift-action fire alarms are essential for chemical laboratories. Fire-fighting equipment in laboratories is usually limited to portable fire extinguishers, sand buckets and fire blankets. Laboratory staff should not be expected to fight fires requiring more extensive equipment but should evacuate the building and await the fire brigade. Fire-fighting equipment should be selected in the light of all likely types of fire, chemical or otherwise. Carbon dioxide extinguishers are particularly useful in chemical laboratories as they will extinguish a wide variety of small fires. Fire involving a restricted range of chemicals cannot be extinguished with carbon dioxide, for example alkali metal fires, and a sand bucket or inert dry powder extinguisher should be to hand where such chemicals are in use. Water extinguishers are unsuitable for many chemical laboratory fires.

Breathing apparatus

Every effort should be made to design laboratory experiments and activities so that breathing apparatus is not routinely required. Where the working is so hazardous that staff must work in face masks, respirators or positive-pressure breathing apparatus for extended periods of time, expert advice must be sought. In general laboratory working use of breathing apparatus is restricted to very short periods for precautionary purposes, or to emergency situations.

Laboratory staff are often very resistant to the wearing of breathing apparatus and look towards face masks and respirators for short-term and emergency use. While this is understandable, the limitations of gas masks must be well understood. Where the hazard potential justifies it, laboratory staff must be trained in the use of positive-pressure breathing apparatus supplied by back-pack cylinders, or air-lines from a pump. Any breathing apparatus provided must be kept in a well-maintained condition.

Chemical spillage kits

Despite all precautions, chemical spillages do occur in laboratories from time to time. It is therefore essential to provide a set of equipment and treatment agents for prompt use following a spill. In any one laboratory the range of chemicals likely to be spilt is often quite restricted, and the spillage kit should reflect this. Proprietary kits can be bought which will cover common problem chemicals such as acids, caustic compounds, flammable solvents, mercury, cyanides and hydrofluoric acid. Liquid spills require the use of an inert absorbent, and reactive chemicals such as acids or alkalis are best neutralized *in situ* before clean-up proceeds. Protective clothing should be provided in spillage kits, and breathing apparatus may be necessary where toxic chemicals are involved. Training in spillage treatment and clean-up is required, and such tasks must be dealt with by laboratory technical staff, not cleaners.

Chemical hazards and first aid

As already indicated, the first line of defence in dealing with potential chemical burns is flooding the affected area for prolonged periods (possible 10 minutes or more) with water from showers, taps, and eyewash bottles. Prompt action in the laboratory is the key to reducing the extent of injuries, and subsequent medical treatment can only ameliorate the problem. A whole variety of subsequent treatments are necessary depending on the nature of the chemical involved. In some cases a preliminary treatment by the first-aider is recommended as useful, but in other cases the burn should just be covered with a dry dressing and hospital treatment sought immediately. First aid kits should contain both reminder information and the necessary materials for dealing with the required procedures. Unless there has been some prior communication and planning, the casualty ward staff of the local hospital will have no specialized knowledge concerning the treatment of specific types of chemical burns. There have been examples of hospital staff initially treating hydrofluoric acid burns as if they were burns from a mineral acid. First-aiders must accompany the injured party to hospital and explain to hospital staff the nature of the treatment required, preferably with written information on hand. Where specialized treatment is required laboratory staff should arrange to carry the treatment chemicals and take these to the hospital with the patient.

Antidotes to chemical poisoning are not normally part of a laboratory first aid kit, with the exception of amyl nitrite cyanide antidote and calcium gluconate gel for HF burns, both of which staff should be trained to administer. Where the nature of the work makes other types of poisoning a distinct possibility, discussions should be entered into with the emergency services concerning the administering of antidotes or emergency oxygen. Where staff have ingested acid or caustic material no attempt should be made to make them vomit, in case of further damage.

Chemical accident first aid treatment should be integrated with general first aid training for recognized first-aiders. Limits on general procedures when chemicals are involved should be stressed, such as the hazards of mouth-to-mouth techniques of artificial respiration where poisoning is suspected. All laboratory workers should be trained in the administering of initial aid (such as eye-washing) as well as procedures for raising the alarm and calling the emergency services.

Health and safety systems with respect to chemical hazards

Well-managed laboratories will have an established system for all health and safety-related aspects of the work which is integrated into the overall programme of activities. From the above comments it is clear that chemical laboratories require a considerable amount of capital and recurrent expenditure to ensure that adequate facilities are available for a good health and safety performance. However, the facilities alone will not ensure satisfactory health and safety standards; as shown by earlier accident cases the way in which workers carry out their activities determines to a considerable extent the overall health and safety performance of a laboratory. A highly efficient fume cupboard is of little value if staff do not use it when working with chemicals emitting harmful vapours. Protective clothing cannot protect staff from injury if it is not worn.

Safety policies and laboratory safety rules

A booklet covering hazards and precautions for the laboratory (or complex of laboratories) should be produced. This should integrate closely with the safety policy, organization and arrangements of the overall working site, whether it is an industrial processing plant, or a university. Chemical hazards and precautions should be an integral part of the laboratory health and safety code. Chemists with expertise in chemical hazards should be asked to vet all paper work covering health and safety management systems. In any country there are likely to be some legal requirements with regard to the safe use of some chemicals. Any booklet should include, under controls and precautions, such matters as the legal and organizational responsibilities of staff at all levels for laboratory safety, planning of experiments, requirements for maintenance of equipment, permit-to-work procedures, safety inspections, accident reporting, emergency procedures and safety training requirements. Consideration of chemical hazards should be integrated into all these procedures.

Emergency planning

Emergencies arise in most laboratory complexes from time to time over the years despite all precautions. The way in which these emergencies are dealt with will depend largely on the extent of prior emergency planning and training. The survey by Dewhurst reported that the state of preparedness of many laboratories against quite foreseeable chemical emergencies was poor. Thus, over 62% of respondents stated that no safety shower was available in their laboratory, despite the fact that nearly 16% stated that at least one accident best dealt with by such equipment had occurred. A total of 189 out of 252 respondents had never received instruction with regard to phenol burns despite the fact that over 50% of the laboratory workers covered by the survey worked with phenol. The widespread nature of this problem of lack of preparedness was also illustrated by responses to a question on the use of hydrofluoric acid. Out of 74 cases where this chemical was regularly used no instruction on appropriate first aid treatment for HF burns had been given in 36 cases, and only written instruction in a further five cases. Undoubtedly, much remains to be done with respect to the preparedness of individual workers to deal with emergencies.

Emergency planning against major emergencies must be carried out in consultation with the emergency services. Both the public and emergency services workers can be put at considerable risk where chemicals are involved in emergencies. A full understanding of the hazards in a particular laboratory will help the emergency services to plan against a variety of emergency scenarios. In the event of an emergency the relevant authorities will then be able to act quickly and securely in dealing with the problem. Laboratory managers must play their part to the full in instructing and training their own staff on how to summon the emergency services and how to liaise with them. Such apparently mundane matters as sensible car parking can become critical issues in an emergency if careless parking causes roads to be blocked to emergency vehicles (such as fire engines when the laboratory is on fire).

Evacuation procedures are especially important with regard to chemical laboratories, where a toxic gas emission or solvent fire can make a whole laboratory a death-trap in seconds. Planning adequate safe means of escape, and ensuring that they remain safe and unblocked, is a key aspect of emergency planning. The raising of alarm, checking that laboratories and side rooms are evacuated, and the switching off of services and equipment, are all vital aspects of emergency procedures.

SPECIAL CONSIDERATIONS WHEN WORKING WITH HAZARDOUS CHEMICALS

Toxic and corrosive chemicals

The importance of identifying as far as possible the hazards of individual chemicals has already been stressed. As far as toxicity is concerned information may be scanty, especially as regards chronic and long-term health hazards, or more subtly harmful aspects than just acute poisoning (such as reproductive hazards). Where positive information is lacking a chemical should be regarded with considerable suspicion, especially if it is similar in some aspects of its chemical structure to known hazardous compounds. Low acute toxicity is no guide as to potential long-term health hazards. Thus vinyl chloride monomer was once considered to be a low-risk chemical because of its relatively low acute toxicity, but is now considered a very dangerous toxic chemical because it was discovered to be a potent carcinogen. This discovery in turn cast suspicion on other low molecular-weight halogenated alkenes, and trichloro- and tetrachloro-ethylene are now thought likely to offer some long-term health risks.

Efforts have been made to define the relative toxicity of chemicals by various routes of exposure. Thus compounds may be assigned acute toxicity gradings according to LD_{50} tests on animals (usually rats), where LD_{50} refers to the single dose in mg/kg of the average body weight of the test animals which will kill half of the animals when ingested. These LD_{50} and LC_{50} (lethal concentration) gradings are shown in Table 7.2 and may offer some guide as to the relative acute hazard potential of chemicals. However, even this apparently straightforward approach to assigning acute toxicity is of very limited value. The test animals may respond in quite different ways to man, the test gives little indication of toxicity effects by other routes of entry to the body, damage to organs which does not reveal itself in terms of short-term mortality (such as significant brain damage) is not revealed, the effects of repeat exposure to lower doses such as might be experienced in the workplace are not revealed, and the test gives us no information about long-term health hazards.

Table 7.2 EEC LD_{50} and LC_{50} requirements for the classification of toxic and harmful substances

Category	LD_{50} oral rat (mg/kg)	LD_{50} cutaneous rat or rabbit (mg/kg)	LC_{50} inhalation rat (mg/litre/ 4 hours)
Very toxic	25	50	0.5
Toxic	25–200	50–400	0.5–2
Harmful	200–2000	400–2000	2–20

Nevertheless, considerations of animal acute toxicity data of this type, plus any evidence from accidental human exposure, can give some guidance as to where extra precautions are necessary to avoid ingestion. Acutely toxic chemicals should be heavily labelled and kept separate from other chemicals in a lockable poisons cabinet with restricted access. For non-volatile toxic compounds accidental ingestion will most commonly occur if mouth-pipetting, eating, and drinking are allowed in the laboratory. These activities should always be forbidden. Poisons have also been transferred to the mouth from contaminated hands (for example, by biting nails). Working with suitable gloves on reduces the risk of hand contamination, although the hands can still become contaminated in removing gloves unless the outsides of these are washed first. Removal of contaminated laboratory coats can also transfer toxic chemicals to the hands. High standards of personal hygiene should be stressed, with frequent hand-washing, especially before eating or drinking. Laboratory coats should be regularly laundered by a specialist service.

Spills of very toxic substances should be urgently and carefully dealt with, and waste chemicals or materials such as waste cleaning papers contaminated with such toxic substances should be placed in well-sealed containers and the containers clearly labelled. As already discussed, it may be necessary to detoxify such chemicals and thus aid disposal. Obviously, such activities can themselves present problems and must be carried out according to safe systems of work.

The above comments about acutely toxic substances can be equally applied to chemicals with potent long-term health hazards. A good deal is now known about the potential of certain common chemicals to cause cancer in man. The evidence derives from epidemiological studies in man, long-term tests in animals, and less directly from mutagenicity tests *in vitro* or structure-activity relationship studies. Some known human carcinogens, such as 2-naphthylamine and benzidine, are banned from use in various countries, and trade unions have been anxious to restrict, as far as possible, the use of known or suspected human carcinogens.

Precautions against contact to the skin with toxic chemicals likely to cause surface damage or penetrate the skin involve the use of protective clothing and procedures which give the least chance of spillage or casual contact with the chemicals. The skin itself provides a protective barrier against the entry of many chemicals into the body. The barrier is broken if the skin is cut or abraded. Unless this type of damage to hands can be protected against toxic chemicals, affected laboratory workers should not be required to work with such chemicals (and preferably not with any chemicals) until the wounds have healed. Puncturing of the skin accidentally with hypodermic syringes containing chemicals is an increasing hazard, particularly in gas chromatographic work, and increased vigilance is required.

Sensible precautions should be taken to avoid spillages in handling toxic or corrosive chemicals, by lifting and carrying with care and not taking risks in pouring from one vessel to another. In particular, minimum quantities should be handled, appropriate funnels should be employed, and drip trays should be placed under vessels to contain splashes and spills.

The most common way for toxic substances to enter the bodies of laboratory workers is via the lungs. Compounds with no smell or colour in the vapour phase are likely to be breathed into the lungs quite unknowingly.

Fumes of certain toxic and corrosive chemicals will actually attack the nasal passages or the bronchial track, but most frequently it is the ability of certain chemicals to penetrate the lungs which gives rise to hazards. Gases, vapours of volatile liquids and very fine solid particles can pass right down into the lungs, damaging the lung cells themselves, or passing into the blood stream to cause damage from there. Toxic substances may attack the blood itself (for example, carbon monoxide or benzene), or the blood may carry the harmful chemicals around the body to vital organs. Attempts have been made to define levels of harmful vapours in the working atmosphere below which no acute or long-term health hazards should arise to workers breathing the atmosphere. The Society of American Governmental Hygienists which an-

133

nually issue a set of 'Threshold Limit Values' for commonly met toxic gases, vapours and dusts has had particular influence in developing this approach. These 'TLVs' are guidelines for maximum workplace exposures to individual toxic chemicals in air, and are based on a 40–hour working week of five 8-hour days. Based on all existing evidence, from accidental exposures, animal tests and *in vitro* tests, these values are thought to represent average levels of exposure which will cause no hazards to the vast majority of workers. Implicit in this concept is the view that there will be a level, however low, where no significant hazard to health will remain. The body does have defence mechanisms for detoxifying some chemicals up to certain levels, so this idea has some validity. On the other hand, it has been suggested that for some substances which cause cancer, such as asbestos dust, there is no 'safe' level, and any degree of exposure presents some risk, even if this is small. The TLV concept also implies that within certain limitations periods of exposure above the TLV can be balanced by periods of exposure below the TLV, provided the average overall exposure is below the TLV. Again, the evidence for this assumption is often challenged.

Although the TLV of a chemical is a useful guide as to potential hazards of breathing some of the substance in laboratory air, it should not be regarded as a 'safe' level indicator. If levels of a substance in the laboratory atmosphere approach or exceed the TLV for significant periods, further efforts must be made to reduce the release of the substance into the air. Average levels should be kept very much below the published TLV, especially if any long-term health hazard is suspected.

In view of the uncertainties involved in attempting to define 'safe' levels of atmospheric exposure it is essential to keep exposure to any breathable substances as low as possible unless they are of proven non-toxicity in every respect.

European readers should note that European Community countries are now increasingly subject to EC directives concerning occupational health and safety. Whereas in the past, countries such as the United Kingdom have largely utilised TLVs in setting national standards, now they are subject increasingly to EC standards, which may differ from American TLVs. Terminology is also changing; UK legislation (and particularly the Control of Substances Hazardous to Health Regulations) now refer to Occupational Exposure Standards rather than TLVs.

Toxic gases, volatile solvents, acid fumes, mercury and toxic dusts are common sources of toxic atmosphere hazards in laboratories. Mixing of two non-toxic chemicals can give rise to a toxic product and all mixing operations should be treated with suspicion. Substances which emit strong odours provide some indication of their presence and a possible hazard, although they may be harmful at levels below the level at which most workers can smell them (for example, benzene). Other substances such as mercury are odourless, and unless they are kept out of the laboratory atmosphere or monitored by atmospheric monitoring, may be creating health hazards for a long time quite undetected.

Since many volatile chemicals are used in the chemical laboratory and some are likely to smell strongly, some indication of the state of the laboratory atmosphere may be given by its 'smelliness'. Consistently smelly laboratories usually indicate poor ventilation and/or careless working practices. Volatile solvents should not be worked with to any extent in the open laboratory. Many well-established practices, such as carrying out solvent distillation or column chromatography on the open bench are no longer acceptable because of the possible long-term health risks involved. Even the repeated pouring of solvents from one container to another may give rise to unacceptable levels of air pollution. Such practices should be carried out in a suitable fume cupboard, and the tops of solvent containers closed if they are left to stand in the open laboratory. No open containers of mercury should be allowed in any laboratory, and any spills must be thoroughly cleaned up.

Toxic gases should only be used in the fume cupboard, and cylinders stored and opened in fume cupboard. Breathing apparatus appropriate to the toxic gas should be kept close at hand in case of emergencies, with a back-up set outside the laboratory.

These precautions should be backed by measurement of atmospheric levels, both 'worst-case' situations where there are likely to be significant levels of pollutants in the atmosphere for short periods, and average 'background' levels of commonly used substances through the working week.

Precautions with flammable chemicals

Non-flammable chemicals should be used in preference to flammable chemicals where a choice is feasible (unless the non-flammable chemical involves even greater risks in other respects, such as toxicity). The quantities of these solvents used in laboratories should be kept to the minimum. Every effort should be made to avoid leaks or spills from flammable liquid containers. If these solvents must be held overnight in laboratories they should be stored in purpose-designed flammable liquid cabinets. These should have good fire resistance and be well labelled as containing highly flammable substances.

The main defence against serious fires (or flammable gas explosions) is to minimize the level of flammable liquids, vapours or gases. Although these require a source of ignition, it is very difficult in a laboratory working environment to ensure that there will never be a source of ignition available. Certainly, the use of naked flames should be minimized, and smoking prohibited. Even so, electrical equipment, sparks from metal tools, or even hot surfaces can provide ignition sources. Electrostatic hazards are often overlooked and can give rise to severe explosions and fires.

135

As for toxic liquids, unbreakable containers, spill trays, aids to pouring and minimum quantities should also be employed where possible with flammable liquids. Volatile flammable liquids should be handled in a fume cupboard suitable for this purpose. The lower explosive limits for the gases and vapours of many flammable compounds will not normally be exceeded where safe systems of work are employed except under accident conditions.

Condenser water cooling failure or insufficiency can lead to distilled vapours not condensing as liquid but pouring from the apparatus as flammable vapour. Such events can cause immediate fires and explosions, or build-up of vapours until a source of ignition finally presents itself. Warning devices against such failures were referred to earlier.

Chemicals vary in terms of the concentration range in air within which they form explosive mixtures. The wider the range the more hazardous they are in this respect (Table 7.3).

Table 7.3 Explosive limits of common laboratory solvents as a percentage in air and boiling points (°C)

Solvent	Lower explosive limit (%)	Upper explosive limit (%)	Boiling point (°C)
Acetone	2.6	12.8	56.5
Butanol	1.7	18.0	80.0
Ethanol	3.3	19.0	78.3
Ethyl acetate	2.2	11.5	77.2
Methanol	6.0	36.5	64.8
Xylene	1.1	7.0	144.4

Appropriate fire extinguishers should be to hand where chemical fires are a significant risk, and staff must be confident in their correct use. (Such confidence can only be gained by 'hands-on' experience of fighting small fires under controlled training conditions.) Fire-risk experiments should not be carried out adjacent to means of escape, or anywhere which could result in workers being trapped in the event of fire.

Precautions against risk of explosion

Obviously every effort must be made to avoid explosions (or implosions) in the design and execution of experiments. Where any likelihood of explosions exists, early experiments should involve minimum quantities, and scale-up should be in careful stages. Just placing experiments behind fume cupboard glass is not a sufficient precaution against explosions. Often the explosion has blown out the front of the fume cupboard and the flying glass has added greatly to the explosion hazard. Purpose-designed screens are available to protect workers and the general laboratory environment against explosion blast and flying glass. Such screens placed in front of experiments on benches located against walls will offer a good degree of protection provided they are large enough and suitably placed. Wherever possible, explosion screens should be secured in position by bolts or screws which are not readily removed. So often explosion screens are provided as part of the 'safe system', but are not in place when an explosion occurs, because they were moved out of place during apparatus adjustment and not replaced for the experiment. Vacuum lines should have screens in place to guard against implosions.

Hazard warning signs should be placed by the equipment and other workers warned to keep away. Those dealing with the experiment should approach the apparatus wearing protective clothing, especially an appropriate face mask. While explosions most often occur during heating of chemicals, many other situations which can give rise to explosion risk were described earlier. Hazard precautions should therefore be maintained until there is complete assurance that no risk of explosion remains. Thus, grinding of solid chemicals together should be carried out behind screens unless there is absolute assurance that no risk exists, and mixing of chemicals is always best performed wearing a face mask. Exothermic reactions are inherently hazardous and full precautions should be taken as a back-up to good cooling and mixing.

Where a continuing significant risk of explosion exists by nature of part of the laboratory work programme, there is a strong case for a properly equipped hazards laboratory. This higher-risk work can then be carried out separately from lower-risk activities. A list of important reference sources follows. These in turn give many references to the vast literature on chemical hazards.

LITERATURE CONSULTED

American Conference of Government Industrial Hygienists (1982). *Threshold Limit Values for Chemical Substances and Physical Agents in the Workroom Environment with Intended Changes for 1982.* (Cincinnati: AGGIH)

Bretherick, L. (1979). *Handbook of Reactive Chemical Hazards*, 2nd edn. (London: Butterworths)

Bretherick, L. (1981). *Hazards in the Chemical Laboratory.* (London: The Royal Society of Chemistry)

Chivers, G.E. (1983). *The Disposal of Hazardous Wastes.* Occupational Hygiene Monograph No. 11. Series ed. Hughes, D. (London: Science Review)

Clayton, G.D. and Clayton, F.E. (1980). Vol. II, *Toxicology*, 3rd rev. edn. In *Patty's Industrial Hygiene and Toxicology.* (New York/London: Wiley Interscience Publishers)

Dewhurst, F. (1983). Accidents, safety and first aid training in laboratories. *Int. Env. Safety*, **4**, 11-13

Fire Protection Association (1974). *Fire and Related Properties of Industrial Chemicals*. (London: FPA)

Gill, F.S. and Ashton, I. (1982). *Monitoring for Health Hazards at Work*. (London: Grant McIntyre)

Harrington, J.M. (1976). MD thesis, London University

Harrington, J.M. and Gill, F.S. (1983). *Occupational Health*. (Oxford: Blackwell Scientific Publications)

Hughes, D. (1980). A literature survey and design study of fume cupboards and fume-dispersal systems. Occupational Hygiene Monograph No. 4. Series ed. Hughes, D. (London: Science Reviews)

Manufacturing Chemists Association (1972). *Laboratory Chemical Disposal Manual*. rev. 2nd edn. (Washington, DC: MCA)

National Institute of Occupational Safety and Health (1977-81). *Manual of Analytical Methods*. (Cincinnati: NIOSH)

National Institute of Occupational Safety and Health and the Occupational Safety and Health Administration (1981). *Occupational Health Guidelines for Chemical Hazards*. (Cincinnati: NIOSH)

Sax, N.I. (1979). *Dangerous Properties of Industrial Materials*, 5th edn. (New York: Van Nostrand Reinhold)

Williamson, G.E. (1978). Labelling of dangerous substances. *Chemistry and Industry*, May, pp. 307-314

8 Safety Measures to be Taken in a Haematological Laboratory

W.L. Ruff

Medical observers have witnessed the evolution of haematology into a broad-based science that encompasses such disciplines as medicine, genetics, biochemistry, immunology, physical chemistry, cell biology and nuclear medicine. Through this evolutionary process the haematologist has acquired an arsenal of tools for the diagnosis and treatment of haematological disorders. Yet the basic approach remains the same – a detailed medical history, a thorough physical examination and laboratory tests. However, additional avenues are available through the judicious application of multidisciplinary aspects/features of haematology to confirm or reject a diagnosis.

A detailed medical history facilitates focusing the physician's search for clues to the most fertile grounds for exploration. For example, ethnic origin and a history of anaemia, jaundice, lymphadenopathy and splenectomy in a male family member may suggest useful clues. Other helpful suggestions from a detailed medical history may include the nature of the patient's diet, what kind of drugs the patient takes and occupational exposure to any of a variety of physical or chemical agents. The physical examination findings do not always suggest haematopoietic system dysfunction. On physical examination a patient may present with a primary finding of congestive heart failure which, on further evaluation, is found to be secondary to pernicious anaemia in relapse. However, there are some physical findings which are highly suggestive of haematopoietic system disorders – sternal tenderness, haemorrhages or spoon nails.

In support of the diagnosis and treatment of patients being evaluated for haematological abnormalities, the haematology laboratory performs a variety of tests. To accomplish this task both manual and automated procedures are used. A primary activity of the haematology laboratory is to help the physician confirm or rule out an anaemia. This begins with the complete blood count (CBC), usually with an automated instrument, including the red cell indices for further classification and evaluation. The next step is the preparation and microscopic examination of the peripheral blood smear to obtain the differential leukocyte count, platelet number and morphology, red cell size, shape and staining characteristics. With the peripheral blood smear and the red cell indices, anaemia can be classified as macrocytic, normochromic normocytic or hypochromic microcytic.

A work-up for macrocytic anaemia should start with screening for vitamin B_{12} or folate deficiency. Serum and red cell lysates are assayed for folate. The red cell folate level is independent of daily intake and thus better estimates the patient's folate status. The macrocytic anaemia evaluation may also include a bone marrow aspiration and biopsy. For this examination the haematologist asks the question: Is the bone marrow megaloblastic? Additional testing for diagnosing macrocytic anaemia may require thyroxine, thyrotropin and thyrotropin releasing factor determinations. Further investigation may include reticulocyte count.

The first test in the evaluation of patients with normochromic, normocytic anaemia is the reticulocyte count. If the count is low, a bone marrow aspiration and biopsy are done to confirm or rule out aplastic or hypoplastic anaemia. If the count is high, haemolysis is suggested. Therefore, haptoglobin, bilirubin, red cell survival, haemoglobin electrophoresis and Coombs test may be indicated, and a bone marrow examination may be necessary.

Tests for patients with hypochromic, microcytic anaemia should include iron and iron-binding capacity (transferrin) to confirm the presence or absence of iron deficiency. To determine the status of iron reserves, serum ferritin and a bone marrow examination are carried out. Ferritin is an especially important test in order to determine the length of treatment, for all symptoms of iron deficiency may cease to exist long before the iron reserves are replenished.

Leukocyte studies represent a major activity of the haematology laboratory. Leukocytes constitute several major subtypes – granulocytes, monocytes and lymphocytes. Abnormalities may occur in single or multiple cell subtypes. In any of the cells the number may be increased or decreased. The total leukocyte count and the relative and absolute concentrations of the various leukocyte forms are determined regularly, and that may facilitate establishing a diagnosis.

In leukaemias the morphological changes are diagnostic. Special stains do help to further classify the acute leukaemias. In other conditions they will confirm or rule out an abnormality. An additional value of leukocyte studies is their use in monitoring the course of a disease, e.g. the toxic effects of chemotherapy and radiotherapy can be recognized by leukopenia.

A haematology laboratory also supports the evaluation of patients with haemostatic or coagulation disorders. In screening for haemostatic abnormalities, the platelet count, bleeding time and tests for platelet function are employed. Screening for coagulation disorders involves PT, PTT, TT and fibrinogen level. When coagulation tests are abnormal, specific factor assays may be required. Sometimes haemostatic and coagulation disorders may coexist. In such cases, all the previously listed tests are helpful.

Considering the spectrum of haematological problems, the haematology laboratory must provide a variety of tests. To do this requires a host of reagents and different types of supplies and equipment. Reagents range from isotonic saline, used as a diluting fluid in electronic cell counters (e.g. Coulter), to organic solvents such as isopropanol used in the denaturation test for unstable haemoglobins, to caustic chemicals such as sodium hydroxide used in screening for the pyruvic kinase enzyme deficiency in hereditary haemolytic anaemia, to radioisotopes used for ferrokinetic studies. Supplies and apparatus vary. They include, but are not limited to: (1) white cell and red cell pipettes for manual cell counts; (2) slides for morphological examinations; (3) sedimentation rate apparatus; (4) waterbaths; (5) thermometers; (6) refrigerators; and (7) sterile lancets for bleeding times. The haematology laboratory equipment comprises manual and automated cell counters, slide stainers, differential counters, clot timers; refrigerators, electrophoresis units, fibrometers, gamma counters, centrifuges, etc.

Table 8.1 Some examples of haematology laboratory safety hazards

		Type of hazard
(1)	Samples	biological (infection)
(2)	Reagents	
	sodium hydroxide	chemical (corrosive)
	methanol, isopropanol	fire (flammables)
	^{59}Fe	radiation
	cyanide	chemical (toxic)
	benzidine	chemical (toxic)
(3)	Supplies and apparatus	
	pipettes	biological (infection)
		physical (cuts)
	electrophoresis units	electrical
	thermometers	chemical (mercury)

Associated with the operation of haematological laboratories are safety implications for both patients and laboratory workers. Some examples of haematology laboratory safety hazards are given in Table 8.1. With respect to patients, the administration of radioisotopes perhaps poses the greatest safety risk. Incorrect dosage, using the wrong isotope and water-soluble isotope given to a patient with compromised renal function are a few potential hazards to the patient. A bone marrow aspiration imposes the risk of infection, bleeding, an occasional allergic reaction to novocaine and mediastinal puncture leading to cardiac or aorta damage.

In the United States, as in other countries, a federal statute mandates a safe workplace. The American law is the *Occupational Safety and Health Act of 1970*, as amended. Besides the federal statute, numerous policies, rules and regulations require a safe working environment. To meet these requirements, the management of the haematology laboratory must give safety a high priority. Moreover, management must provide the leadership and support needed for an effective safety programme. The promotion of safe laboratory practices is accomplished most frequently through a structured safety programme. The components of a safety programme usually include a safety officer or representative, a safety manual, safety education and training programmes, periodic inspections and medical surveillance monitoring.

The safety officer or representative is a person with special training and interest in safety. This training may consist of lectures, seminars, workshops, conferences, etc. Thus, the safety representative is a resourceful person directly responsible for implementing safety policies. Some of his/her duties include: coordination of safety activities between one haematology laboratory and other safety units, distribution of safety materials and information, participation in safety inspections, accident data analysis and reporting. To be effective the safety representative cannot operate in a vacuum. He/she must work closely with other safety units (internal and external) to facilitate problem-solving and to prevent potential problems.

A safety manual is the cornerstone of the laboratory policy. The document should clearly and concisely address the:

1. managerial commitment to safe laboratory practices;
2. structure of the safety organisation;
3. laboratory inspections;
4. actions to take and forms to be completed in case of an accident or fire;
5. safety education and training of laboratory workers;
6. fire safety and loss prevention;
7. personal protection;
8. electrical safety;
9. chemical hazards;
10. biohazards;
11. waste disposal;
12. flammable solvents; and
13. radioactive hazards.

SAFETY MANUAL

Managerial commitment

Safety is everybody's business. This includes employees and employers. Employers are required by law to create and maintain a safe working environment. Employees are advised to follow the policies and procedures. To implement its commitment to employee safety, employers develop safety manuals containing written policies and procedures for the laboratory. Typically the safety manual specifies the organizational structure used by management to maintain the working environment. A safety organization usually consists of at least a safety committee and safety officer. It is through the vehicle of the safety organization that management expresses its support for safety. The effectiveness of the safety programme can only be assured with full managerial support. Contravention of the policy, as defined in the safety manual, should not be tolerated. Wilful violation of the policy should be sufficient grounds for the employee's dismissal.

Safety organization

The safety manual lists the members of the safety organization and their duties. Usually, the organization consists of a safety representative/officer and safety committee. Depending on its size, there may not be a safety committee. A safety committee is more likely to be found in a large laboratory than a small one. A typical organization may look as shown in Figure 8.1. Ultimately, the laboratory director is responsible for safety in the laboratory. However, he or she may delegate the authority to the safety officer/representative to make and enforce such rules, policies and regulations as may be required to ensure a safe workplace.

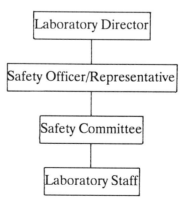

Figure 8.1 A typical safety committee

Laboratory inspections

Periodic inspections should be held in each laboratory. The frequency of the inspections should be as often as necessary, but on not less than a quarterly basis. Inspections are perhaps the best means for continuous monitoring of safety practices, and increases the visual activity of the inspector and of the inspected laboratory staff. Through this process potential hazards are recognized and corrective action taken. Moreover, inspection heightens the safety-consciousness level of the inspector and the laboratory. Hence, with time, laboratory hazards are permanently eliminated. A short inspection checklist is given in Table 8.2.

Table 8.2 Short safety inspection checklist haematology laboratories

	Inspector:_____Date:_____	Yes	No
	Physical Facilities		
(1)	Is the laboratory clean and free of clutter?	____	____
(2)	Are the aisles obstructed?	____	____
(3)	Are there tripping hazards?	____	____
	Fire Safety		
(1)	Is a fire blanket present?	____	____
(2)	Is a fire extinguisher present?	____	____
(3)	Do the laboratory staff know how to use them?	____	____
	Personal Protection		
(1)	Are gloves, protective eye gear and aprons available when needed?	____	____
(2)	Are there adequate hand-washing facilities and supplies?	____	____
(3)	Is there medical surveillance monitoring of employees who habitually do not follow safe laboratory practices?	____	____
(4)	Are mouth pipetting, eating and smoking prohibited in the laboratory?	____	____
	Specimen Collection and Handling		
(1)	Are samples clearly labelled with the appropriate precautions?	____	____
	Reagent Handling		
(a)	Inflammable solvents		
(1)	Are inflammable solvents present?	____	____
(2)	If inflammable solvents exceed 10 gallons, are they stored in approved storage cabinets?	____	____
(b)	Radioisotopes		
(1)	Are radioisotopes used?	____	____
(2)	Is radioactive waste properly discarded?	____	____
(3)	Are personnel using radioisotopes wearing radiation exposure monitoring devices?	____	____

Table 8.2 (continued)

	(4)	Is there a log that lists the type of isotope, date of receipt, chemical form, activity and supplier?	_____	_____
	(5)	Have all personnel using radioisotopes received the proper training?	_____	_____
(c)		Carcinogenic and corrosive chemicals		
	(1)	Are corrosive chemicals used?	_____	_____
	(2)	If corrosive chemicals are used, are safety showers and eye wash units available?	_____	_____
	(3)	Are carcinogenic or potentially carcinogenic chemicals used? If so, are there specific handling requirements defined in the policies and procedures manual?	_____	_____

Statutory and Regulatory Requirements

(1)	If radioisotopes are used, is there a licence by the appropriate licensing agency?	_____	_____
(2)	Is there a written chemical hygiene plan?	_____	_____
(3)	Are material safety data sheets available?	_____	_____

Miscellaneous

(1)	Is there documentation to show that safety deficiencies from previous inspections have been corrected?	_____	_____

Recommendations:_____

_____

Action(s) Taken:_____

_____

Action to be taken in case of accident or fire

Everyone in the laboratory, through training, should be prepared for an accident or fire. Both accidents and fires are often unpredictable. Despite emphasis on prevention, they still occur. Time may be crucial. Therefore, the laboratory staff must know what to do in the event of an accident or fire.

In case of an accident or fire, personnel safety is of paramount importance. Concerns of property damage are secondary. For accidents, first aid is administered immediately. Cuts or wounds should be treated promptly by the health service (Employee Health or Emergency Room). For minor cuts or wounds it is permissible to clean them with water and apply a bandage and then make a report to the health service. Acid or alkaline spills or splashes which contact the skin should be doused with copious quantities of water. Special care must be taken when there is eye involvement. Special eyewash stations should be used to minimize the risk of eye damage associated with a high water pressure. Generally, all injuries should be reported to the health service.

Usually within 24 hours of an accident, a written report must be filed with the appropriate safety authorities. A copy of the report is retained by the safety representative. Pertinent information found in a report includes the name of the victim, the date, the nature of the accident and where it occurred, personal injury and property damage, place and type of treatment and the name of the person giving the treatment.

In case of a fire, priority one is patient and personnel evacuation to safety. It is the duty of the safety representative or other designated person to ensure that contingency plans are in place if there is need for personnel egress from the immediate danger area. Then, the person discovering the fire should sound the alarm, notify the switchboard operator of the location of the fire,. close all windows and doors, turn off electricity and fight the fire with a proper fire extinguisher. If the fire gets beyond control, laboratory personnel should evacuate the site and leave the fire fighting to the professionals. Clothing fires should be smothered in a fire blanket or with heavy towelling. When the fire is extinguished, complete the written report making sure the safety representative gets a copy.

Education and training

To be effective, a safety programme must have an education and training component. Safety should be a part of each new employee's orientation. During the orientation the employee is briefed on the laboratory's safety organization, safety manual and safety programme. The briefing ought to provide preliminary practical information: how to use a fire extinguisher, fire blanket and eyewash units. Upon reporting to the assigned work station, additional specific safety information is furnished. The laboratory workers are told of the nature of the specific work hazards, the requirements for protective clothing, safety glasses, etc. It is through these activities that the laboratory staff is made safety-conscious. Indeed, it is easier to avoid an accident or injury if there is an awareness of the work-associated hazards.

Periodically, supplementary safety information should be provided to all staff. Conferences, workshops, seminars, etc. are good vehicles for disseminating this information. Regular safety education and training programmes promote the development of positive attitudes towards accident prevention. It is through this framework that maintenance of a safe workplace occurs.

Fire safety and loss prevention

In recent years there have been many changes in fire and building codes applicable to laboratories. The result has been to sharply reduce the number of fires and the associated losses. One of the changes has been the require-

ment for installation of automatic fire extinguishing systems in newly constructed facilities. For economic reasons older buildings are exempt from this
standard. However, retrofitting of the buildings with automatic fire extinguishing systems is recommended when funds are available. Laboratories
with automatic fire extinguishing systems should be separated from surrounding health care areas by one hour rated fire doors and fire resistive
construction. With the improved fire prevention and control measures, the
number of fires has declined. Moreover, personal injury and property losses
have dropped. Yet the risk of a fire persists.

As long as the components of a fire are present, the risk is there. The
components of a fire may be thought of as forming a triangle, with oxygen on
one side, fuel on one side and heat on one side. Remove any one of the three
parts of the triangle and the fire goes out if already started, and fails to start
if not already initiated. An understanding of these interactions may reduce
the risk of a fire. Moreover, safety programmes further reduce the risk of fire
by promoting safety consciousness.

The principal objective of a fire safety programme is prevention and
containment. Prevention begins with safe laboratory practices and following
laws, rules and regulations. Strict adherence to fire laws and voluntary
compliance with safety standards are essential elements. In the United States,
the National Fire Protection Association (NFPA) has issued two principal
standards for fire prevention and control in medical laboratories. The standards are the *Life Safety Code (NFPA 101)* and *Laboratories in Health Related
Institutions (NFPA 56C)*. Other organizations such as the American National
Standards Institute (ANSI) and the National Committee for Clinical Laboratory Standards (NCCLS) also issue voluntary consensus standards.

The *Life Safety Code* specifies the location of fire alarms within the
laboratory or in close proximity to it. Moreover, it specifies that the fire bell,
public address system or other alarm system must be audible from anywhere
in the laboratory. The safety standard for laboratories in health related
institutions imposes the requirement for emergency procedures, orientation
and training of personnel, building construction, equipment use, ventilation,
fire extinguishing systems, storage limits and use of inflammable solvents, etc.

The laboratory staff must be aware of potential fire hazards: smoking,
inflammable liquids, faulty electrical equipment, etc. At least once annually,
fire drills should be held on each work shift. Smoking should not be permitted
in the laboratory.

Inflammable liquids should be used in a well-ventilated area and stored as
recommended by NFPA 99 (as revised or other recognized safety standard).
Thus inflammable liquids or gas cylinders should be positioned well away
from open flames or heat sources. Faulty electrical equipment should be
taken out of service or retired immediately.

Fire containment is achieved by suitable selection and proper use of an
extinguisher. The type of extinguisher employed should depend on the kind

of fire. For firefighting purposes, it is convenient to consider the classification of fires:

Class A   Fires involving ordinary combustible material such as paper, textiles and wood.
Class B   Fires involving inflammable liquids, gasoline, solvents, greases, etc.
Class C   Fires involving electrical equipment.
Class D   Fires involving combustible metals; sodium, titanium, magnesium, etc.

Classification is important because there are different types of fire extinguishers. Hence, the laboratory worker must have available the appropriate fire extinguisher for a given fire. Choose an extinguisher based on the class of fire. Fire extinguishers are classified as follows:

Class A   water
Class B   dry chemical foam, carbon dioxide
Class C   multipurpose dry chemical
Class D   dry powder

Generally the class of fire's letter designation should correspond to that of the fire. Fire extinguishers should be checked periodically to see that they are in good working order. The staff should know how to use them properly. The extinguisher should be located close to likely hazards. A class B fire extinguisher is the most common one found in a haematology laboratory.

Personal protection

Safety in the laboratory requires not only a managerial commitment, but also a personal one. Laboratory workers must assume some responsibility for their own safety. This means obeying the laboratory policy forbidding smoking, eating, drinking and applying cosmetics. A 'no smoking' policy protects laboratory staff from hand to mouth transmission of toxic and infectious agents. Moreover, the policy also helps to reduce the risk of fires. Smoker carelessness in a laboratory may contribute to a fire.

Appropriate attire *must* be worn at all times. This includes laboratory coats and skid-resistant shoes. Open-toed shoes, tennis shoes (or trainers) and clogs should not be permitted in the laboratory because they offer little if any protection against acid or alkaline spills. Hair length should be adjusted to keep it from becoming contaminated. Protective gear must be worn as required - safety glasses, laboratory coats, aprons, etc. Moreover, food should be stored only in refrigerators earmarked for that purpose. The use of laboratory glassware for food and drink is not advisable. When using corro-

148

sive, toxic, caustic or other materials, wear a safety shield or goggles to protect your eyes. Protective aprons are useful at times, they prevent skin penetration by harmful agents.

The wearing of gloves and frequent handwashing afford some protection against hazardous agents. Biological samples and chemical substances are two examples of agents that may pose a safety risk. Pipetting of reagents and samples should be forbidden. With the ready availability of pipetting aids, mouth pipetting is not necessary.

Electrical safety

Shock, fire and the ignition of inflammable gases and vapours are some potential electrical hazards in the laboratory. Any equipment which produces a tingle should be reported promptly and removed from service until it is repaired. 'Shorts' are especially dangerous because they have a tendency to become progressively worse. When a person simultaneously makes contact with a shorted electrical device and metal (e.g. exhaust hood or sink) or a damp floor, conditions are favourable for electrical shock.

Unusual noises or odd smells in electrical equipment may be indicative of overheating. Any electrical equipment which overheats may lead to ignition of the electrical insulation or other combustible material resulting in a fire.

Inflammable solvents stored in ordinary refrigerators and freezers may accrue enough vapours to ignite and explode. Similarly, these solvents stored in enclosures which contain heaters, motors, light switches, or lights may ignite and explode.

Using certain safety precautions, the laboratory worker can reduce the chances of injury and/or property damage from electrical hazards. Some precautions are:

1. Only use equipment which has been tested and certified to meet the standards by a recognized testing laboratory.
2. *Prior to use*, and periodically thereafter, have each piece of electrical equipment inspected. The inspection should be carried out, in a safe area, by a person qualified to service electronic equipment. Any faulty equipment should be removed from service.
3. Have all fixed electrical receptacles checked for grounding integrity at least annually.
4. Have all laboratory appliances and instruments adequately grounded and checked for current leakage at least once a year.
5. Never unplug a piece of equipment by jerking the power cord. To do so may break the ground connection and create a potential hazard when the equipment is used again.
6. Unplug instruments prior to servicing.

7. Never handle electrical equipment with wet hands or feet or while standing on a wet floor.

8. Ensure that all equipment is properly grounded in accordance with a standard such as the National Electric Code.

9. Replace a fuse with one of the same output and never replace one without first unplugging the instrument.

10. Turn off any electrical equipment which emits noises and odours. Then unplug them from the outlet. Remove the equipment from service until it has been checked and approved for continued use by an electronic engineer or other skilled electrical expert.

11. Store inflammable solvents in approved storage cabinets. Never store inflammable solvents in refrigerators or freezers unless they are explosion-proof. Ordinary refrigerators generally have higher temperatures than the flashpoints of some inflammable solvents stored in them. Hence, the conditions are favourable for ignition and explosion.

12. Use inflammable solvents in well-ventilated areas.

Chemical hazards

In response to the threat to the health and safety of workers exposed to hazardous chemicals, the United States Occupational Safety and Health Administration (OSHA) promulgated a Hazard Communication Standard also known as 'Right to Know' legislation. Basically, the Hazard Communication Standard states that employees have a right to know about known and suspected health hazards associated with the workplace, so that they make informed decisions about their employment, how to protect themselves, etc. An integral part of 'Right to Know' legislation is the requirement for assessment of chemical hazards in the workplace, and employer provided information to workers through hazard communication training programmes. These programmes should include: review of Material Safety Data Sheets (MSDS), training in the hazards and uses of chemicals, labelling information, etc. Increasingly, inspectors are looking for a written chemical hygiene plan that defines the safety procedures to be followed for each hazardous chemical used in the laboratory.

Over a year laboratory workers are exposed to single or multiple hazardous chemicals in the workplace. These chemicals are potential physical or health hazards. Physical hazards result if the chemical is a combustible liquid, explosive, inflammable, compressed gas, oxidizer, organic peroxide, etc. Health hazards, which may be acute or chronic, include the effects of chemicals which are corrosives, carcinogens, hepatoxins, reproductive toxins, neurotoxins or other toxic or highly toxic agents. Some of the agents may produce pulmonary tissue damage or irritation. In fact, prolonged exposure to hazardous chemicals may be associated with cardiomyopathy, renal and pulmonary impairments, carcinomatosis, infertility, etc.

Toxicity refers to the ability of an agent to cause body tissue injury by direct chemical action. Agents which are toxic comprise a spectrum of chemical substances from irritants to known carcinogens. Whatever their *modus operandi*, toxic agents interfere with normal cell function. The nature of the interference varies with the substance.

Chemical agents which are toxic may act in an acute or chronic manner. Acute toxicity is a condition resulting from brief exposure to a harmful agent. Chronic toxicity results when the duration of exposure to the toxic agent is prolonged. The exact time frame for both acute and chronic toxicity is ill-defined. Toxicity studies are performed on animals and the results extrapolated to humans. The classification of toxic agents is achieved, in part, by administering them to test animals through four exposure routes – swallowing, skin and eye contact, injection and inhalation. The units of toxicity worthy of note are:

LD_{50} — Lethal dose which kills 50% of the test animal population. This is expressed in mg/kg of body weight.

LC_{50} — Lethal concentration which kills 50% of the test population (expressed in minutes or hours of exposure).

TLV — Threshold limit value is an estimate of the average safe airborne concentration of the toxic substance for all day, every day exposure (expressed in ppm).

Carcinogens are a class of substances that cause malignant disease or statistically increase the risk of neoplasia. Since there are many agents that are involved in carcinogenesis, they have been classified into four classes by the United States Occupational Health and Safety Administration (OSHA): Class I – confirmed carcinogens; Class II – suspected carcinogens which require medical monitoring; Class III – substances under study by OSHA; and Class IV – substances not subject to OSHA regulations.

In humans, carcinogens are discovered largely through epidemiological studies. When such studies show that the incidence of tumours in a group exposed to a given agent is increased significantly over the control, the substance is given a carcinogen label. For an up-to-date list of known or suspected carcinogens the reader is referred to the *Registry of Toxic Effects of Chemical Substances*.

Hydrochloric, sulphuric and nitric acids, sodium, potassium and ammonium hydroxide solutions are a few common corrosive substances found in the laboratory. Corrosive chemicals are agents which are injurious to body tissues. The injury may be major or minor. The degree of injury depends on the concentration of the substances and the duration of exposure.

A safety shower and eyewash solution are the prime pieces of equipment required to contain this type of hazard. They are essential to meet safety requirements. Both the safety shower and eyewash solution must be in good working condition and should be checked regularly. For an additional measure of safety, the wearing of protective goggles is recommended whenever solutions of corrosive chemicals are being prepared.

Good laboratory practice, coupled with a knowledge and understanding of the use and handling of chemicals are essential for worker safety. In addition, guidelines for use of various chemicals should be followed rigidly. Moreover, medical surveillance monitoring and safety training are useful adjuncts.

BIOHAZARDS

The risk of infection is a real one in the haematology laboratory. Body fluids handled and analysed in the laboratory are potential vectors of hazardous agents. To reduce the risk(s), laboratory personnel must have an awareness of the hazards and use prudent (safe) laboratory practices. Eternal vigilance must be the motto! In addition to internal controls, the haematology laboratory must verify the presence and effective utilization of external controls.

Internal controls

From the time a sample arrives in the laboratory to the time it is analysed, results reported and the sample waste discarded, prudent practices must be observed. All samples must be checked for valid identification – name, date, location, tests requested, priority status (STAT or Routine), infectivity, etc. Biohazard warnings on the label may be general such as 'Blood Fluid Precaution' or it may be specific, e.g. 'Hepatitis'. Although all specimens should be regarded as potentially infectious, some deserve special handling. Specimens from patients with hepatitis or acquired immunodeficiency syndrome (AIDS) are in this category. These samples should have a special label, preferably one that is colour-coded. Moreover, other high-risk patient samples should be handled with caution: tuberculosis, haemodialysis, drug addiction, etc.

External controls

External controls are those measures taken, prior to samples reaching the laboratory, to reduce the biohazard risk(s). Perhaps the first step is to ensure that phlebotomists are properly trained not only in the principles and practice of phlebotomy, but also in safety considerations. Thus, all samples should be properly labelled to include appropriate biohazard warnings, as indicated.

Remove needles from syringes! Exercise extreme caution if samples are transported to the laboratory through a pneumatic tube system. In such cases, ensure that the samples are protected from breakage. If breakage does occur, carefully remove the glass and place it in a suitable container specifically earmarked for broken glass. Usually, samples transported to the laboratory via carrier, pose a low risk if the transport device is made for that purpose. This reduces the risk to others.

Personal hygiene

Eat, smoke, drink and apply cosmetics only in designated areas: not in the laboratory! Wear laboratory dress such as an apron, coat/jacket and gloves while working in the laboratory. Do not wear them to the cafeteria or lunch room! Remove them before you leave the room. Wash your hands, as required, with an antiseptic soap. The use of foot pedal controlled faucets is recommended. Clean and disinfect your work area daily or whenever a spill occurs! A variety of effective germicidal agents are commercially available. However, chlorine bleach type disinfectants are satisfactory. For best results, prepare them fresh daily in carefully cleaned containers.

Radiation hazards

Radiation hazards pose a special risk to the laboratory worker. The hazards are often insidious but real. A major hazard is the potential interaction of radioactive emissions and body tissues to produce deleterious health effects. Although the emissions may be of many kinds, alpha, beta and gamma are the most common. These differ in their ability to penetrate various kinds of matter. Thus, a knowledge and understanding of the formation and disintegration of radio-isotopes are helpful in formulating and effective implementation of a good radio-isotope policy.

Everyone who works with radio-isotopes should be knowledgeable about their use and handling. The background for this should derive from courses, seminars, workshops, on-the-job training, etc. The background should be comprehensive enough to include the kinds of radioactivity and their detection. Prior to use, all affected personnel should have read the applicable federal, state, local and institutional radiation safety manuals.

Radioisotopes must be used only in designated areas. Accurate records must be kept of their receipt, use, storage and disposal. Information found in the records must include the type of isotope, quantity, chemical form (solid, liquid, or gas), location, date of receipt, name of person making the entry, etc. At no time should the possession limits for the isotope(s) be exceeded. Segregate radioactive and non-radioactive waste prior to disposal. Only use the institutionally approved disposal procedure.

With the approval of the appropriate US regulatory agency, low level (< 10 μCi/week) water-soluble, radioactive waste may be released into the sewer system followed by copious amounts of water. Non-soluble waste should be collected in solvent waste containers with due concern for both toxic fumes and fire hazard. This waste, properly labelled, is stored in a separate area adjacent to the non-radioactive solvent storage area. Collect solid waste in containers specially lined to eliminate leakage. Label the container and seal fully before disposal. For the exact disposal protocol, the reader is referred to the Radiation Safety Manual.

In case of a spill of radioactive material, steps must be taken to (1) prevent the spread of contamination, (2) minimize the evaporation of the materials into the room atmosphere, and (3) prevent other persons or objects from being contaminated. Some suggested actions to take are: apply absorbent materials (e.g. vermiculite) to the spill, block the flow of the spill with physical barriers such as vermiculite, putty, etc., check personnel for contamination, turn off air supplies, close doors and windows, seal and evacuate the area and notify the radiation safety authorities.

Periodically, all personnel working with radio-isotopes should be monitored for exposure to radiation with devices such as film badges. The records of such monitoring should be maintained in accordance with institutional policy. To limit the exposure of persons entering the area when radio-isotopes are used, appropriate signs should be displayed bearing the radiation caution symbol and words like: 'Caution, Radioactive Materials' or 'Caution, Radiation Area', etc. All waste containers must be marked with similar signs.

Waste disposal

Waste disposal is rapidly becoming a big problem! Horror stories were aired almost daily after the chemical accident at Bhopal, India. Moreover, in the United States there have been many negative press reports relating to the association of toxic waste dumps with birth defects. Hence, there are frequent heated debates on the issue of waste disposal. With respect to the haematology laboratory, waste disposal may be divided into four categories – physical, chemical, radioactive and biohazardous (infectious). Some methods of waste disposal according to their category, are listed below:

Physical waste

Glass and plastic syringes, broken pipettes and other glassware, scalpel blades, hypodermic needles, paper, etc. may be classified as physical waste. Syringes should be autoclaved prior to disposal. Broken glassware should be placed in special marked containers to protect workers who handle it. Sharps (scalpel blades, hypodermic needles, etc.) should be secured in puncture-proof containers suitably marked. Recapping and bending are not recommended for sharps. Such practices, if instituted, drastically increase the risk of physical injury and infection. Incineration, burial in a landfill, if available, and recycling, are among the most common disposal methods; perhaps the procedure with the fewest environmental objections and which has the broadest public support is recycling. This is especially true for glassware. Any physical waste that is contaminated with infectious materials/agents should be autoclaved.

Chemical waste

The mode of disposal of chemical waste is dependent on its classification as non-hazardous or hazardous. A non-hazardous chemical is one that is not regulated as a pesticide or polychlorinated biphenyl and is not listed as a hazardous waste by the Environmental Protection Agency. Hazardous waste is that which, because of its physical, chemical or biological properties, may pose a threat to human health or the environment when improperly treated, disposed of, transported, stored, or managed.

Chemicals classified as non-hazardous may be disposed of in the sanitary sewer system. It is recommended that the quantity of chemicals disposed of by this route be limited to no more than 2 kg per chemical. Before using this method, laboratories should check with local authorities to find out any regulatory prohibitions. Further, the disposal should be carried out, using copious amounts of water. Hazardous chemical waste disposal is usually subject to fairly stringent regulations with a view to protecting public health. Basically, there are four common modes of hazardous chemical waste disposal: (1) burial in an approved landfill, (2) biological or chemical degradation, (3) incineration, and (4) recycling. Incineration is the method of choice, if it is available. In order to ensure complete combustion, the temperature of the combustion chamber must be high enough for a sufficient period of time. The incinerator must be maintained properly and adequacy of combustion verified at regular intervals. Moreover, special attention must be paid to the incinerator effluent, to safeguard against the release of hazardous substances into the environment. Failure to do this will make incineration environmentally unacceptable.

Burial in an approved landfill may be used in the absence of statutory or regulatory constraints. Liquid waste should be absorbed on Fuller's earth, vermiculite, etc. Incompatible wastes should not be placed in the same container. Most laboratories do not have the resources to incarcerate their own hazardous chemical waste. Hence, a commercial disposal firm must be contracted to do the job. Frequently, manifests must accompany the waste.

Degradation, whether chemical or biological, is used to convert hazardous chemicals into less innocuous substances for disposal in a landfill and, sometimes, in a sewer system. Chemical degradation consists of oxidation-reduction reactions, neutralization, hydrolysis, precipitation, etc. Biological degradation consists of enzymatic treatment to convert the waste into other products. Care should be exercised to minimize the risks of property or bodily damage, and only experienced chemists should use this procedure.

Recycling, if available, is the disposal procedure which is least objectionable environmentally. Salvageable waste is harvested and converted into useful products.

Literature consulted

Barnes, D.E. and Taylor, D. (1963). *Radiation Hazards and Protection*. (London: George Newnes)

Biohazards Safety Guide (1974). National Institutes of Health, US Department of Health and Human Services, Washington, DC

Casarett, A. (1968).*Radiation Biology*. (Englewood Cliffs: Prentice Hall)

Daziel, C.F. (1971). Deleterious effects of electric shock. In (N.V. Steere, ed.) *Handbook of Laboratory Safety*. p. 521. (Boca Raton: CRC Press)

Department of Health, Education and Welfare (USA) (1978). Guidelines for the laboratory use of chemical substances posing a potential occupational carcinogenetic risk (revised draft). Laboratory Chemical Carcinogen Safety Standards Subcommittee of the DHEW Committee to Coordinate Toxicology and Related Programs. (Washington, DC: DHEW)

Eckardt, R.E. and Scala, R.A. (1978). Toxicology: assessing the hazard. *J. Occup. Med.,* **20**, 490–493

Forrey, A.W., Delancy, C.J. and Ruff, W.L. (1982). Safety. In Faulkner, W.R. and Meites, S. (eds.), *Selected Methods of Clinical Chemistry,* Vol. 9, pp. 43–56. (Washington, DC)

Hartree, E. and Booth, V. (1971). *Safety in Biological Laboratories*, Spec. Publ. 5 (London: Biochemistry Society)

Hawke, W.A. and Hoeltge, G.A. (1983). Safety in the medical laboratory. *Clin. Lab. Med.,* **3**, 467–484

Henry, R.J., Olitsky, I., Lee, N.D., Walker, B. and Beattie, J. (1976). *Safety in the Clinical Laboratory*. (Van Nuys, California: Bio-Science Enterprises)

Laboratories in Health-Related Institutions, NFPA 56C. (Quincy, MA: National Fire Protection Association)

Life Safety Code, NFPA 101. (Quincy, MA: National Fire Protection Association)

Manufacturing Chemists Association (1972).*A Guide for Safety in Chemical Laboratories*, 2nd Edn. (New York: Van Nostrand, Reinhold)

Occupational Safety and Health Act (OSHA), Public Law, 91–596, US Department of Labor, Washington, DC (1970)

Pecsok, R.L., Chapman, K. and Ponder, W.H. (1975). *Chemical Technology Handbook*. (Washington, DC: American Chemical Society)

Safety and Health Manual (1948). The National Institute of Environmental Health Sciences, US Department of Health and Human Services, NIH Publication No. 70-1848, Research Triangle Park, NC

Shotwell, H.P. (1982). Safety in the clinical laboratory.*Am. J. Med. Technol.,* **48**, 61–63

Simmons, N.A. (1980). Safety in clinical laboratories.*J. Hosp. Infect.,* **1**, 92–94

Steere, N.V. (1971). *Handbook of Lab Safety*, 2nd edn. (Cleveland, Ohio: Chemical Rubber Publ. Co)

Steere, N.V. (1980). Physical, chemical and fire safety. In Fascaldo, A.A., Erlick, B.J. and Hindman, B. (eds), *Laboratory Safety: Theory and Practice*. (New York: Academic Press)

US DHEW Public Health Service Bureau of Radiological Health (1970). *Radiological Health Handbook*. (Washington, DC: Govt. Printing Office)

Wang, Y. (1969). *Handbook of Radioactive Nuclides*. (Cleveland, Ohio: Chemical Rubber Publ. Co)

Wintrobe, M.W., Lee, G.R., Boggs, D., Bithell, T.C., Foerster, J., Athens, J.W. and Lukens, J.N. (1981). Original and development of the blood and blood forming tissues. *Clinical Hematology*, 8th edn, pp 35–74. (Philadelphia: Lea & Febiger)

9 Health Hazards in Microbiology

C.H. Collins

INTRODUCTION

Although there have been problems of health and safety in microbiology laboratories since the days of Pasteur and Koch there was little concern until the 1970s, when a high incidence of hepatitis B was noted among laboratory workers[1]. There were two incidents involving smallpox laboratories[2,3], and some scientists expressed fears about the possible hazards of recombinant DNA research[4]. As a result there was a renewed interest in the published accounts and surveys of laboratory-acquired infections which revealed that in the previous 50 years there had been nearly 4000 such infections of which about 160 had proved fatal[5]. Moreover, the routes and modes of such infections and methods for preventing them had been thoroughly investigated and were fully documented[6].

This sudden interest in laboratory-associated disease provoked several reactions. There was an immediate increase in the number of publications on the subject, both scientific and journalistic, and a proliferation of committees which were set up to investigate the problems and to make recommendations. There was a wider interest in the excellent microbiological safety manuals of the Centers for Disease Control[7] and the National Institutes of Health[8,9], codes of practice for the handling of pathogenic micro-organisms were formulated in the United Kingdom[10,11]; and the World Health Organization introduced its *Special Programme on Safety Measures in Microbiology*, published its *Memorandum on Emergency Services* for dealing with the escape of dangerous pathogens and its *Laboratory Biosafety Manual*[12,13].

In addition, some learned societies in the United Kingdom published guidelines for microbiological safety[14], and others initiated investigations into the incidence of infections among laboratory workers[15-22].

Since 1983 the Centers for Disease Control and NIH have produced a new

159

book on biosafety[23] and in the United Kingdom the Advisory Committee on Dangerous Pathogens and Health Services Advisory Committee have up-dated parts of the *Code of Practice for the Prevention of Infection in Clinical Laboratories*[24-26]. An independent and simplified version has also been published which contains a set of check lists[27].

It is my intention in this chapter to indicate those courses of action that may be taken by laboratory managements to fulfil their legal obligations (duty of care), and by laboratory workers to avoid infections.

It is not possible, however, to include all aspects of laboratory-acquired infections and their prevention, and more detailed information can be obtained from other publications[11,13,28,29].

THE RESPONSIBILITIES OF MANAGEMENT

In most developed countries there are regulatory bodies that are concerned with the health and safety of the inhabitants. It is obviously necessary for laboratory management to conform with the requirements of such bodies. This may not in itself be sufficient, however, because laboratory activities may affect other authorities, national or local. These may include postal and transport services if micro-organisms are to be moved within the state and across its borders, and the disposal of waste material or its discharge into drains and sewers.

In view of the complexity of some regulations affecting microbiological and other laboratory work it is often desirable for management to appoint one or more persons to ensure that there are no infringements which might lead to litigation or criminal proceedings. Such individuals would be members of the safety staff.

Safety staff

In several countries there are legal requirements for the management to appoint safety officers and safety committees. Unfortunately, although many formulae have been postulated for the ideal safety organization few have been successful in practice. Except in very large institutes or companies the safety officer will have other work to do and there may be a conflict of interests. As no one individual can be expected to be familiar with all aspects of laboratory and industrial safety it follows that different individuals may have to be appointed, e.g. as microbiological safety officer, chemical safety officer, etc. and that their spheres of influence will have to be agreed. They will frequently need to consult one another.

Other problems may arise: if a safety officer is a very senior person then he may be regarded as a 'management man' by his subordinates; if he occupies a junior position he may lack experience and may be ignored by his superiors. Furthermore, if safety committees are too large, and meet too often, they are regarded as bores; busy scientists, who may have much to offer, do not bother to attend. There may also be problems with safety committees. Many have started well but have either foundered or become militant nuisances. There is no simple or easy solution but some successes in safety organization have been achieved in those institutes where the safety officer is a middle-aged member of middle management and is still involved in day-to-day laboratory work. The best possible kind of safety committee is the small one that meets only when there is something urgent to discuss. A management might also consider the appointment of an independent safety advisor from outside the institute or company.

Duties of safety officer

As indicated above advising management on its legal obligations and duties is an important task for a safety officer. He should also be involved in formulating any policy statements that may be required by national or local regulatory bodies. In this, he and management may be able to obtain assistance from professional scientific or learned societies.

Internally, one of the most important duties of the safety officer is the drawing up of local rules and codes of practice for the safe handling of micro-organisms and the protection of other workers. Again, assistance may be obtained from several sources: various guidelines and codes have already been published[11,13,23,27,28,29]. These are all susceptible to modification for local use. The implementation of any codes or guidelines is an obvious task for a safety officer and is best done by persuasion rather than by coercion. Success, therefore, may depend upon his personality.

It is obvious that a microbiological safety officer should acquaint himself with all microbiological activities and techniques within his province. For example, in a laboratory where dangerous pathogens are handled, he needs to know the whereabouts of all cultures and what every scientist is doing with them. The organization of training in safe microbiological techniques certainly comes within a microbiological safety officers' province but it merits separate treatment here.

TRAINING IN SAFE MICROBIOLOGICAL TECHNIQUES

It is commonly believed that any scientist or technician who has obtained a qualification in microbiology has been trained in the safe handling of pathogenic microbes. This is quite untrue: many new graduates have only sketchy ideas of good techniques and few seem to have acquired any useful practical skills. It must also be remembered that the recent enlargement of the horizons of microbiology has necessitated the employment of specialists in other fields, such as biochemists, molecular biologists and geneticists, who are required to handle micro-organisms but who have had no experience of the techniques and hazards involved.

If laboratory workers are to avoid infecting themselves, their colleagues and their families it is important that they are taught some of the facts about the mechanisms of such infections and about host-parasite relationships. This should be followed by illustrations of the faulty techniques which allow microbes to 'escape' from their containers and of the various routes by which they may enter the human body. Training should continue with information about how primary barriers may be placed around the organism to prevent their escape into the laboratory during manipulations, secondary barriers around the worker to prevent their entry into his body, and should these measures fail, inside the worker to minimize ill effects.

In the UK, as distinct from the USA, such courses of instruction are now rare, but syllabuses and protocols have been published[13,29], and there are individuals, apart from local safety officers, who are qualified to teach and who possess the necessary 'visual aids'. The problem of instruction may, therefore, be easily overcome in large institutes or companies. Smaller ones could band together to hold seminars or to persuade a local college of further education to oblige. Advice and information may be obtained from the World Health Organization Geneva (Special Programme on Safety Measures in Microbiology) and from the author of this chapter.

No great expense need be involved in such enterprises and they may very well be cost-effective in terms of good health and confidence among the staff as well as freedom from possible litigation and conflict with regulatory bodies.

THE ASSESSMENT OF RISK

In a microbiological establishment the health hazards to which the staff are exposed are largely determined by the nature of the micro-organisms that are being examined or grown. If these organisms are relatively non-pathogenic and do not have a history of infecting those who handle them then the risks are minimal and the safety precautions may be adjusted accordingly. If, on the other hand, the organisms do have a bad record then the risks are greater and safety precautions should vary from the strict to the stringent.

Unfortunately, it is popularly supposed, even by some scientists, that micro-organisms may be clearly divided into those that cause disease and those that are 'harmless', and that no precautions need be taken by people who work with the 'harmless' varieties. In fact, reports of infections in man and animals, arising from such organisms, have become frequent features in medical journals. It is true, of course, that some of these infections arise from the entry into the body of large numbers of the organisms, possibly by unusual routes, but these are just the conditions that might obtain in microbiological laboratories, especially those that are engaged in mass culture work. There is also an increasing number of individuals in the general population whose resistance to infections has been impaired by medication or exposure to steroids and immunosuppressants.

In addition, a laboratory that confines its activities to the culture of 'harmless' micro-organisms may unwittingly grow pathogens that the staff might not recognize. Much depends on the composition and pH of the culture media and the incubation temperature. Many pathogens grow on ordinary media at pH 5.5 to 8.0 and between 20 and 40 °C. Such organisms are frequently present in raw materials such as food, animal feedingstuffs, fertilizers, natural water and soil. They may also gain access to cultures from the worker's hands, mouth, nose, bowel and skin lesions. Many pathogens are widely distributed in the environment, albeit in numbers too small to constitute and infective dose, but they are easily and rapidly concentrated into many infective doses by common laboratory procedures.

Material imported into teaching laboratories, e.g. blood, tissue cultures, organs, dead or living animals, may contain pathogenic micro-organisms. Great care is needed in the selection of such specimens and in ascertaining their provenance.

Laboratories that examine clinical material have a more immediate problem because they have no control at all over the microbiological content of the specimens they receive. This uncertainty emphasizes the need for extra vigilance in pathology departments.

There are, however, well-documented and easily available records of the risks attached to many individual organisms, in terms of the number of infections that they are known to have caused among laboratory workers[5,29,30]. For example, between 1930 and 1974 *Serratia marcescens* was responsible for five infections, but *Brucella* species (including vaccine strains) for 423; adenoviruses accounted for 10, but hepatitis virus for 234; rickettsial pox for five, but Q fever for 278. A continuing survey of infections in British laboratories[20-22] identifies other hazardous agents.

Classification of micro-organisms on the basis of risk

These records of infection have allowed the organisms concerned to be graded or categorized according to the likelihood that they will infect laboratory workers, and, if they escape from laboratories, the general public. This was first done in the United States and later by the World Health Organization[32] and in the UK[24]. These all follow the same principles, differing only in their wording. They are shown in Table 9.1. Similar classifications have also been introduced in the Netherlands[33] and Germany[34]. The WHO system is used in this chapter.

Table 9.1 Classification of micro-organisms on the basis of hazard

United States[7]	WHO[13]	United Kingdom[24]	EFB*
Class 1 ...no or minimal hazard under ordinary conditions of handling	*Risk Group I* low individual limited community risk	*Hazard Group 1* ...most unlikely to cause human disease	*EFB Class 1* ...have never been identified as causative agents of disease ...offer no threat to the environment
Class 2 ...ordinary potential hazard... may produce disease of varying severity... by accidental inoculation	*Risk Group II* moderate individual, limited community risk... can cause human or animal disease but is unlikely to be a serious hazard to lab workers	*Hazard Group 2* ...may cause human disease... might be a hazard to lab workers, but unlikely to spread in the community	*EFB Class 2* ...may cause disease in man... might offer hazard to laboratory worker. Unlikely to spread in environment
Class 3 ...involving special hazard or derived from outside the US	*Risk Group III* high individual, limited community risk... usually produce serious human disease, but does not normally spread from one person to another	*Hazard Group 3* ...may cause serious human disease and present a serious hazard to lab workers. May spread in community... effective treatment and prophylaxis is available	*EFB Class 3* ...offer a severe threat to health of lab worker but small risk to population at large. Prophylactics availble, therapy effective
Class 4 ...extremely hazardous to lab personnel, and may cause serious epidemic disease	*Risk Group IV* high individual and community risk... usually produces serious human or animal disease... may be readily transmitted from one person to another	*Hazard Group 4* ...can cause serious human disease and is a serious hazard to lab workers... may present high risk of infection in community... usually no effective treatment or prophylaxis	*EFB Class 4* ...cause severe illness in man. Offer serious hazard to lab workers. Prophylactics not available, no effective treatment known.
			EFB Class E (Environmental risk) ...offer a more severe threat to environment than to man. May be responsible for heavy economic losses. Already subject to regulations.

* European Federation of Biotechnology[35]

These classifications are all intended for use in clinical laboratories and may not serve the purposes of biotechnology.

The European Federation of Biotechnology (EFB) has, therefore, formulated a system that includes a group for organisms that offer a greater threat to the environment than to man35. This is also shown in Table 9.1.

Individual countries must, of course, draw up their own lists within each class or group as no one list is likely to apply universally because of the following variables: (1) pathogenicity of the organisms; (2) modes of transmission and host range; (3) existing levels of immunity; (4) presence and control of vectors; (5) prevailing standards of hygiene; (6) available preventive and therapeutic measures.

Lists of organisms in each risk group may be obtained from governments and professional organizations: for example, in the United Kingdom, the Health and Safety Executive; in the United States, the Center for Disease Control; in West Germany, the Deutsche Gesellschaft für Hygiene und Mikrobiologie; and in Holland, the Dutch Society for Microbiology.

CLASSIFICATION AND DESIGN FEATURES OF LABORATORIES

The concept of risk groups introduces that of levels of containment – where the word 'containment' embodies all the precautions necessary to prevent the escape of the organisms. These are influenced by the design of laboratory premises, and the World Health Organization[13,32] proposed three kinds of laboratory: Basic, Containment and Maximum Containment, but in the USA and the UK four 'Biosafety Levels' or 'Containment Levels' are defined. Again, they are similar, and are shown in Table 9.2. Containment conditions for the EFB groups are being codified. Recommendations are made for the construction, engineering facilities, such as ventilation and other services, and for security arrangements. Several countries have adopted these or modified them to suit local conditions. They are too detailed to review fully here but specifications have been published[13,29]

Table 9.2 Classification of laboratories for classes and groups of hazardous micro-organisms

Class, risk or hazard group		WHO[13]	United States[23] biosafety level	United Kingdom[24] containment level
I	(1)	basic	1	1
II	(2)	basic	2	2
III	(3)	containment	3	3
IV	(4)	maximum containment	4	4

Basic, levels 1 and 2 laboratories

In outline, basic laboratories need no particular design features apart from

165

the sensible construction to give reasonably comfortable conditions for work and the avoidance of stress. Two features that should be mentioned, however, are the provision of efficient autoclaves and, in each workroom, of handbasins.

Containment, level 3 laboratories

These are intended to protect the workers from micro-organisms that have low infective doses, particularly by the airborne route (see below). They, therefore, need microbiological safety cabinets to protect the worker, and ventilation facilities that prevent the dispersal of contaminated air to other rooms. They are usually maintained at a lower air pressure than other rooms and corridors to ensure that air passes from 'clean' to 'dirty' areas and not *vice versa*. Their position within the building, therefore, requires careful consideration[29]. Containment laboratories may require their own autoclaves. Handbasins are essential. As a general principle, materials and cultures used in these laboratories should not be removed from them until they have been decontaminated or sterilized.

Maximum containment level 4 laboratories

These are designed on the same general principles as containment laboratories but the requirements are more stringent. They are provided with the most sophisticated kinds of safety cabinets and double-door – single-pass autoclaves so that no material leaves the laboratory without being sterilized. All effluents from sinks, handbasins and lavatories must be decontaminated. These laboratories are usually licensed by governments and subjected to inspection.

Table 9.3 Relation of UK containment levels for work with natural pathogens and for genetic manipulation

Pathogens (ACDP[24])	Genetic manipulation (GMAG[36,37])
1	GMP*
2	I
	II
3 }	III[†]
4 }	
	IV

* GMP - Good Microbiological Practice
[†] Includes some of the requirements for ACDP levels 3 and 4. From *Guidelines for Microbiological Safety*, [14]

The terminology used above is not universal. In some countries, basic laboratories may be described as P1 and P2 laboratories, where 'P' stands for physical containment. Similarly, containment laboratories may be known as P3 laboratories and maximum containment laboratories as P4 laboratories.

The Physical Containment (P) system was originally used in the USA to define levels of containment deemed necessary for different kinds of genetic manipulation, depending on the nature of donor and recipient organisms, but it has now been harmonized with the Biosafety Levels, so that the USA has only one general system for classifying containment in laboratories. In the UK, on the other hand, two separate systems persist[36,37] at present. The relationship between the classifications for work with 'natural' and 'genetically manipulated' organisms is shown in Table 9.3[14].

General design features

Laboratories at any level should be designed for the safety and convenience of those who work in them. These two factors must be considered together because errors in design may predispose accidents which may lead to infections as well as physical injuries[6,13]. Design errors may also indirectly cause accidents by imposing unnecessary stresses on the workers. Common errors include: (1) inconvenient bench heights, too high for sitting (most microbiologists sit) and which necessitate high stools (the latter are a recognized cause, not only of sprained ankles, but of dropped and broken cultures); (2) inadequate lighting, above and behind the worker so that he casts a shadow over his work; (3) poor ventilation and defective air conditioning which may be responsible for a variety of minor ailments and loss of productivity – the 'sick building syndrome'; (4) ceiling heating which leads to cold feet and to the use of unauthorized and dangerous electric and gas heating devices; (5) insufficient services, necessitating long trailing electricity cables and gas tubing[29].

Poor design may also mean that cultures have to be carried or conveyed on trolleys for long distances, even along public corridors, with the increased risks of breakage and dispersal of contents.

Unfortunately, some quite spectacular and expensive errors have been made in the design of laboratories, almost entirely because management and designers have failed to consult users and regulatory bodies.

Housekeeping

It is now accepted that some accidents and infections are related to certain kinds of equipment[6,13,29]. Such equipment varies from large items such as safety cabinets, autoclaves, centrifuges and mechanical devices that might disperse aerosols, to glassware that breaks or chips easily but is kept in circulation, leaking hypodermic syringes, poorly made bacteriological loops, and microscope slides with sharp edges or which break easily. The particular hazards associated with these are discussed below, but as the provision of such equipment is a function of management some general observations are relevant here. Two factors influence the choice of equipment. One is cost. This is a universal problem and no objections can be made to a genuine desire to save money. The cheapest is rarely the best, however, and may well not be 'cost-effective' in the long run. The other factor is the willingness of the purchasing officer, who is rarely a scientist, to co-operate with those who know more about equipment and its hazards than he does. In the provision of equipment of all kinds consultation with the users is as important as it is in design.

Housekeeping also includes day-to-day maintenance. Floors need to be kept clean (with non-slip materials!) and should be cleared of clutter that might trip people who are carrying cultures or other hazardous materials.

Clean overalls, towels and soap should always be available, and when lights fail or equipment breaks down there should be no delay in repairs.

MICROBIOLOGICAL SAFETY CABINETS

These essential pieces of microbiological equipment are intended to protect the worker from inhaling any infectious particles that are released in the course of his work. They will only do so, however, if he works well within the cabinet and then only if he is using good microbiological techniques. They will not protect him from spillages or contamination of the skin.

Two warnings are necessary before these essential pieces of equipment are discussed.

1. They are not fume cupboards and should not be used as such. Similarly, fume cupboards should not be substituted for safety cabinets.
2. 'Laminar flow cabinets' are not necessarily microbiological safety cabinets. In some laminar flow cabinets clean air flows over the work, out into the room and at the operator's face. He will, therefore, inhale any particles which are released during the course of his work. While these cabinets may be useful in preventing the contamination of inanimate culture media during tubing and pouring, they should not be used for dispensing tissue culture cells or any other living materials. Even 'sterile' cell cultures may contain slow viruses or oncogenic agents without showing any sign of contamination.

Detailed information about the construction, performance, installation, testing and decontamination of safety cabinets, as well as their limitations, has already been published[11,13,29,38-41]. Cabinets that do not satisfy the appro-

168

priate standards should not be purchased. Only brief details will be given here.

There are three classes of microbiological safety cabinets:

Class I

These have open fronts through which the operator inserts his arms. He observes his work through a glass screen. Air is extracted from the room through the open front at 0.75-0.85 m/s. It entrains any particles, infective or otherwise, and carries them into the high efficiency particulate air (HEPA) filters which retain most, but not all, of them (few filters retain more than 99.997% of a challenge of small particles). The effluent, which may therefore still contain a few particles, is dumped to atmosphere outside the building where it is so diluted that it is innocuous. The extract fan is at the far end of the installation to ensure a negative pressure in the trunking. Any leaks will be into the trunking and not into the room. Class I cabinets protect the operator and may, subject to certain aerodynamic constructions, protect the work from contamination. A class I cabinet is illustrated in Figure 9.1.

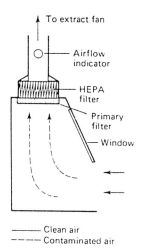

Figure 9.1 Class I microbiological safety cabinet (Figures are reproduced from *Collins and Lynes' Microbiological Methods.,* 6th edn. Eds. C.H. Collins, P.M. Lyne and J.M. Grange, by permission of Butterworths Publishers Ltd., London)

Class II

These also have open fronts and glass screens. Air passes through a HEPA filter and descends vertically through the cabinet (laminar flow) at about 0.5 m/s. It entrains any particles released during the work. At the same time it

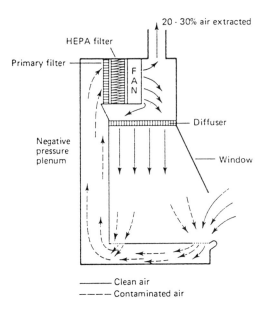

Figure 9.2 Class II microbiological safety cabinet

forms a curtain across the open front which prevents particles from entering or leaving the cabinet. This contaminated air passes through slots at the front and rear of the cabinet and after passing through the HEPA filter about 70% of it is recirculated through the cabinet. The remaining 30% is dumped to atmosphere as with class I cabinets. An equal volume of air passes almost vertically from the room through slots in the front of the cabinet floor, forming an additional barrier to the passage of particles into and out of the working area. Class II cabinets protect the operator and also protect the work from contamination by room air. Figure 9.2 shows a class II cabinet.

Class III

These are the ultimate in safety cabinet engineering. They are totally enclosed and are gas-tight. The operator works with his hands in gloves that are sealed into the front panel and views his work through the glass window. Air enters through a HEPA filter at the rear or side of the cabinet and is extracted to atmosphere through one or more such filters. Class III cabinets give maximum protection to the operator and his work. Figure 9.3 illustrates a class III cabinet.

Class I cabinets are used mainly in clinical and veterinary laboratories that handle those risk group III organisms which cause infection by the airborne

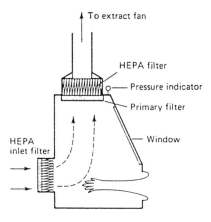

Figure 9.3 Class III microbiological safety cabinet

route, e.g. tubercle bacilli and brucellas.

Class II cabinets also protect the worker from risk group III organisms but are more expensive to purchase and maintain. They are of particular value, however, in virological procedures such as work with tissue cultures and eggs because of the protection they afford to the work as well as to the worker. There is an official but quite unscientific objection to class II cabinets in the United Kingdom, based on work done over 10 years ago. It has been quite clear, however, for several years now that class II cabinets constructed to national standards afford the same level of protection as class I cabinets.

Class III cabinets are rarely used outside maximum containment (level 4) laboratories where particularly hazardous viruses are investigated.

The choice of microbiological safety cabinets should reside with the people who are going to use them, and who will be at risk.

Installation can cause problems. In the design of new buildings the siting of safety cabinets in rooms, and the position of the rooms themselves in the building, should be considered at a very early stage because the degree of protection afforded by any cabinet is impaired by cross-draughts, ventilation, movement of people and by lengthy and tortuous trunking. The point of discharge is usually the concern of regulatory bodies. The manufacturer, as well as the user, should be consulted. Afterthoughts can be very expensive and unsatisfactory. In old buildings, again, advice should be obtained from the manufacturer as unusual problems may arise. Indeed, some manufacturers prefer to sell installations, not isolated cabinets; they do not care to accept responsibility or discredit for other people's work which may result in poor performance.

Attempts by designers to recirculate cabinet effluents to the room on aesthetic grounds or because of design errors should be resisted, whatever their arguments. Even with the best maintenance (which may well fail), particles which escape the filters may soon build up into an infective dose in a room. I have never met an advocate of this practice who is prepared to accept the effluent into his own room. Another problem is the decontamination of cabinets that do not exhaust to atmosphere. This must be done regularly and certainly before the filters are changed. Formaldehyde is used (see p.182) and this offers a hazard to health. Either the whole room must be treated or temporary trunking erected to duct the gas to the outside of the building – very difficult in premises that have no openable windows.

Safety cabinets require expert maintenance; air flows and filters should be tested regularly and the latter replaced when air flows fall below the recommended national standards.

Work in safety cabinets should be done in the middle to rear of the working surface and never near to the front. Bunsen burners and large pieces of equipment should not be placed in cabinets as they disturb the airflows and the resulting turbulence may lead to the escape of infectious particles into the room.

ROUTES OF INFECTION

In the laboratory micro-organisms may enter the body in several different ways. They may be ingested, inhaled, gain access through wounds or small lesions in the skin or through the eye. Natural infections may be initiated in the same way, of course, but not infrequently the routes differ for any one organism. For example, laboratory-associated brucellosis is usually contracted by inhaling airborne brucella cells, but outside the laboratory it is usually a result of drinking infected milk. In addition, there are many more opportunities in the laboratory for large numbers of various organisms to enter the body at any one time.

Ingestion

The most obvious, and regrettably the most frequent, way in which micro-organisms may be ingested is mouth pipetting. Mostly this occurs when the infectious material is actually sucked into the mouth, but pipettes which have become contaminated while lying on the bench are also possible vehicles. Although mouth pipetting has been banned in many laboratories it still occurs, particularly among recruits who have had little or no training in microbiological techniques (and even among some who have). In some laboratories in the United States two infringements of the 'no mouth pipetting' rule will earn dismissal! Other vehicles by which organisms are conveyed to the mouth include fingers, contaminated with spilled cultures or by minute droplets released during various techniques, and articles such as cigarettes, pipes and food which have been contaminated, directly, or by the fingers.

Inhalation

A significant fact that emerged during a series of investigations in the fifties and sixties was that in only about 20% of laboratory-acquired infections could the actual cause be identified as, e.g. aspiration (mouth pipetting), accidental inoculation, wounding by broken glass, animal bites[5,6]. Investigations revealed that many ordinary laboratory techniques with micro-organisms result in the release into the laboratory air of large amounts of aerosol, i.e. minute droplets of liquid containing one or a few organisms. Large droplets settle rapidly (and contaminate surfaces), but the smaller aerosol droplets evaporate, leaving the organisms as 'droplet nuclei'. These remain suspended in air for long periods and are easily moved about a room or a building by quite small air currents. If these particles are less than 5 μm in size and are inhaled they pass into the lungs and may cause infections. Larger particles are filtered off in the nasal passages and destroyed by local body defences.

Activities that release airborne particles include: using bacteriological loops; spreading cultures on slides; blowing out pipettes; mixing cultures by bubbling; using hypodermic syringes and needles; opening screw-capped bottles, or culture tubes which have wet stoppers; opening lyophilized cultures and cultures containing fungal spores; pouring cultures or bacterial suspensions, even into disinfectant; centrifuging fluids in uncapped tubes, especially in angle centrifuges; breakage of tubes in the centrifuge; blending and shaking infected materials; and slide catalase tests. These hazards have been investigated by a number of different scientists; their work has been reviewed by Darlow[42] and Collins[29].

Through the skin

This is the so-called percutaneous route. The obvious accidents are stab wounds with infected hypodermic needles ('needlestick'). These have been responsible for many infections[43]. The sampling probes of certain automated equipment also offer a hazard, as do stab wounds from Pasteur pipettes, cuts from broken pipettes and broken culture tubes and bottles. But the apparently unbroken skin, especially of the hands, usually has many barely visible or microscopic cuts and abrasions and these will permit the entry of micro-organisms from surfaces that have been contaminated as a result of spillage, splashing or the settling of larger aerosol droplets.

Through the eye

Micro-organisms may enter through the conjunctivae. They get there in two ways: rubbing with contaminated fingers and in splashes of culture fluids.

Much information has accumulated over the last 30 years on the incidence of infections acquired by various routes. A review, with an extensive list of references has been published[29].

EXAMPLES OF LABORATORY ACQUIRED INFECTIONS

It is not easy to select a few incidents from the 400 or so reports of about 4000 laboratory-acquired infections, but the following are salutary inasmuch as they reflect different kinds of hazard and varying degrees of responsibility of management, scientist or neither.

About 290 cases of typhoid fever, contracted in laboratories, were reported between 1930 and 1974[5]. Most of them appear to have been associated with mouth pipetting. In 1979 and 1980, however, about 30 cases occurred, all associated with quality assurance material issued to laboratories in the United States[44,45]. Precise details of the way in which each infection occurred are not available, but it is most likely that in most of them it was the hand-to-mouth route. Some of them, therefore, could have been due to the contamination of hands from apparatus or bench and to insufficient attention to hand-washing.

There were about 230 known infections with hepatitis B virus between 1930 and 1974[5]. They occurred as single cases and as common source outbreaks. It is significant, however, that after an outbreak in Edinburgh in the late sixties which attracted much attention, the number of laboratory-acquired cases notified in the United Kingdom fell from 17 in the period 1970–72 to six in the years 1977–78 and to none in 1979–80[1,19]. This dramatic decline could be attributed to publicity and to the realization, on the part of laboratory workers, that infection arises from contact between infected blood and the skin and mucous membranes. As a result there was greater care in the handling of blood, in the wearing of gloves and in the avoidance of mouth pipetting. Since 1980, however, there has been a slight increase in the numbers reported[19-22].

Airborne infections have frequently been responsible for outbreaks involving a number of people. Brucellas have the distinction not only of being the most frequent cause of laboratory-acquired diseases but of infecting a large number of people as a result of single incidents. Thus in one building 45 clinical cases and 49 subclinical infections were associated with a massive aerosol release from a single centrifuge operation[46]. The organisms were dispersed around the building, possibly on the ventilation system. It is possible that better siting of the centrifuge and an improved ventilation system could have avoided this unfortunate occurrence. Another incident in which ampoules of freeze-dried Venezuelan equine encephalitis were dropped and broken on a laboratory stairway after collection from a basement store resulted in the infection of 24 people in the same building[47]. The agent was probably dispersed by the ventilation system – or lack of it. This case highlights the problems of where infectious material should be stored and how it should be transported around the laboratory.

According to Pike[5] accidents with needles and syringes accounted for about one quarter of 700 known infections, although it is not clear how many of these were due to needlestick. Two incidents are worth including here: two workers contracted Rocky Mountain spotted fever after accidental inoculations[48], and another nearly died after a small prick with a needle infected with Ebola fever virus[49]. Others have been reviewed recently[43].

Finally, a splash in the eye from a culture of meningococci resulted in a fatal infection[50]. This might have been avoided by the wearing of safety spectacles. A number of other eye infections have been reported[29].

Of course, many of the 4000 infections that have been reported occurred before the hazards were fully appreciated; others would not be serious now because prophylactics and chemotherapeutic agents are more freely available. But they indicate quite clearly that there is no cause for complacency.

MINIMIZING INFECTION HAZARDS

The risks of infection that arise in work with micro-organisms may be related to techniques, to equipment, or to both. Even with the best techniques, poor equipment will introduce hazards; the best possible equipment will not protect the careless or untrained worker.

The precautions outlined below provide primary barriers around the organisms. Those concerned with protection against the dispersal or aerosols are particularly important; these hazards can never be reduced to zero and any operations with risk group III micro-organisms should always be done in a safety cabinet.

Bacteriological loops

Loops that are larger than 3 mm in diameter or are imperfectly closed shed their loads easily, creating infectious aerosols and droplets. Loops with long shanks vibrate and are also likely to discharge their contents. Heavily charged loops placed in ordinary bunsen flames frequently spatter living material around the bench. Hooded bunsens and microincinerators effectively prevent this. Plastic disposable loops overcome all the above problems and should be discarded into disinfectant pots. They are particularly useful in safety cabinets where bunsens are undesirable (see above).

Preparation of slides for microscopy

Cheap slides have sharp edges, are easily broken and may injure fingers with a consequent risk of infection. Vigorous rubbing of charged loops in saline on a slide will release aerosols and droplets that contaminate the bench. This hazard may be reduced by replacing saline with a saturated solution of mercuric chloride.

Pipettes

There should be a total ban on mouth pipetting, even of water. This avoids the dangers both of aspiration and of introducing potentially contaminated articles into the mouth. There are many different kinds of rubber teats and mechanical pipetting devices and the worker himself should exercise the choice. Not all devices suit all workers or all kinds of work. The devices need regular inspection and maintenance and do not last for ever. Some training in their use is essential. Pipettes with cracked or chipped ends should be discarded; they may injure fingers, allow the contents to leak, and damage pipetting devices.

Violent pipetting and violent discharge of contents should be avoided: both produce bubbles, which burst and release aerosols. 'Delivery' pipettes are safer than 'container' pipettes: with these it is not necessary to blow out the last drop - a fruitful source of infectious airborne particles.

Glass Pasteur pipettes frequently cause stab wounds and cut fingers. They should be replaced by disposable soft plastic varieties.

Hypodermic syringes and needles

The laboratory use of these should be minimal. Infections arising from needlestick are frequently reported[43]. For many purposes, especially in virological procedures, the needles may be replaced by cannulas. Syringes and needles should not be used instead of pipettes unless it is absolutely necessary, e.g. for removing the contents of rubber-sealed containers. This activity requires special precautions to avoid the dispersal of infectious materials when the needle is withdrawn through the cap. Aerosols are released by the disruption of a fine thread of liquid that is formed when the needle is drawn through the cap, and also by the vibration of the needle. The needle should be withdrawn through a pledget of cotton wool soaked in alcohol and held firmly on the cap. It is safer to remove septum caps with the commercially available gadgets and to use pipettes.

Other hazards arise from leaks between plungers and barrels of syringes, leading to contamination of the hands. Aerosols and splashes may be produced if the needle flies off its butt when pressure is applied to the plunger.

There are serious differences of opinion between those who advocate removing the needle from the syringe after use and those who think that it is safer to discard syringe and needle as one unit. In any case hypodermic syringes and needles should be discarded into stout containers which can be autoclaved and/or incinerated. Several varieties are on the market, but those made of thin card should be avoided: their sides are easily penetrated by needles which may then stab anyone who handles the containers. Precautions against needlestick have been reviewed[43,51].

Culture containers

These should be robust. Thin glass tubes, bottles and Petri dishes are easily broken, resulting in the dispersal of infectious material and possibly causing personal injury.

Opening culture containers

There is frequently a film of liquid between the neck and the stopper of a culture tube or bottle and between the rim and the lid of a Petri dish. When this film is ruptured by opening the container an aerosol is produced. It is difficult to overcome this hazard, except by ensuring that tubes and bottles are always stored upright and by opening them in a safety cabinet. Some plastic Petri dishes have nibs which raise the lid from the rim. Although designed to ventilate the dishes this also minimizes the formation of the wet film. Plastic Petri dishes are preferable to those made of glass; they do not break when dropped and, therefore, do not disperse their contents so widely.

Hazardous airborne particles are released by some procedures that do not involve the production of aerosols. Infectious material may dry around the stoppers and rims of culture tubes and is dispersed when these are disturbed. Lyophilized material is also easily dispersed and care should be taken when ampoules of freeze-dried cultures are opened. Curators of culture collections usually issue instructions on how to open ampoules safely. Directions have also been published in at least two books[11,29]. Cultures of some fungi contain large numbers of spores which are released into the air when the tubes or Petri dishes are opened.

Pouring infectious material

Although pouring liquid cultures is usually regarded as bad practice, decanting supernatant fluids after centrifugation seems to be a normal procedure. It is commonly believed that centrifuging a suspension of organisms removes them from the supernatant fluid. Many people also believe that it is quite safe to pour cultures and bacterial suspensions into disinfectants. Neither of these beliefs has been supported by experiment. Some organisms do remain in supernatant fluids. Splashes and droplets bounce off the surface of disinfectants and may contaminate the surrounding area.

A funnel should be placed over a discard jar so that it is supported by its rim, and its outlet is just below the surface of the disinfectant. The supernatant fluid should then be poured into the funnel. A drop of fluid often remains on the lip of the tube. This should be wiped off with a piece of filter paper which is then discarded into disinfectant.

Centrifugation

Centrifugation of fluids in unstoppered tubes is a common but undesirable practice. If the fluid nearly fills the tube, if the centrifuge is started or stopped abruptly, or if an angled rotor is used some of the fluid is likely to be ejected. It will be aerosolized by impact with the centrifuge bowl and will emerge in the ventilation airstream. Breakage of tubes within a centrifuge results in a massive release of aerosol.

It is good practice to stopper all centrifuge tubes and if the liquid being centrifuged contains risk group III pathogens it is essential to use sealed centrifuge buckets (known also as safety cups). Those with polycarbonate caps allow the user to see broken tubes before the bucket is opened. All such buckets should in any case, be opened in a safety cabinet. Windshields and sealed rotors are not as efficient as sealed buckets. They may leak after they have been in use for some time, and if a tube breaks all the contents and the rotor must be decontaminated instead of a single bucket.

There is little point in placing the centrifuge inside a microbiological safety cabinet in the hope of containing airborne particles; the velocity of air leaving the ventilation ports is about 200 times greater than that of the air entering the cabinet.

Shaking and blending

These operations generate aerosols and need special precautions. Even the least violent macerating by hand in a Griffith's tube can be hazardous: if a tube breaks the hand may be cut with infected glass. These tubes should be

178

held firmly in a thick pad of cotton, and if the specimen is thought to contain risk group III organisms the operation should be done in a safety cabinet.

Materials that require mechanical shaking should be in tightly stoppered containers, which, as an added precaution, may be placed in sealable plastic bags. High-speed homogenizers and blenders should be chosen with care. Domestic models always release aerosols. Some models marketed for laboratory use may become unsafe if they are not properly maintained: their lids work loose and they develop leaks around the spindle shaft. Aerosols under pressure are generated in these instruments and released violently when the lids are removed. Special kinds of Waring blenders have been designed that overcome all these problems. The Seward 'Stomacher' in which materials are homogenized in strong plastic bags, and which produces no aerosols, can be recommended. Other devices, such as sonicators, should always be covered when in use by large Perspex boxes.

Catalase tests

A positive catalase test produces bubbles of oxygen which disperse aerosols as they burst. Slide catalase tests should therefore be abandoned in favour of tube tests which contain the aerosols.

PERSONAL PROTECTION

Accidents happen, even with the best techniques and equipment, and secondary barriers around the individual are just as important as primary barriers around the organisms. There are four kinds of secondary barriers that afford personal protection: (1) protective clothing and equipment; (2) immunization; (3) medical supervision; (4) personal hygiene.

Protective clothing and personal equipment

These are intended to protect normal clothes, skin, eyes, nose and mouth from micro-organisms that might be released during laboratory work. Clothes are considered first because they cover the larger part of the worker's body and could be the means of transmitting infection, not only to him, but to his associates.

Most employers provide overalls or coats of one kind or another, but persuading people to wear them properly, i.e. fastened, may be a problem. No solution can be offered here and employers must decide for themselves what sanctions to use. The traditional white coat is not particularly effective: it gapes at the front and at the knees when the wearer is sitting and it fails to protect the exposed parts of the neck, wrists or lower arms or clothing that may cover them. It is better than nothing, however, in those places where there are objections to the more sensible kinds of protective clothing that are currently available[11,29].

Gloves, preferably the disposable kind used by surgeons, should be provided and always worn for handling blood and materials that may contain viruses (e.g. hepatitis B) or bacteria that can cause serious infections if they enter the body through small cuts and abrasions on the skin of the hands. It is often argued that gloves decrease manual sensitivity and slow up the work. Certainly there is no case for wearing them all the time, but risks must be weighed against discomfort and loss of speed.

Eye protection is offered, and even insisted upon, in many chemical laboratories. Protection of the eyes from splashes of infected material is no less important. The 'safety spectacles' worn by chemists are recommended: they have side shields and they fit over ordinary spectacles.

The wearing of surgeons' masks is controversial. They are intended to protect the patient, not the surgeon, and those in common use in hospitals offer no barriers to the passage of micro-organisms (e.g. in aerosols) at the levels that may be encountered in laboratories. There are masks made of rigid fibres, however, that mould to the face and which do afford a considerable degree of protection against the inhalation of infectious particles. They may also be worn to protect the work, e.g. tissue and egg cultures, from oral and nasal sprays that arise during coughing, sneezing and conversation.

Immunization

It is by no means possible, or even sensible, to try to immunize all laboratory workers against all organisms that they might encounter in the course of their work. In developed countries most individuals are immunized against tuberculosis, poliomyelitis, diphtheria, tetanus and, if they are inclined to travel, typhoid fever. Certainly, those who work with tubercle bacilli should have received BCG or have a positive skin test, and consideration should be given to the vaccination of scientists who are exposed to hepatitis B virus. Otherwise, immunization should be restricted to individuals at special risk, e.g. scientists who are working with certain viruses. As policies vary between countries it is desirable to obtain advice from state health authorities. See Chapter 5.

Medical supervision

Medical supervision of staff is obviously more important in maximum containment units than in basic laboratories. As pointed out above, however, unexpected hazards may arise in work with organisms in the lower risk groups and the occupational health staff should be aware of them.

In many countries it is usual, and in some it is mandatory, for staff who are in contact with risk groups III and IV pathogens, and also those who work in clinical laboratories, to carry cards stating this fact. If such a worker is ill he is expected to show the card to his physician who will then be alerted to the possibility of an unusual or laboratory-acquired infection. The cards should bear the name, address and telephone number of a designated member of the laboratory medical staff.

Although there is no great risk to those who work with other micro-organisms they would be well advised to inform their family doctor of the nature of that work.

It is generally agreed that scientists who work with tubercle bacilli should have annual chest X-rays, but for other workers, even those who have occasional contact with tuberculous material, an X-ray taken every 3 years would be a satisfactory compromise. Unnecessary exposure to X-rays should be avoided, especially in women of childbearing age.

Pregnant women are at special risk from certain viruses, especially during the first trimester. This fact should be made known to all women of childbearing age and private counselling should be offered. Women who are working with rubella virus or cytomegalovirus should be transferred to other duties as soon as they suspect they are pregnant. See also Chapter 5.

PRECAUTIONS AGAINST SPECIFIC INFECTIONS

Work with certain infectious agents which have a bad reputation for infecting laboratory workers may require specific precautions. These include *Salmonella typhi*, *Mycobacterium tuberculosis* and hepatitis B virus. To these one must add human immunodeficiency (AIDS) virus (very few cases of laboratory-acquired infection to date) and the agents of spongiform encephalopathies, although evidence that these are hazardous is inconclusive. Space here does not permit a discussion of such precautions but information may be found in several publications[11,25,27,29,52,53].

DECONTAMINATION

In the context of this chapter the word 'decontamination' is used instead of 'sterilization' and 'disinfection' because in some circumstances it may not be necessary, or even possible, to achieve sterilization – which is the complete destruction or removal of all living matter. On the other hand, disinfection, defined as the destruction of pathogens, frequently fails because of poor techniques and a lack of understanding of its principles.

The object of decontamination is to render non-infectious: (1) all used cultures and discarded materials so that they may be disposed of safely into the public refuse or sewarage systems; (2) all re-usable equipment and laboratory surfaces. Full reviews of methods applicable to microbiological safety have been published[29,54].

The old custom of dumping all discarded materials and cultures into a bucket of disinfectant of uncertain age and concentration, leaving them there for an unspecified time and then washing them or throwing them away has been superseded by safer and more reliable procedures.

In principle, all discarded materials should be autoclaved before they leave the laboratory. They may then be incinerated, but incineration should not be regarded as an alternative to autoclaving unless the incinerator is under strict laboratory control. There have been many accounts of infectious material that has by-passed incinerators and found its way on to rubbish tips. The ensuing publicity is unwelcome, even when the health risks are slight.

Chemical disinfectants, properly used, serve three purposes in laboratories: (1) as discard jars – repositories for small articles used at the bench and which will subsequently be autoclaved (the exceptions are graduated pipettes); (2) the decontamination of surfaces; (3) the treatment of spillage.

Autoclaves

Care is needed in the choice of these expensive items of equipment. Glossy advertisements, the blandishments of salesmen and the advice of individuals who never actually use them should be viewed with suspicion. It is best to consult practising microbiologists who have had experience with the various different models. For the effective decontamination of cultures and equipment 'mixed load' autoclaves are required, not pharmaceutical, dressing or instrument sterilizers. Autoclaves used for discarded materials should not also be used for sterilizing culture media which may require quite different treatment. The choice of autoclaves may lie between a single, large and sophisticated machine and two or more simpler and smaller models. The more complicated an autoclave the more often it will need maintenance. An autoclave that is out of commission can disrupt the work of a laboratory, may necessitate the storage of infectious material under hazardous conditions and may lead to unsafe 'short cuts' in disposal. The important feature of an autoclave is that the load should reach 121 °C in a very short time. The temperature in the drain, which is usually recorded on the gauge or the chart, is irrelevant. Very often the drain temperature reaches 121 °C while that in the load is still under 100 °C. Indeed, the load temperature may never reach 100 °C during the holding time, which is usually 15–20 minutes. Many microorganisms may therefore survive. Higher temperatures (134 °C) are necessary for the safe disposal of material containing the scrapie and Creutzfeldt-

Jakob agents[29,53].

Autoclaves should be commissioned and then tested frequently by placing thermocouples at various points in the load, and also under 'worst load' conditions. External recording devices are not expensive and thermocouple wires are thin enough not to interfere with the door seals of autoclaves that do not have suitable access ports.

Autoclaves should be loaded in a sensible manner. Even efficient machines are unlikely to sterilize a load that is packed so tightly that steam cannot circulate and expel all air.

Containers for autoclaving discarded cultures, etc. may be of metal or heat-resistant plastic, but should not fit tightly in the chamber. They should not be more than about 25 cm deep so that steam can easily penetrate their contents. The contents should not be tightly packed and any lids that are used to cover the contents during transport from laboratory to autoclave room should be removed and autoclaved at the same time as the containers. If autoclavable plastic bags are used to hold discarded materials they should be supported in rigid containers; otherwise, if they are full of heavy articles, they may burst and cause serious local contamination. The bags may be closed with plastic ties during transport to the autoclave, but even if it is claimed that they are pervious to steam they should be opened for autoclaving. Detailed and useful information on the use of autoclaves is given by Gardner and Peel[54].

Incinerators

Problems and failures may occur with incinerators even if they are under laboratory control. If they are packed too well or are left unattended some of the material may never be burned. Infectious particles may be carried up the flue and into the open air by the updraught before the flames and heat reach them. Smoke production can lead to conflicts with local authorities and neighbours. The best models are those that have after-burners and consume their own smoke.

There is an increase in the laboratory use of containers made of cardboard and thin metal for used disposable syringes, needles and small bench equipment. These containers are purpose-made and are intended to be incinerated. Their use is recommended.

Disinfectants

Only those disinfectants that have proved their worth in other microbiological laboratories should be used. Rideal-Walker coefficients and similar discredited figures should be disregarded, as should pleasant smells. Clear phenolics, hypochlorites and glutaraldehyde are the obvious choices where pathogens are handled. Not all of them are effective against all organisms, however, and some care is necessary in their choice and use. In general, phenolics are active against most fungi, bacteria and lipid viruses but not against spores and non-lipid viruses. Hypochlorites are not particularly effective against fungi but are effective against bacteria, spores and both kinds of virus. Glutaraldehyde is effective against all of these, but is not all that active below 20 °C. There are, of course, other considerations: all of these disinfectants are inactivated to some extent by protein (especially hypochlorites), by natural and man-made materials (phenolics) and by hard water. If they are to be used in conjunction with detergents it is advisable to ask the manufacturers if they are compatible. In addition, they are all toxic to some degree: phenolics to skin and eyes, hypochlorites and glutaraldehyde to skin, eyes and lungs. If they are used intelligently and according to the manufacturers' instructions, however, the hazards are minimal.

For laboratory use disinfectants should be diluted accurately to the manufacturers' recommended use-dilution for the worst or dirtiest situations. Phenolics and hypochlorites should be made up daily and not stored diluted. Some glutaraldehydes, however, have a life of 7 days or more after activation, as long as they are not abused.

Abuse of disinfectants is all too common an occurrence. Discard jars on benches are emptied infrequently and are often overloaded with protein, paper and small items which rapidly inactivate the disinfectant. Some articles may not even be completely immersed. Such misuse can lead to laboratory-acquired infections.

Plastic discard jars are safer than those made of glass. They should be large enough to allow all the small waste that accumulates in one day's work to be completely covered. The jars should be emptied daily by pouring their contents through an autoclavable sieve or colander held over a sluice or sink connected to the public sewer (large amounts need special arrangements with local authorities). The sieve or colander containing the solid material should then be placed in a suitable container and autoclaved.

In some laboratories these disinfectant jars are being replaced by the card and metal bins mentioned above which are incinerated with or without prior autoclaving.

The only articles that may be recycled after disinfection and without heat treatment are graduated pipettes. These should be left, completely submerged, in disinfectant for at least 18 hours and then washed in very hot water. Gloves should be worn for this work.

If there has been a spillage of infectious material the area should be covered with absorbent cloth or paper soaked in the appropriate disinfectant. More disinfectant should be poured over the absorbent material and the whole left undisturbed for at least an hour before the debris is removed with gloved hands and the area swabbed again. A serious spillage or breakage involving risk group III organisms will need the immediate attention of the safety officer: aerosols may have been dispersed. The room may have to be evacuated, and possibly decontaminated (see below).

At the end of the day's work the bench and any other surfaces that may have been contaminated without the knowledge of the worker should be swabbed down with a suitable disinfectant. Glutaraldehyde is probably the best for this purpose, as phenolics may leave sticky residues and hypochlorites may attack metals. Glutaraldehyde should be used if the spillage has occurred inside a centrifuge bowl or in similar equipment.

Microbiological safety cabinets require regular disinfection of surfaces, preferably with glutaraldehyde. It is also necessary to decontaminate the whole cabinet, filters and trunking at regular intervals, depending on the amount of use and certainly before the filters are changed. Formaldehyde gas is used for this purpose and is generated by boiling formalin or heating tablets of paraformaldehyde. Most cabinet manufacturers provide equipment and instructions for this purpose but as the gas is very toxic certain precautions must be taken. The cabinet should be sealed before the gas is generated and it should not be fully opened until the gas has been dispersed by running the fan. There is usually provision for allowing some air to enter the cabinet before the front is removed. The manufacturers' instructions should be followed and various techniques for the decontamination of safety cabinets have been published[11,29,38].

Only rarely is it necessary to decontaminate whole rooms, e.g. after major spillage or aerosol release of risk group III or IV organisms. The technique which necessitates sealing the room and the expert use of respirators and formaldehyde gas, is beyond the scope of this chapter but is given in detail elsewhere[29]. It is similar to that used in the terminal disinfection of hospital wards and cubicles.

For more information on the use of disinfectants in laboratories and elsewhere see Collins[29], Gardner and Peel[54] and Ayliffe et al.[55].

CONCLUSIONS

The hazards of working with micro-organisms are real but should not be regarded as alarming. As with many other pursuits, if the risks are appreciated and appropriate techniques are used, casualties are few. The incidence of laboratory-acquired infections may be minimized and they may be almost entirely prevented by good laboratory design, correct equipment properly used, good housekeeping and training in careful technique. The sum of all these may be described as good laboratory practice.

REFERENCES

1. Grist, N.R. (1975). Hepatitis in clinical laboratories; a three year survey. *J. Clin. Pathol.*, **28**, 255-9
2. Report (1974). *Report of the Committee of Enquiry into the Smallpox Outbreak in London, March and April 1973*. Cmnd. 5626. (London: HMSO)
3. Report (1980). *Report of the Investigation into the Causes of the 1978 Birmingham Smallpox Occurrence*. House of Commons Paper 79-80. (London: HMSO)
4. Berg, P., Baltimore, D., Boyer, H.W., Cohen, S.N., Davis, R.W., Hogness, D.S., Nathans, D., Roblin, R.O., Watson, J.D., Weissman, S. and Zinder, N.D. (1974). Potential hazards of recombinant DNA molecules. *Science*, **185**, 303
5. Pike, R.M. (1976). Laboratory associated infections. Summary and analysis of 3921 cases. *Arch. Pathol. Lab. Med.*, **102**, 333-6
6. Phillips, G.B. (1961). *Microbiological Safety in US and Foreign Laboratories*. Technical report no 35. US Army Chemical Corps. (Washington, DC: US Army)
7. Centers for Disease Control (1974). *Lab Safety at the Centers for Disease Control*. (Washington, DC: Government Printing Office)
8. National Institutes of Health (1974). *Biosafety Guide*. (Washington, DC: Government Printing Office)
9. National Institutes of Health (1978). *Laboratory Safety Monograph, Supplement to the NIH Guidelines for Recombinant DNA Research*. (Washington, DC: Government Printing Office)
10. Department of Health and Social Security (1976). *Control of Laboratory Use of Pathogens Very Dangerous to Humans*. (London: HMSO)
11. Department of Health and Social Security (1978). *Code of Practice for the Prevention of Infection in Clinical Laboratories and Post-mortem Rooms*. (London: HMSO)
12. World Health Organisation (1980). Guidelines for the management of accidents involving micro-organisms. A WHO Memorandum. *Bull. Wld. Hlth. Org.*, **58**, 245-56
13. World Health Organisation (1983). *Laboratory Biosafety Manual*. (Geneva: WHO)
14. Microbiological Consultative Committee (1986). *Guidelines for Microbiological Safety*. 3rd edn. (Reading: Society for General Microbiology)
15. Grist, N.R. (1976). Hepatitis in clinical laboratories 1973–74. *J. Clin. Pathol.*, **29**, 480–83
16. Grist, N.R. (1978). Hepatitis in clinical laboratories 1975–76. *J. Clin. Pathol.*, **31**, 415–17
17. Grist, N.R. (1980). Hepatitis in clinical laboratories 1977–78. *J. Clin. Pathol.*, **33**, 471–73
18. Grist, N.R. (1981). Hepatitis and other infections in clinical laboratory staff, 1979. *J. Clin. Pathol.*, **34**, 654–58
19. Grist, N.R. (1983). Infections in British clinical laboratories 1980–81. *J. Clin. Pathol.*, **36**, 121–26
20. Grist, N.R and Emslie, J.A.N. (1985). Infections in British clinical laboratories 1982–83. *J. Clin. Pathol.*, **38**, 721–25
21. Grist, N.R. and Emslie, J.A.N. (1987). Infections in British clinical laboratories 1984–85. *J. Clin. Pathol.*, **40**, 826–29
22. Grist, N.R. and Emslie, J.A.N. (1989). Infections in British clinical laboratories 1986–87. *J. Clin. Pathol.*, **42**, 677–81
23. Centers for Disease Control and National Institutes of Health (1988). *Biosafety in Microbiological and Biomedical Laboratories*. 2nd edn. (Atlanta: Centers for Disease Control)
24. Advisory Committee on Dangerous Pathogens (Health and Safety Executive and Health Departments) (1984). *Categorisation of Pathogens According to Hazard and Categories of Containment*. (London: HMSO)
25. Health Services Advisory Committee (Health and Safety Commission) (1985). *Safety in Health Service Laboratories: Precautions to Minimise the Risk of Infection from Specimens*

Known or Suspected to be Positive and in Testing of Specimens for the Presence of Hepatitis Antigens and Antibodies. (London: HMSO)

26. Health Services Advisory Committee (Health and Safety Commission) (1986). *Safety in Health Service Laboratories: the Labelling, Transport and Reception of Specimens.* (London: HMSO)

27. Collins, C.H. (ed.). (1988). *Safety in Clinical and Biomedical Laboratories.* (London: Chapman and Hall)

28. Collins, C.H., Lyne, P.M. and Grange, J.M. (Eds.) (1989). *Collins and Lynes' Microbiological Methods.* 6th edn., (London: Butterworths)

29. Collins, C.H. (1988). *Laboratory-Acquired Infections: History, Incidence, Causes and Prevention.* 2nd edn. (London: Butterworths)

30. Pike, R.M. (1979). Laboratory associated infections; incidents, fatalities, causes and prevention. *Ann. Rev. Microbiol.,* 33, 41-66

31. Centers for Disease Control (1974). *Classification of etiologic agents on the basis of hazard.* (Washington, DC: Government Printing Office)

32. World Health Organisation (1979). Safety measures in microbiology; minimum standards of laboratory safety. *Weekly Epidem. Rec.,* No. 44, 340-2

33. Nederlandse Vereneging voor Microbiologie. *Richtlijnene voor Veilig Microbiolisch Werk.* Maart

34. Laboratoriumssicherheit (1981). Vorläufige Empfehlungen für den Umgang mit pathogeenen Mikroorganismen und für die Klassifikation von Microorganismen und Krankheitserregern nach den im Umgang mit ihnen auftretenden Gefahren. *Bundesgesundheitsblatt,* 24 (22), 30 October 1981

35. Report (1985). European Federation of Biotechnology Safety in Biotechnology Working Party. Safe biotechnology: General considerations. *Appl. Microbiol. Biotechnol.,* 21, 1-6

36. Genetic Manipulation Advisory Group (1978). Genetic manipulations: new guidelines for UK. *Nature,* London, 276, 104-8

37. *The Third Report of the Genetic Manipulation Advisory Group* (1982), Cmnd 8665. (London: HMSO)

38. Clark, R.P. (1983). *The Performance, Installation, Testing and Limitation of Microbiological Safety Cabinets.* Occupational Hygiene Monograph No.9. (Northwood: Science Reviews)

39. National Sanitation Foundation (1984). *Standard No. 49. Class II (Laminar Flow, Biohazard Cabinetry.* (Michigan: Ann Arbor)

40. British Standards Institution (1979). *Specification for Microbiological Safety Cabinets.* BS 5726. (London: British Standards Institution)

41. Standards Association of Australia (1980). *Biological Safety Cabinets (Class I) for Personal Protection.* Australian Standard 2252. (Sydney: Standards Association of Australia)

42. Darlow, H.M. (1972). Safety in the microbiological laboratory: an introduction. In Shapton, D.A. and Board, R.G. (eds.), *Safety in Microbiology.* Society for Bacteriology Technical Series No.6, 1-20. (London: Academic Press)

43. Collins, C.H. and Kennedy, D.A. (1987). Microbiological hazards of occupational needlestick and 'sharps' injuries. *J. Appl. Bacteriol.,* 62, 385-402

44. Centers for Disease Control (1979). Laboratory associated typhoid fever. *Mortal. Wkly. Rep.,* 28, 44

45. Blaser, R. and Feldman, R.A. (1980). Acquisition of typhoid fever from proficiency testing specimens. *N. Engl. J. Med.,* 303, 1481

46. Huddleson, I.F. and Munger, M. (1940). A study of an epidemic of brucellosis due to *Brucella melitensis. Am. J. Pub. Hlth.,* 30, 944-5

47. Slepushkin, A.N. (1959). An epidemiological study of laboratory infections with Venezuelan equine encephalitis. *Prob. Virol.,* 4, 311-14

48. Centers for Disease Control (1977). Fatal Rocky Mountain Spotted Fever. *Morb. Mortal.*

Weekly Rep., **26**, 84
49. Edmond, R.R., Evans, B/. Bowen, E.T. and Lloyd, G. (1977). A case of Ebola virus infection. *Br. Med. J.*, **2**, 541-4
50. Anon (1936). Obituary: Bacteriologist dies of meningitis (Anna Pabst). Death attributed to meningitis contracted while conducting experiments in the laboratory. *J. Am. Med. Assoc.*, **106**, 109
51. Kennedy, D.A. (1988). Needlestick injuries: mechanisms and control. *J. Hosp. Infect.*, **12**, 315–22
52. Advisory Committee on Dangerous Pathogens (Health and Safety Executive and Health Departments). (1986). *LAV/HTLV III - The Causative Agent of AIDS and Related Conditions - Revised Guidelines*. (London: Health and Safety Commission)
53. Department of Health and Social Security (1984). *Management of Patients with Spongiform Encephalopathies*. (London: Department of Health)
54. Gardner, J.F. and Peel, M.M. (1986). *Introduction to Sterilization and Disinfection*. (London: Churchill)
55. Ayliffe, G.A.J., Coates, D.A. and Hoffman, P.A. (1984). *Chemical Disinfection in Hospitals*. (London: Public Health Laboratory Service)

10 Safety Measures in a Clinical Chemistry Laboratory

J.H. Smith

The aims of a hospital clinical chemistry laboratory are not dissimilar to those of other industrial analytical laboratories. That is, the quantitation of different substances using techniques and instrumentation which will provide accurate and precise results.

Where it differs, is that the sample material comes from the human population, and represents a potential infection risk to those who handle it. The degree of risk may be unknown at the time of analysis and only later may further information reveal the nature of the hazard involved.

A clinical chemistry laboratory must adopt the standard safety measures adopted in other analytical laboratories and already discussed in this book. For example, eating, drinking and smoking must only take place in an area specifically set aside for that purpose.

This chapter will focus attention on those safety measures and hazards which are particularly pertinent to the functions of the hospital clinical chemistry laboratory in its handling of patient specimens.

GENERAL

As in any other laboratory, clinical chemists rely heavily on services (heat, light, gas, water, electricity) and instrumentation, but it is the staff who are crucial to the operation of an effective safety policy, incorporating the appropriate procedures. A major priority must be to avoid personal injury and, secondly, to avoid damage to equipment, property and records. Although fire is a major hazard, it is currently less so in clinical chemistry. Cigarette smoking is not allowed in the laboratory, and it is rare to see a Bunsen burner in use. There remain the flames of emission and atomic absorption spectrophotometers, which are enclosed by a hood. Nevertheless, because flame photometers may remain switched on for most of the day it is easy to forget the presence of a naked flame.

The handling of inflammable solvents is not a frequent daily occurrence, such that whenever a member of staff does use one they should check their surroundings for heat sources.

In the author's experience the most serious incidents have been the breakage of a large bottle of liquid chemical resulting in a dangerous spillage. The consequences may be burns to anyone nearby, damage to equipment and a rapid spread of poisonous fumes which could also be inflammable. The laboratory area must be evacuated since staff can be rapidly overcome by poisonous vapour.

It may be possible, depending on the chemical involved, to contain and/or neutralize the spillage and there are a number of products for this purpose. Nevertheless, the spillage of a Winchester containing 2.5 litres of fluid can be difficult to handle, and there is still the problem of getting rid of the waste material.

The local fire service are usually well equipped to deal with such a problem and are prepared to respond urgently, to what they regard as a 'special service call'. They will need advice at the scene, but are more likely to be better equipped, have the appropriate protective clothing and breathing apparatus to cope with the situation.

Protective clothing

The traditional white coat is still worn as protection in most clinical chemistry departments. There are now available wrap-over style white coats which offer greater protection and can be removed quickly in the event of spillage. It is also necessary to make available auxiliary items such as gloves, plastic aprons and safety spectacles to deal with particular situations. Such items must be seen to be readily available rather than stored away at the back of a cupboard.

Pipetting

As in any other laboratory mouth pipetting of reagents must be avoided. As far as clinical chemistry is concerned the mouth pipetting of any biological material must be prohibited. There are available, numerous devices for the accurate pipetting of volumes as different as $5\,\mu l$ to 2 ml. Most of them use tips of glass and plastic which should be carefully disposed of, and some incorporate ejection of the tip without handling by the operator.

It is quite common in the laboratory for recent school leavers, research graduates, doctors and experienced scientific officers to be working alongside each other. It must be seen that safety rules apply to everyone. The appointment of the Safety Officer of the laboratory must be a person who carries the respect of all departmental staff and has sufficient authority to ensure that rules and guidelines laid down, are followed.

THE BUILDINGS

Many hospitals in various countries were built in the early part of the twentieth century. At that time, planned laboratory accommodation was not envisaged as a necessary requirement.

Although new laboratories have since been built, many departments are still faced with working in premises not specifically designed for the purpose. Also it is not uncommon for new departments to have deficiencies, since unexpected cash restraints force compromises to be made in order to complete the building programme. Therefore, when planning a new laboratory or occupying other types of premises, it is essential to establish safety priorities, in order that certain activities occupy areas which give some physical separation from the general laboratory. Examples of these areas are given below.

Out-patients reception

Patients should not enter the laboratory for the purpose of blood collection or the issuing of instructions. The author once observed a blind patient with her guide dog waiting in the laboratory prior to her blood test. In the meantime, the activity of the laboratory was conducted around her including the carrying of inflammable solvents.

Specimen reception

This area should handle the receipt and centrifugation of all specimens including blood and urine. Any samples which are of a high risk nature will be dealt with here, but by separating this area from other parts of the laboratory the risk of spreading infection to all members of staff, will be minimized.

The office

Apart from the usual secretarial work normally undertaken, it is possible that this area may be used to prepare work lists and record patient information from the request form. Care should be taken to exclude patient specimens from such areas, particularly when the handling is performed by non-technical staff. Under such circumstances it is inevitable that there will be an exchange of information between the staff in Specimens Reception and the Office, so care must be taken when handling what may be contaminated request forms. It is inappropriate for the office staff to be exposed to the possible hazards which may be present in the laboratory.

Radioisotope laboratory

Most clinical chemistry departments undertake some radioimmunoassays. The activities handled are usually less than $1\ \mu Ci$, but again contamination is possible and equipment should be set aside to be used only in this area.

Faecal analysis

It may be necessary to prepare, analyse and dispose of faecal specimens from a variety of analyses. Due to the risk of infection and odour, this should be performed in an area apart from the main laboratory. There should be the facility to dispose of faeces and urine via a sluice of some kind. The staff toilet facilities must never be used for such a purpose.

This list is not exhaustive, since laboratories may undertake work of a particular speciality, or they spend a greater proportion of their time undertaking tasks where a separate area is advantageous, for example, liquid chromatography involving a variety of solvents.

To achieve separation of activities may be difficult, given the layout of the premises with accommodation on different floors or even in different buildings. The hospital engineer can be helpful in rationalizing decisions where to situate certain functions, although it must be remembered that they too must work with the services at their disposal.

The hospital clinical chemistry laboratory serves the hospital, the community and above all, the patients. It is important to remember that the siting of laboratory services ensures effective access between itself and the consumer.

THE RECEIPT OF SPECIMENS

The laboratory must design request forms and issue collecting tubes and bottles for the various types of specimen they are likely to receive. The different containers must be selected such that they can be handled safely by laboratory staff and those who collect and deliver the specimens. This includes nurses, doctors, porters and patients.

It is important to stress that what appears safe and acceptable within the laboratory, may generate unexpected handling difficulties by hospital staff and patients alike. Most laboratories ensure that the accompanying request form and specimen are not in physical contact since this reduces the risk of infection to the secretarial staff who handle the form. This can be achieved using the dual plastic bags shown in Figure 10.1.

Another approach is to use an envelope type request form (Figure 10.2) which will contain the specimen. It is usually easy to identify leakage and locate that particular package, and the system avoids the sample becoming separated from the form and being mislaid.

Sample containers

Sample containers must be supplied for clotted blood and anti-coagulated specimens. Most laboratories prefer a screw-top container rather than the stopper variety since this avoids the production of aerosols. It is important to ensure that they do not leak even when subjected to rigorous testing. Some containers need to be opened and mixed more than once in the laboratory, and under these circumstances it can be difficult to prevent seepage around the cap. Also available are evacuated blood tube-collection systems in which venous blood is drawn under vacuum directly into the appropriate tube, thus avoiding the distribution of blood from a syringe and reducing the risk of infection to the phlebotomist.

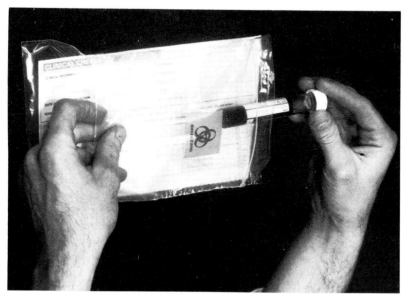

Figure 10.1 Double pocket plastic bag

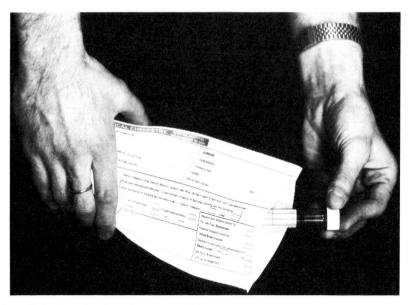

Figure 10.2 Preprinted envelope request forms

In the United Kingdom some containers have 'Kite Marked Approval' which is an indication that they have passed the standards set down by the British Standards Institute (Figure 10.3).

Urine

Similar standards must also apply to urine containers where normally a standard 25 ml screw-top Universal container is used and the 24 h urine collection bottle. The latter presents a number of problems since it must be used for collection by both sexes, and be used on wards, but perhaps more importantly for urine collection by patients at home. This may necessitate carrying 1.5 litres of urine safely back to the laboratory. Quite often the bottles are distributed containing chemicals for the preservation of the urine which are potentially harmful, e.g. hydrochloric acid.

At the very least the bottle must be leakproof. Can it be inverted without leaking fluid? It should also have a carrying handle. There are a number of containers which incorporate features such as a funnel and re-sealing devices that claim to be completely safe and free from leakage, but the presence of different designs would suggest that no-one has yet found the complete answer.

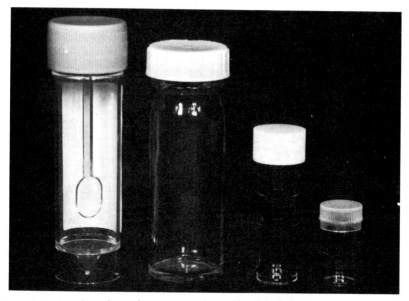

Figure 10.3 A variety of containers commonly used in clinical chemistry

Faeces

The collection of faeces may require collection of all stools passed over 3 or up to 5 days. This is usual for fat analyses and may be accommodated using a robust polythene bag inserted inside a plastic tub (Figure 10.4) such that the patient may pass the specimen directly into the container. A single sample of faeces, for say, occult blood or porphyrin analysis, may be achieved by a small plastic tube incorporating a plastic spatula.

All containers must be leakproof and whilst they must be capable of being handled safely by the laboratory, their ease of use by doctors, nurses and patients is also important.

Specimen reception

It is necessary for this area to be separate from the routine analytical work of the laboratory to reduce the possible spread of infection from particular specimens to all members of the laboratory.

The working surfaces should be of an impervious material and capable of being washed daily with disinfectant. Space must be available for siting centrifuges, a wash-hand basin and laboratory sink. There should be refrigerator facilities for the storage of specimens at 4 °C and a deep-freeze for some specimens at –20 °C. There must be adequate bench space to carry out a variety of paper work as well as serum/plasma separation, since it is

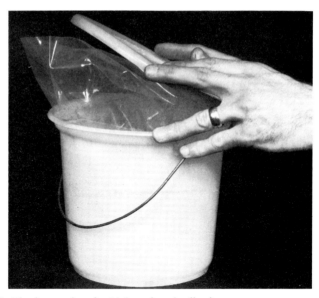

Figure 10.4 Plastic container for 24–hour faecal collection

necessary for most laboratories to pack up some samples prior to despatch to other laboratories for certain analyses.

The separation of serum from blood clots used to be performed using a teat and glass Pasteur pipette, but this has been superseded by an all-in-one plastic disposable device (Figure 10.5). This avoids the difficulty of washing and/or disposal of an awkward piece of glassware which can be prone to breakage. The introduction of this device has reduced, considerably, the number of cut fingers and it can, of course, be used for other types of separation.

The centrifuge chosen for serum/plasma separation should have an internal windshield or better still sealed buckets (Figure 10.6). This will prevent the spread of aerosol from the centrifuge, during operation, into the surrounding atmosphere. All tubes should be centrifuged with caps in place, but even in these circumstances it is still possible to observe marks around the internal rim indicating leakage of specimen. It is, therefore, necessary to clean all centrifuges, at least weekly, to reduce contamination and afford regular inspection. Glutaraldehyde may be used, but not bleach since it is corrosive to certain metals.

The centrifuge may undergo excessive usage in this area and regular servicing by the manufacturer at 6-monthly intervals is essential to avoid mechanical stress and possible serious accidents.

Since the staff working in this area come into contact with all blood specimens, they are exposed to the greatest risk of infection from potentially hazardous specimens. As in any other area of the laboratory, cuts and abrasions must be covered and some laboratories insist that gloves be worn at all times in this area. This can be difficult to achieve in practice, and much depends on the quality of the gloves in use and the ability to change them at frequent intervals.

The department must have a recognized policy for the handling of hazardous specimens and this is referred to elsewhere. Samples from any patient may be hazardous since the medical staff may be unaware of an underlying clinical disorder.

It can be quite common for some departments to centrifuge and separate over 300 blood samples a day. There can be a tendency to regard blood as just another 'substance' which may lead to a casual approach. Staff must be educated to treat all patient specimens with caution. Any spillages should be wiped up with disinfectant immediately, and close attention given to personal hygiene such as frequent washing of the hands.

If all specimens are received in this area much responsibility rests on the shoulders of the staff involved. The use of computers to document and record the tests required has eased some of the administrative work of this area. Nevertheless, one must ensure that safety protocols are adhered to, in order to avoid problems which may spread to the rest of the laboratory.

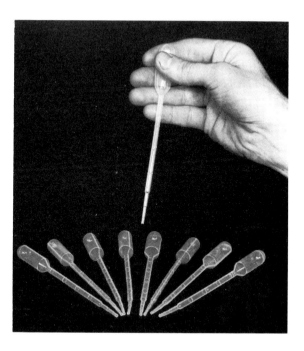

Figure 10.5 Disposable plastic pipette

197

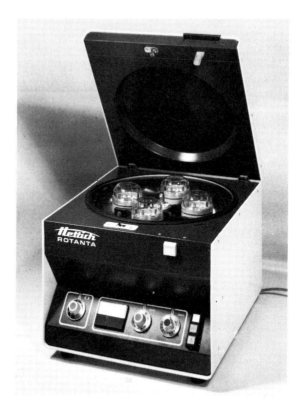

Figure 10.6 Centrifuge fitted with sealed buckets (courtesy A.R. Horwell)

The handling of high-risk specimens

It is not unusual for a department to receive 200 blood specimens a day on which 2000 different analyses may be performed involving 10 different people. This illustrates the nature of the problem in avoiding transmission of infective agents to laboratory staff.

In 1969–1970 there was an outbreak of hepatitis in the Renal Unit of the Edinburgh Royal Infirmary which resulted in 11 deaths. This included clinical and laboratory staff as well as patients.

This tragic occurrence resulted in a thorough appraisal of the handling of high risk specimens in every laboratory. The incident probably led to a serious examination of all aspects of safety in the clinical laboratory.

In 1972, *Safety in Pathology Laboratories* was published, there followed a report under the chairmanship of Lord Rosenheim in 1972, which was specifically related to hepatitis and the treatment of chronic renal failure. It was apparent, however, that apart from the clinical areas, it was not always possible to identify high risk specimens without subsequent testing in the laboratory. In 1978 the *Howie Report* was published which proposed Codes of Practice for the prevention of infection in clinical laboratories.

It would be inappropriate to reiterate the contents of these detailed reports, but they were extremely valuable in providing information and advice in the handling of human biological material.

It is now nearly 20 years since the Edinburgh outbreak and many of the proposals in the publication were adopted. Attitudes changed to regarding *all* specimens as potentially hazardous with particular attention on those with a known risk.

There are those who believe that although the incidence of hepatitis has dropped sharply – no case of laboratory-acquired hepatitis was reported in 1979 – the evidence to support the extensive and sometimes expensive precautions taken was not entirely substantiated. For example, it was once thought the aerosols generated by specimens could be infectious but as Grist[1] points out, there is no evidence to support this.

AIDS specimens

In September 1981, a review by Howie dealt with the implementation and adaptation of the Howie Report. Since then, another major hazard has appeared which poses a serious threat, namely, Acquired Immune Deficiency Syndrome (AIDS). The AIDS virus is less easily transmitted than Hepatitis B to staff who are unfortunate enough to receive accidental inoculation injuries. The consequence for those who become infected is very serious, although not all will develop AIDS which, to date, has invariably proved to be a fatal disease. The risk of acquiring the virus from handling samples from patients with AIDS *are virtually zero* when Hepatitis B precautions are carried out[2]. Many laboratories have adopted an increased level of safety by treating all specimens as 'high risk' since AIDS may be undiagnosed and unsuspected in some patients. This is particularly relevant in epidemic areas and where large numbers of specimens are received from high risk groups such as drug addicts.

Inactivation of AIDS specimens – The addition of β-propiolactone (BPL) to body fluids, giving a final concentration of 0.25%, has been shown to inactivate the virus. Such treatment can significantly interfere with laboratory analyses although, in the case of blood, this can be minimized by treatment of serum/plasma after separation rather than addition to whole blood. It is important for each laboratory to establish the degree of interference in its own methodologies. For example, the treatment of serum interferes with the enzymatic measurement of paracetamol. A further problem is the suspected carcinogenic properties of BPL.

Heat treatment of specimens at 56 °C for 30 minutes has been shown to reduce the infectivity of AIDS specimens to undetectable levels, although experiments on specimens with high titres has shown that infectivity was still detectable. The use of inactivation procedures will depend upon the type of instruments being used. Some equipment affords better separation between specimens than others. Difficulties remain, however, with instruments such as blood gas analysers and their decontamination. Some centres have set aside specific equipment for high risk specimens.

The spread of AIDS has generated alarm and controversy. It was perhaps fortunate that laboratories were compelled to take stricter safety measures following the hepatitis outbreak in the 1970s. As a result they were better prepared for the AIDS problem.

The publications referred to are detailed and contain much information. The revised guidelines in relation to AIDS is particularly helpful. A short series of general recommendations to avoid accidental infection from all laboratory specimens, are listed below:

1. Avoid cuts from glassware and needles;
2. Avoid breakages and contaminating leakages, particularly in association with equipment;
3. Minimize contamination by working tidily, carefully and cleanly;
4. Protect the skin from contamination by using disposable gloves. Any skin abrasions must always remain covered;
5. Clean up working surfaces frequently with disinfectants; and
6. Regard all specimens as potentially hazardous.

Handling semen and sputum

It is very rare for this type of specimen to be used in a routine clinical chemistry laboratory. There is a potential risk of infection from both of them, and the level of risk could depend upon clinical information available from the patient. This may result in a decision to handle the specimens in a safety cabinet. The latter is not standard equipment in clinical chemistry and the advice of the microbiology department should be sought.

Fresh semen, although initially viscous becomes less so on standing, and pipetting should not present a problem. Sputum, however, is always mucoid, sometimes stained with pus and virtually impossible to pipette. One answer is high speed centrifugation at 50 000 **g** when the resultant supernatant can be pipetted.

Storage for subsequent testing will depend on the analyses to be undertaken which, for enzymes, may necessitate a temperature of -20 °C.

ANALYTICAL EQUIPMENT

The clinical chemistry laboratory is totally reliant on instruments and machinery, much of which is complex and expensive. Most analyses are completed by using such instruments, and their situation in the laboratory depends on many factors. The decision to perform certain analyses in different areas can relate to the volume of work, the degree of urgency, the frequency of usage, and the availability of the various services required to complete the task. Instruments rely on an electrical supply, some on an industrial gas source, others may require a drain or sink in close proximity.

Electrical socket outlets should be plentiful to avoid using multi-socket adaptors. It may be necessary to have separate circuits capable of tolerating a higher than normal load as, for example, with some refrigerated centrifuges.

The department must also be able to conduct some of its work at any time of the day or night throughout the whole of the year. Hospitals are often protected against an unexpected loss of electrical supply. Internal problems may occur in old hospitals where increases in power consumption over several years are not followed by adjustments to the main switch gear. Many hospitals have a standby generator for such emergencies, and it may be possible for the laboratory to identify certain sockets and overhead lighting which would remain live under these circumstances. In the event of an accident it is essential that everyone knows the location of the mains switch isolator.

It is important that all instruments are electrically safe. Technical staff do correct minor problems with certain equipment. This may involve removal of protective panelling whilst the instrument is connected to the mains supply! Obviously this is dangerous, but instruments will often be clearly marked where certain components are live. Much equipment is imported and it is essential to ensure that it does not contravene established codes of electrical safety. It may not be apparent on cursory inspection of a piece of equipment that the instrument is switched on, unless a warning light is illuminated.

Many of the instruments used involve moving parts such as pumps, and this involves the movement and transfer of chemicals and serum which is potentially hazardous.

Continuous flow analysers

Many laboratories have continuous flow single channel and multi-channel analysers with up to four separate pumps (Figure 10.7). A variety of reagents are pumped through the instrument and there are a considerable number of interconnections which may result in leakages. Spillages must be cleaned up immediately since some reagents are strongly acid or alkaline and may cause

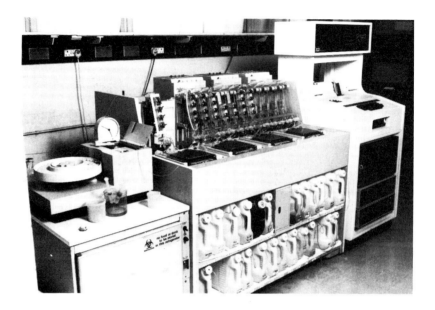

Figure 10.7   A continuous flow multi-channel analyser

burns to the fingers as well as corrosion to the instrument. Staff must be conscious of the dangers of trapping items of clothing in such moving machinery, the possibility of allowing liquid to reach electrical contacts and the spurting of liquid under pressure from a leaking tube. Whilst an on/off switch may be close by, additional assistance may be essential to avoid injury should a problem arise. There may be 25–30 different reagents being pumped through the system, all of which must be eventually led away as effluent. There is a facility on the instrument to dilute this effluent with tap water in order to reduce risk of dangerous chemical reactions (Figure 10.8).

Many different specimens of patient's sera are run through the instrument, and this is likely to include high-risk hepatitis specimens. It may not be possible to isolate such specimens and analyse them separately, but after each day's run the instrument should be washed through with distilled water, followed by a cleansing agent to kill harmful bacteria and prevent reagent and protein deposition, and again with water. The choice of a cleansing agent is not a simple one since some chemicals will adversely affect certain analytical channels particularly dialysis membranes.

In the author's laboratory we pump molar sodium hydroxide through reagent and sample lines and have found this satisfactory. In other laboratories proprietary detergents are used and 1% sodium hydrochloride solution.

All continuous-flow analysers require the dialyser membrane to be

202

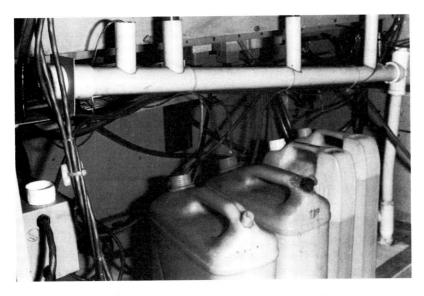

Figure 10.8 Rear view of multi-channel analyser showing waste pipe. Tap water is continuously fed down the length of pipe

changed at intervals. The membrane should be discarded carefully, wearing gloves, into an autoclavable bag to avoid risk of infection.

In recent years, there has been a move away from this type of instrumentation to a more discretionary approach, an example being centrifugal analysers. The main dangers are probably the moving arms of sample pick-up and delivery systems with risk of fingers getting in the way.

The most commonly occurring instruments in clinical chemistry laboratories are those which measure light absorption in a variety of solutions. They vary in their degree of sophistication, but are usually of robust construction and unlikely to lead to problems in that their circuitry is usually well protected from spillage of solutions.

Electrophoresis tanks are another example where, although the voltage may be small, they involve the use of buffer solutions in conjunction with electrical currents so it is helpful to have safeguards which avoid receiving any electrical shock.

Another commonly used piece of equipment is the *flame emission photometer* for measuring sodium and potassium in body fluids. It is used frequently, routinely and urgently day and night, requires a gas supply which is commonly propane and compressed air, and usually has a pump to dilute specimens. Gases should be piped to the instrument from a protected external location. This can be expensive, particularly in older buildings and may mean reduced flexibility in the siting of the instrument. The cost of piping-in of gases may be prohibitive which may necessitate the use of gas cylinders within the laboratory. It is important that they are accessible, but sited away from sources of heat (e.g. radiators). After using the equipment, the gas supply should be turned off at the main cylinder valve. It is possible to switch off the flame photometer which automatically cuts off the propane supply to the burner. There is, however, a risk of failure or leakage in the various regulators and filter devices which occur after the main cylinder.

The equipment mentioned is certainly not exhaustive, but all manufacturers must make clear in their instrument manual where safety precautions must be taken. Instrument manuals should be available to all staff and not locked away for safety!

Major instrument manufacturers offer service contracts of various kinds. The kind of contract undertaken will depend on a number of factors such as its importance in maintaining an analytical service, the degree of complexity, the potential for recurring problems and the replacement of components. For some apparatus, it may be adequate to ensure that insulation of electrical wiring and visual inspection is adequate. But for major items of equipment, particularly those with moving parts or involving the use of inflammable gases, they should be inspected at least annually by the manufacturer and any defects remedied.

Some simple servicing is possible by laboratory staff, and they should be encouraged to visually inspect equipment for signs of wear and keep it free from dirt and reagent contamination.

THE USE OF RADIOACTIVE SUBSTANCES

There can be a wide variety of diagnostic tests using radioactive substances within the hospital. Some of these involve the administration of such substances to patients, but this work is often undertaken outside the laboratory.

Radioactive isotopes are used to measure the concentration of various hormones and proteins in the blood using a technique called radioimmunoassay. This involves labelling, for example, a hormone with ^{125}I. The latter is added to the patient's serum which contains the unlabelled hormone. The addition of a specific antibody which will combine with both forms and subsequent separation of the free-from the antibody-bound fraction, enables the concentration of hormones in the patient's serum to be quantified.

There are a number of kits available which provide all the materials necessary to make the technique simple to perform. The activity of ^{125}I used will be low. For example, this laboratory performs approximately 1200 thyroid tests a month and the total activity of ^{125}I does not exceed $200\,\mu\text{Ci}$.

Where tests are performed under such circumstances it is still important to maintain good working practices associated with the use of radioactive isotopes.

The radioactive material must not be inhaled or come into contact with the body in any way. This will involve the use of safe pipetting devices, trays to contain spillages, gloves and other protective clothing. It is sufficient to perform such analyses on the laboratory benches, with non-absorbent tops or disposable covers, but the area where radioisotopes are used must be clearly defined and set aside specifically for that purpose. The floor of the area must also be covered with impervious material.

Items such as protective clothing and apparatus should be used only in this area and not circulated through the laboratory.

Some laboratories may carry out labelling of proteins previously referred to. If ^{125}I is used, this will mean the purchase of concentrated sodium iodide at say 100 mCi/ml the labelling procedure commonly uses 1 mCi/10 μl.

The limit of intake set by the International Commission on Radiological Protection is 54 μCi by inhalation which is contained in 0.5 ml of this solution, and 27 μCi by ingestion. The handling of such activities represents a much higher risk and consequently a fume cupboard must be used since it is the dose received which may cause harm. There are well recognized precautions which must be taken to reduce the risk. They are, lead shielding, increasing the distance between the radioactive source and the operator, and minimizing the time taken to complete the procedure.

There are other radioactive substances which may be used in clinical chemistry departments, particularly if it is involved in research. In these circumstances it is essential to contact the local radiation protection officer who can advise on the appropriate methods of handling different radioactive substances. In most hospitals all radioactive substances must be ordered and received through a designated radiation protection officer such that the range of incoming radioactive substances can be monitored.

An incident was reported where americium-241 in acid solution was stored for a long period of time in a cupboard. It was subsequently discovered to have 'disappeared' by leakage. This isotope has a long half-life and is classified as highly toxic. Contamination was widespread in the laboratory and was detected in some of the homes of people who worked there. Such an event might not have occurred if the ordering system had been appropriately monitored, and adequate records kept.

The precautions necessary in this particular area are not detailed here since they are referred to elsewhere in this book. There are also many excellent publications to guide all grades of staff in the use of radioactive isotopes.

The radiation protection officer has already been referred to, and in the United Kingdom there are established Regional Radiation Protection Services to control, monitor and issue guidelines on the use of radioactive substances. Their help is invaluable on all aspects, from setting up a new laboratory, drawing up local rules and the choice of an appropriate contamination monitor, all of which can save time and money. Consultation should be established at an early stage since they will inspect the premises at intervals to ensure that nationally agreed codes of practice are upheld.

EMERGENCY WORK OUT OF NORMAL LABORATORY HOURS

It is necessary for most departments to perform analyses outside the usual working hours of 9.00 a.m. – 5.00 p.m., Monday to Friday. This can also occur on public holidays and usually means that one person may be working alone in the laboratory. Under these circumstances it is necessary to assess what risks there are to staff when performing certain analyses, since assistance will not be immediately available should an accident occur. It may be necessary to adjust the type of method used under these circumstances, or even question whether the analysis is necessary at that time. The situation is often made more difficult since many laboratories may be some distance from ward areas in the hospital if emergency assistance is necessary.

The analysis of paracetamol in serum is often conducted out of normal hours. One method involves evaporation of inflammable solvent whilst another avoids this entirely. It is arguable that, although the latter may not be as accurate, its precision is satisfactory and it avoids the risk of fire. Where it is necessary to perform techniques with similar risks while working alone, staff should be experienced in good laboratory practice and be clearly instructed in the correct technique. They should also be aware of what steps to take in the event of an accident. Such staff involved should have had experience or at least have seen the operation of a carbon dioxide fire extinguisher, since it can be alarming when used for the first time.

As in any other laboratory, the provision of first aid boxes, eye wash stations, and instructions is essential. Different countries have statutory requirements as to the contents of the box and careful thought must be given to its location. The degree of first aid applied in the department will vary according to the hazards involved and the proximity of expert attention. In some hospitals it is mandatory for every accident, however slight, to be treated in the Accident and Emergency Department, and reported.

At the very least, cyanide antidote and dressings to cover minor cuts and abrasions must be available. In the event of a serious incident or accident the first duty of any person is the preservation of life.

WASTE DISPOSAL

Any chemical laboratory has a wide variety of waste substances which necessitate separation into different categories. The clinical chemistry department must incorporate such procedures, and in addition make provision for the disposal of all biological specimens.

The responsibilities of ensuring safe handling of waste does not end once it has left the department, and the department has a duty to ensure safe handling by all those who may come into contact with such material.

Chemical waste

This may be generated from analytical work and be an end-product of a particular technique. Most analytical techniques in clinical chemistry are conducted on a small scale such that the volumes of waste generated rarely exceed a litre.

The types of chemical waste may vary considerably, and the route by which they are disposed of must be considered carefully. Different countries will adopt varying legislation and controls which may be monitored by a local authority. Since the volumes of most acids and alkalis generated are not excessive it may be appropriate to dispose of them separately and with plentiful dilution down the drain. Where volumes are excessive it may be necessary to enlist the help of a contractor or authority with the appropriate means to dispose of the material safely.

The drainage system of the laboratory must be constructed with some thought to the chemicals likely to be used in the department. It would not be possible to give space to all the chemicals used, but mention is made of those which are commonly used in most diagnostic laboratories and which carry some risk.

Picric acid

Used as a saturated solution in water for the analysis of creatinine. Picric acid is known to be explosive when dry and, hence, care must be taken to ensure adequate flushing of any waste material.

Toluene

Used as a solvent base in liquid scintillation counting processes to measure certain radioisotopes. Toluene is highly flammable, has a harmful vapour and if it is contaminated with other chemicals, including radioisotopes, advice should be sought from the local authority as to the appropriate means of disposal. It may be possible to burn off the toluene is suitably controlled conditions.

Diethylamine

Used in the analysis of calcium in continuous-flow systems where it usually contains a small quantity of sodium cyanide. The reagent has a strongly ammoniacal vapour which is irritating to the skin, eyes and respiratory system. Since it contains cyanide the reagent must, under no circumstances, come into contact with acid since this can result in the release of hydrogen cyanide which is extremely poisonous. It is usual to ensure that the waste is diluted with water.

An accident occurred in the author's laboratory which resulted in the spillage of 2 litres of diethylamine. This necessitated evacuation of the laboratory, but it was not realized until the area was cleared, that diethylamine is also extremely inflammable and the accident had occurred immediately adjacent to water distillation units. This drew our attention to the need for, and reference to, a descriptive compendium of chemicals to ensure that one is aware of all possible harmful effects.

Phosphoric acid/sulphuric acid

These chemicals are used in conjunction with ferric chloride in the analysis of urea on continuous-flow systems. Again the waste should be diluted with water. This method, and that of calcium and creatinine previously mentioned, are often run together in large multi-channel analysers. There is, therefore, an increased risk of an inappropriate mixing of these reagents unless appropriate precautions to dilute them are taken.

Diethyl ether

Used in a variety of extractions such as porphyrin analysis, faecal fat and chromatographic methods. The reputation of ether in terms of its inflammability is well known to most laboratory workers. Some may not be aware of its ability to form explosive peroxides on exposure to light.

It is unusual to see a naked flame in a clinical chemistry laboratory, but staff may be blissfully unaware of a flame photometer in use near an ether extraction test.

Disposal of biological waste

This will consist of patients' samples which may be in glass or plastic containers. It may be whole blood, serum or plasma, urine, faeces and other fluids such as pleural aspirate and cerebral spinal fluid.

The need to treat all biological material with caution has been stressed elsewhere. The manner of disposal may depend, to some extent, on the volume of fluid involved and its container.

Whole blood

Clinical chemistry departments conduct analyses on large numbers of serum or plasma specimens separated from blood which has been collected in glass or plastic tubes. This could mean a total of at least 300 blood tubes per day. Also, there may be several tubes of anticoagulated blood.

It appears to be common practice to treat such containers as 'disposable'; that is, they are used only once before being thrown away.

All such specimens should leave the department in readily identifiable bags as being infective, and be incinerated. Some hospital sites may not possess incineration facilities and, even if they do, it is necessary to ensure that the incinerator has the capability of handling glass and plastic.

Any transportation to a distant site must ensure that such containers are carried safely and not mixed with general rubbish. Local authorities may assume responsibility for the movement of waste from the site and its disposal, but again the laboratory must ensure that such samples will be incinerated. Incidents have been reported in the United Kingdom of children discovering blood specimens on refuse tips. It has been the policy in this hospital that all such specimens are autoclaved before transport from the site to avoid infectious hazards in the event of leakages.

Whilst it is possible to re-use such tubes, emptying and cleaning is a difficult and unpleasant job with the attendant risk of infection.

Serum or plasma

Serum or plasma is stored prior to analysis in a variety of containers which may be glass or plastic. It is often convenient to use containers which can be inserted directly onto a piece of equipment.

When no longer required they should be placed in a plastic bag set aside for the purpose. Autoanalyser cups may be disposed of in this way without their original capping device. Since the volume of serum left over might be 0.5 ml and 500 can be used in a single day, the bag must be sufficiently leak-proof to retain, say, 200 ml of patients' serum. Such bags should be removed from the laboratory daily and incinerated.

Glass containers used in this way can be treated similarly, but there is a greater risk of breakage with consequent puncturing of the bag and, hence, leakage. Therefore, a greater degree of care is necessary during transportation to the incineration site.

Urine

The laboratory may receive urine specimens in the traditional 25 ml screw-top universal container. After analysis they may be disposed of in a manner similar to that described for serum or plasma.

Other urine specimens sent to the laboratory are the outputs from 24 hour collections. The volume of the collection may vary from 300 to 3000 ml, although the average volume is about 1200 ml.

The urine should be disposed of, wearing gloves, via a sluice which can be flushed with water. Laboratory sinks must not be used or staff/patient toilets. The containers must be disinfected before re-issuing.

Faeces

A portion of the faecal specimen may be sent in a screw-top container for some analyses. This may be disposed of by incineration.

Other faecal analyses require all faeces passed to be sent to the laboratory for analysis. This may result in the disposal of several litres of liquid faeces which should be poured down a sluice, whilst wearing gloves, additional protective clothing and possibly a face mask.

It is desirable to use disposable containers for handling faecal material which can subsequently be incinerated.

The laboratory may receive other biological fluids for testing, but most of them can be disposed of in the ways just described.

The use of disposables considerably reduces any infectious hazards to washing-up staff, but the need to prevent spillages and ensure safe handling prior to disposal are paramount.

Disposal of glass and sharps

Broken glassware must be segregated from other waste and placed into clearly identifiable containers. Before disposal one should attempt to ensure that it carries no risk of infection or is contaminated with dangerous chemicals.

'Sharps', such as syringe needles and blood lancets for capillary blood samples must be disposed of in separate containers which are resistant to puncturing. Containers can be purchased specifically for the purpose (Figure 10.9), but it may be possible to use cardboard boxes which have been used for deliveries to the hospital. Prior to disposal they must be sealed and a label fixed to the outside clearly indicating that the contents are medical sharps.

A variety of waste will leave the clinical chemistry laboratory, much of it

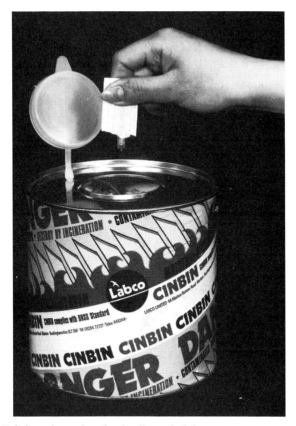

Figure 10.9 Reinforced container for the disposal of sharps

potentially infective. It is an advantage if all infective or potentially infective material is incinerated on the hospital site. Different types of waste should be segregated, and it is the duty of the laboratory to ensure that transport of the waste from the department is conducted safely.

Disinfectants

Although many of the items used in the laboratory will be 'disposable' there will be containers, apparatus and areas of the laboratory which must be free of bacterial or viral contamination.

Hypochlorite

A disinfectant widely used in the laboratory. Solutions of 10 g/l are said to be effective against bacteria, but solutions rapidly lose their 'free chlorine' and should be prepared daily from concentrated stock solutions. Since it is corrosive to some metals it should not be used on items such as centrifuges.

Glutaraldehyde

This is effective against viruses at a concentration of 20 g/l and is non-corrosive to metals. It may be used to disinfect autoanalyser modules but some staff find the vapour irritating.

LEGISLATION

Since the introduction in the United Kingdom of the *Health and Safety at Work Act 1974*, which was applicable to government agencies as well as private industry, much attention has been focused on all aspects of safety.

Visits by the Health and Safety Inspectorate, which were formerly confined to factories and offices, have now been broadened to include hospitals. In the event of serious deficiencies an 'Improvement Notice' may be served on a hospital to correct such deficiencies within an agreed time limit.

Much of the health and safety legislation is concerned with the words 'as far as reasonably practicable'. This may be interpreted in terms of a risk/cost ratio. That is, if a particular hazard in the laboratory is considered to be small and the cost of correcting it high, it should receive a low priority.

Money to support building alterations, even of a minor nature, is difficult to obtain so the laboratory must clarify its priorities for such safety improvements very carefully. The visiting Health and Safety Inspectorate can be very helpful in arriving at an agreed programme.

POLICIES, PEOPLE, PROTECTION, PUBLICITY

In spite of stringent policies and codes of operating, accidents do happen in the most safety-conscious of laboratories.

Such accidents are usually a result of human fallibility. Safe-working must depend on the attitudes adopted by every member of staff. Failure of the Head of Department to foster safe-working practices will quickly lead to indifference by other staff. The staff of a clinical chemistry department may vary widely in its experience, but the research worker of long standing must demonstrate to junior colleagues a regard for safety awareness.

Where the turnover of staff is high, this may pose greater problems due to inexperience. But in a laboratory where there is a stable staffing situation another problem arises – that of complacency.

It is difficult for many of us to be enthusiastic about safety. We all need reminders, for example, a fire lecture at least once a year, the display of posters around the laboratory reminding one of the possible dangers. It can be a salutary experience, but a helpful one, to be inspected by a colleague from a laboratory in another hospital who may identify problems which one has failed to notice.

Despite all the measures taken, regrettably an incident or near-miss is often necessary to re-emphasize the need for safety vigilance.

The safety problems pertinent to clinical chemistry are largely related to the handling of biological material whose degree of infectivity may be unknown. Such hazards are not visible and specimens may come to be regarded as 'just another fluid'. The encouragement of high standards of personal hygiene in the individual and tidiness in the workplace will do much to reduce laboratory accidents and dangers from infection.

References

1. Grist, N.R. (1981). Hepatitis infection in clinical chemistry. *Med. Lab. Staff Sci.*, **38**, 103-9
2. Geddes, A.M. (1986). Editorial: Risks of AIDS to health care workers. *Br. Med. J.*, **292**, 711-12

Bibliography

DHSS (1972). Safety in Pathology Laboratories. (London: HMSO)

DHSS. Hepatitis and the Treatment of Chronic Renal Failure. *Report of the Advisory Group 1970-72.* (London: HMSO)

DHSS (1978). Code of Practice for the Prevention of Infection in Clinical Laboratories and Post-Mortem Rooms. (London: HMSO)

DHSS (1981). Code of Practice for the Prevention of Infection in Clinical Laboratories and Post-Mortem Rooms. Bulletin No. 2. (London: HMSO)

Report (1972). Code of Practice for the Protection of Persons against Ionizing Radiations arising from Medical and Dental Use. (London: HMSO)

DHSS (1986). LAV/HTLV III – The Causative Agent of AIDS and Related Conditions – Revised Guidelines. (London: HMSO)

Report (1986). Safety in Health Service Laboratories: The Labelling, Transport and Reception of Specimens. (London: HMSO)

11 Safety Precautions in a Clinical Cytogenetics Laboratory

B. Czepulkowski

INTRODUCTION

Clinical cytogenetics has advanced considerably over the past decade and is moving ever closer to the rapidly developing field of recombinant DNA technology. DNA laboratories are currently being integrated into some existing cytogenetic departments and the training of laboratory workers now includes both disciplines. The DNA work is normally allocated space and personnel of its own, though there may be some rotation of staff for training purposes. Thus, the safety procedures in this part of the laboratory will differ from and extend beyond those in the cytogenetic section. However, health and safety procedures for the recombinant DNA technologist merit more attention than is appropriate in this chapter on cytogenetics. We have, therefore, confined our attentions to the 'pure' diagnostic cytogenetic laboratory.

SPECIMENS DEALT WITH IN A CYTOGENETIC LABORATORY – THE POTENTIAL RISKS

It is hoped that clinics will make every possible effort to inform the laboratory of any risks that may be associated with the samples they send. This information should be made clear on the request form, and the sample labelled with the appropriate hazard warning sticker so that the laboratory can process it in accordance with the regulations relating to the particular pathogen involved. In practice, however, it should not be assumed that in the absence of such warning a specimen is without risk.

Samples from the following patients constitute the highest risks that are likely to confront the cytogeneticist, and these should always be dealt with by experienced staff in accordance with the strictest precautions:

1. Intravenous drug abusers. These are in high risk groups for both HIV and HB_sAg;
2. Homosexual and bisexual men. At risk for HIV;
3. Haemophiliacs. At risk for HIV;
4. Persons who have returned from sub-Sahara Africa during the last 5 years. At risk for HIV;
5. Sexual partners and babies of the above. At risk for HIV;
6. Patients who are Australia antigen positive;
7. Down's syndrome patients who are institutionalized. At risk for HB_sAg due to immunosuppression;
8. Other immunosuppressed patients. At risk for HB_sAg;
9. Unscreened patients from renal units. At risk for HB_sAg;
10. Patients with suspected infective diseases of the liver. At risk for HB_sAg; and
11. Babies with diarrhoea and vomiting. May be due to virulent pathogen.

The pathological specimens dealt with by most cytogenetic laboratories include blood, amniotic fluid, abortus material, chorionic villi, skin biopsy and some post-mortem material, mostly from babies. Some laboratories also process bone marrow, buccal smears, tumours, testicular biopsies, spleen, lymph nodes and pleural effusions. Specimens sent for chromosome investigation are all potentially infective since they are received unfixed. Not all tissues, however, carry the same degree of risk.

Blood

Blood is a major source of potential infection. It is a particularly efficient transmitter of many pathogens, especially HB_sAg and HIV. All blood specimens, including separated blood, should be handled with particular caution.

Bone marrow and leukaemic blood

Granulocytopenia due either to the leukaemia itself or as a result of cytotoxic therapy is the most important factor increasing the risk of infection to these patients. Fungal and bacterial infections are those most commonly observed. Furthermore, damage to natural barriers from cytotoxic therapy, and invasive procedures carried out to aid diagnosis and administer treatment can produce routes for infection. Immunological impairment also occurs due to the effects of drugs or disease.

Over half of the documented infection in patients with leukaemia are due to hospital-acquired organisms. Virus infections rarely occur in patients with neutropenia. Herpes simplex, disseminated herpes zoster, severe herpes virus pneumonia, and cytomegalovirus infection are also a major problem in transplantation patients.

The leukaemic patient may be transfused with blood products. Although these are now screened for the presence of HIV, the risks presented by these patients as a result of transfusion should be regarded as similar to the situation for haemophiliacs.

Epstein–Barr Virus

The supernatant from an Epstein–Barr Virus (EBV) producing cell line B95–8 is utilized in B–cell malignancies and for transforming lymphoblastic cell lines. It is a tumour promoter. Filtration is required prior to use, and this must be done under the strictest safety conditions. A class 1 safety cabinet must be used for all cultures which have been in contact with EBV.

Amniotic fluid

Some amniotic fluid specimens may be contaminated with maternal blood, and these carry the same risks as blood specimens. It is important to remember that some specimens may not be obviously bloodstained, but after centrifugation will show a small amount of blood in the pellet. For this reason, uncentrifuged amniotic fluid should be treated as potentially bloodstained and the appropriate precautions taken. Apart from this, there is little risk of infection from an uncontaminated amniotic fluid specimen.

Chorionic villus samples (CVS)

CVS samples are nearly always contaminated with maternal blood. In addition, there is a small risk that contaminants from the cervix and vagina may be present.

Abortus material and stillbirths

The main risks of infection from this type of specimen are due to contact with maternal blood and body fluids. In some cases, spontaneous abortions may have occurred as a result of infection in the fetus, which may in turn present a risk of infection to the laboratory worker. Examples of such infections are syphilis, toxoplasmosis, cytomegalovirus, herpes simplex type II, rubella, rubeola. For this reason, all products of conception should be treated with particular caution.

Skin biopsy, testicular biopsy, and post-mortem tissues

All of these tissues have been in contact with blood and other body fluids and are, therefore, capable of transmitting many pathogens, especially if the patient has died of an infection. However, since most of these samples (apart from testicular biopsy) will have come from babies, such material is a comparatively minor risk in the cytogenetic laboratory.

Lymph nodes, effusions, tumours, thymus, spleen

Contact with any malignant tissues requires stringent handling procedures. The aetiology of most malignancies is as yet unknown. However the isolation of human T-cell–lymphoma–leukaemia virus (HTLV) from patients with T-cell leukaemia, sezary cell leukaemia and mycosis fungoides is the most direct evidence of a possible viral causation of human leukaemia. It should be borne in mind that vectors of malignant diseases may be present, but as yet undiscovered, and extreme caution should be exercised when handling potentially malignant material.

Pleural effusions carry a high risk of tuberculosis, and should be handled with extreme caution by experienced staff who have a positive Mantoux reaction.

Buccal smears

Unfixed buccal smears are potentially capable of transmitting infections, especially when these cells have been in contact with infected sputum, but are of comparatively minor risk. This is the only type of sample that can be transported to the cytogenetic laboratory already fixed, and clinics should be provided with the appropriate fixative for this purpose.

THE COLLECTION, PACKAGING AND TRANSPORT OF SPECIMENS

The collection of specimens for chromosome analysis is normally performed by clinicians, nursing staff or phlebotomists, on whom the cytogeneticist relies to take reasonable precautions to protect himself from the risk of infection from the sample. It is, therefore, advisable that the laboratory should supply clinics and wards dealing with cytogenetic specimens with a concise protocol which should be regularly updated and shown to new members of staff. It would be advantageous, where possible, to encourage clinics to follow the procedure by supplying them with suitable containers, plastic bags and boxes which will help them to remember to use these items. When devising a protocol, the following points should be considered.

Containers

The use of plastic containers instead of glass for fluid specimens eliminates one of the most dangerous situations: that of broken glass contaminated with potentially infective material. Virtually all pathogens can be introduced through a wound. Most laboratories have now adopted the use of plastic containers.

Specimen containers should be leak-proof, easy to open and close securely without danger of infecting the operator. Snap-on plug closures should be avoided as these produce a fine spray when opened. It is important to use containers which have a cap that does not trap part of the specimen between itself and the wall of the container. If a screw-cap is used, the thread should be on the outside of the neck of the container.

There are several designs of heparinized tube commercially available for the collection of blood samples, suitable for cytogenetics. We would recommend the use of plastic screw-capped vessels and the avoidance of glass tubes with rubber bungs or snap-on plugs. Standard plastic screw-capped Universal containers are adequate for most other fluid samples. It is a good idea to seal the rim of these containers with parafilm if the sample is to be transported any distance.

Many cytogenetic laboratories receive entire fetuses from late abortions. These are best transported in the sweet 'jar' type of container or in a plastic bucket-style container such as in Figure 10.4.

Packaging

1. All containers should be transported in a sealed, leak-proof bag; this is of particular importance when the specimen is fluid. Any leakage while in transit will be contained, thereby preventing potentially infective material from penetrating the outer packaging and exposing non-laboratory staff to the risk of infection.

219

2.   When two or more specimens are to be sent in the same box, they should be sealed in separate plastic bags to prevent any cross-contamination.
3.   Specimens in plastic bags should be packed in a strong box and padded tightly with absorbent material such as cellulose wadding or absorbent cotton wool. The box should be securely fastened, and preferably wrapped in a stout envelope or padded bag.
4.   Hazard warning labels must be used where appropriate.

Request forms

Clinical staff should be asked to fill in request forms either before taking the specimen or after washing their hands having already taken the sample. This avoids contamination of request forms with potentially infective material. Similarly, specimen containers should not be handled when a sample is being taken. If possible, the labelling of containers and completing of request forms should be done beforehand, or by a colleague.

Request forms should never be put into the plastic bag with the specimen, or stapled to it, as these will become contaminated if the specimen should leak. Plastic bags designed to hold the form in a separate compartment are available commercially (as illustrated in Figure 10.1) and these could be supplied to clinics with the containers and forms.

Clinics must always be informed immediately if a specimen arrives wrongly or badly packaged, and every effort should be made to correct the mistakes of those people who habitually send material in this way.

RECEPTION OF SPECIMENS

A specimen which has been collected, packaged and transported properly should pose few problems for the recipient. The only precautions necessary in this case would be the receipt of the specimens by a trained person in a specifically allocated area of the laboratory. Specimen containers must only be opened in the appropriate safety cabinet. The following points should be considered when a specimen is received in a potentially dangerous condition.

Leakages

Laboratory coats and protective surgical gloves must always be worn when dealing with contaminated items.

Leakage contained in a plastic bag

It is a good idea to have a stock of disposable trays or similar receptacles on which leaking plastic bags and boxes can be placed inside the safety cabinet. If the entire specimen has leaked out of the container, the whole bag should be disposed of. If, however, some of the specimen has remained in the container and can be salvaged, it can be transferred into a fresh container. This is best achieved by getting a colleague to hold a new container ready so that when the leaking container is opened the remainder of the specimen can be transferred into the new container with a syringe or pipette. This avoids contamination of the new container. The bag, container, tray and gloves can then be disposed of.

Leakage not contained in plastic bag

If potentially infective material has penetrated the outer packaging, all persons likely to have been in contact with the package must be informed immediately. The sender must also be notified as soon as possible. The package should be placed on a disposable tray, opened inside the safety cabinet and treated as for a contained leakage.

Leaking involving broken glass

The glass must not be touched once the package has been opened, but disposed of in the appropriate hazardous waste container.

Specimen container contaminated with specimen

The container should be treated as for 'contained' leak and the specimen transferred to a fresh container. The old container should be disposed of safely.

Request form contaminated with specimen

Details should be copied out onto a fresh form, and the old form discarded in the appropriate hazardous waste container.

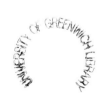

PROCESSING THE SPECIMENS

The principal ways in which unfixed pathological material can be brought into contact with the skin or mucous membranes are by:

1. The formation of aerosols and droplets;
2. Spillage and splashing;
3. Accidents involving sharp objects which may themselves be contaminated with the specimen, or which cause wounds through which pathogens may enter the body.

The reader is also referred to the section on 'Routes of infection' in Chapter 9.

Safety precautions relating to the handling of pathological material are, therefore, designed to minimise the occurrence of such situations. They should also serve to provide adequate protection to the laboratory worker should such situations occur.

Most of the procedures used to prepare a specimen for chromosome analysis involve centrifugation, removal and replacement of supernatant and other reagents, resuspension of cell pellets, mixing and then fixation, after which the specimen ceases to be an infection risk.

General precautions

1. All unfixed material must be dealt with in a microbiological safety cabinet using full aseptic technique. The different classes of microbiological safety cabinets and their uses are discussed fully in Chapter 9.

   Most specimens received in the cytogenetic laboratory can be handled in a Class 2 cabinet. However, for some higher risk specimens such as HIV or HB$_s$Ag a Class 1 cabinet should be used. *High risk material should not be dealt with by a laboratory that does not possess, or have access to, the appropriate safety cabinet.*
2. Laboratory coats and protective surgical gloves should be worn when dealing with all unfixed pathological material.
3. The hands must never be brought into contact with the eyes, nose or mouth during the handling of any biological material.
4. If it is necessary to answer the telephone, or attend to other such matters during the processing of a specimen, the gloves should be first removed and discarded. A fresh pair of gloves should be put on when processing is resumed.
5. Plastic containers, culture vessels and other utensils should be used in preference to glass, to avoid accidents involving infected broken glass.

6. Care must be taken to ensure that the tips of dispensers, wash bottles etc., are not brought into contact with the unfixed specimen or contaminated containers when adding reagents to cultures.

7. Syringes should be used without needles where possible. An example of this is the aliquoting of a blood sample from a heparinized tube to a culture vessel.

8. Replacing a contaminated needle in a sheath is extremely dangerous if done hastily. It is preferable to remove the needle from the syringe and discard it in a 'sharps' bin. If the sheath must be replaced, this should be done very carefully.

9. Centrifugation should be carried out in plastic tubes which are securely stoppered. Sealed buckets should be used, if possible, since these are more efficient than sealed rotors. The buckets should be opened in the safety cabinet if unfixed material has been centrifuged.

10. Operations requiring mechanical blending (such as mixing of blood with hypotonic solution by means of a 'Whirlimix') should be done in tightly stoppered tubes. Even mixing by hand requires tightly stoppered tubes.

11. Pouring liquid cultures and supernatants should be discouraged even if carried out in a safety cabinet. Spillage is likely to occur from time to time, especially if the operator is an inexperienced trainee.

12. If suction pumps, etc. are used for removal of supernatant (e.g. removal of hypotonic solution from blood culture), the expelled air (containing potentially infective aerosol particles) must be filtered and exhausted with the outflow from the cabinet. Most safety cabinets are designed to facilitate the incorporation of an outflow pipe from a pump into the exhaust system.

Incubation

Cultures which are grown in an 'open' system (i.e. allowing the circulation of CO_2) require that the caps of the vessel be loosened by a turn of the thread. Overfilling of these vessels should be avoided since leakage of contaminated medium can easily occur. Some designs of Leighton tube are especially prone to this, particularly if they roll over when accidentally knocked. It is good practice to stack culture vessels in racks or on trays which can be removed from the incubator and decontaminated. This prevents contamination of incubator shelves should leakage occur.

Some cytogenetic procedures require the addition of hazardous reagents during the incubation period. These are discussed in detail in a later section.

DISPOSAL OF CONTAMINATED WASTE

Every hospital or institution dealing with pathological material will have strict regulations regarding the disposal of infected or potentially infected waste, and every laboratory worker must be familiar with these procedures. The decontamination of waste pathological material is dealt with extensively in Chapter 9, and information applicable to the cytogenetic laboratory is also discussed in Chapter 10. We will not, therefore, reiterate this at great length. However, to summarize briefly:

Hypodermic syringes and scalpel blades

'Sharps' and broken glass can normally be placed in commercially available boxes or containers with imperforate, not readily penetrable, walls, which can be autoclaved and incinerated. An example is the 'Cin-Bin' illustrated in Figure 10.9.

Discarded specimens, cultures, contaminated disposables

These should be placed in metal or heat-resistant plastic containers and autoclaved before leaving the laboratory. They should then be incinerated. Large volumes of fluid may be emptied into a sink or sluice connected to the public sewer (these will be specially designated as such), or treated with a disinfectant such as hypochlorite or glutaraldehyde. If solid tissue is disinfected overnight it should be poured through a sieve over the sink so that the liquid can be washed down and the solid tissue autoclaved and incinerated.

Disinfectants

Clear phenolics should be used for most organic matter other than blood. This is suitable for disinfecting metal instruments after setting up tissues for culturing, since phenolics do not attack metal. Hypochlorites should be used for blood, including those which may be at risk for HB_sAg, but should never be used for equipment with metal parts (such as centrifuges or work surfaces of safety cabinets) since hypochlorites attack metal.

SAFETY PRECAUTIONS TO BE TAKEN WHEN HANDLING CHEMICALS AND REAGENTS

All chemicals and reagents used in the cytogenetic laboratory must be

224

handled with caution, even if there is no particular known risk associated with a specific substance. Protective clothing and gloves should be worn whenever chemicals are to be handled. Before dealing with the different chemicals commonly used in the cytogenetic laboratory, it is necessary to draw attention to the following general safety precautions.

1.   Mouth pipetting of *all* chemicals, reagents and specimens should be strictly forbidden.
2.   All chemicals and reagents should be clearly labelled and bear the relevant international standard hazard warning symbols.
3.   *Both* hands should be used when carrying large bottles containing chemicals and reagents, one hand being used to support the bottle from its base.
4.   Large bottles of chemicals should be transported in carriers specifically designed for this purpose, with one hand free to give support.
5.   When solutions are prepared in large flasks, the flask should not be held by the neck and rotated, since breakage could easily occur.
6.   Chemical solutions should never be poured from a container being held above eye level. The recipient container should be held firmly on the bench while the solution is being gently poured into it.

Corrosive chemicals – acids and alkalis

Corrosive fluids should be stored on low shelves, or preferably in an 'inflammables' store if this is appropriate. Bottles containing strong acids should be opened with extreme caution, in a fume cupboard. Protective safety spectacles should also be worn while dealing with these corrosive substances. Since an exothermic reaction occurs when water is added to strong acid, dilutions must only be produced by adding measured amounts of the acid to the water slowly, mixing them until the desired amount of acid has been added. Acids and alkalis can be disposed of down the sink as long as they are thoroughly diluted, and the water is run for a few minutes afterwards.

The following corrosive chemicals are those commonly used in cytogenetics:

Glacial acetic acid

Acetic acid is in constant use in the cytogenetic laboratory, since it is mixed with methanol (1:3) to make the fixative used for processing all samples. Although considered a weak acid, acetic acid in glacial form is highly corrosive. This acid must always be handled in a fume cupboard since harmful vapours are produced, and it must be kept away from heat, naked flames and sparks.

Hydrochloric acid (HCl)

Concentrated HCl may be used with 70% ethanol for the cleaning of cover-slips or slides which are used for culturing, but 0.2 N HCl is the strength more commonly used for C-banding. If a laboratory uses this acid in both strengths, it is a good idea to buy the 0.2 N strength commercially, rather than prepare the dilution from concentrate, thus minimizing the need for handling the more dangerous concentrate. Concentrated HCl is corrosive, poisonous and produces a harmful vapour which readily destroys the mucous membranes, producing violent irritation of the upper respiratory tract.

Sodium hydroxide/potassium hydroxide/barium hydroxide

These are extremely corrosive substances. Barium hydroxide is particularly toxic. This is used in C-banding and care should be taken when weighing out this substance.

Inflammable chemicals

Alcohols and solvents may be toxic as well as inflammable. All highly in-flammable chemicals must be stored in a metal cabinet with a secure lock at a suitable level such that access is not impaired. This cabinet must be clearly marked with the appropriate hazard warning label. These chemicals should be handled within a fume cupboard.

Large stocks of solvents must be kept outside the laboratory in a cool fire-proof store, and when they are brought in from such a cool store, the stopper must be loosened cautiously. Any solvent stocks to be stored within the laboratory must be stored in metal containers in a cool place.

Since solvent vapours can travel a long way they may cause 'flashback' from a distant bunsen burner. All burners must, therefore, be extinguished prior to the use of a solvent, or be kept in a separate room.

Care should be taken in the collection of solvents to avoid incompatible reactions; indeed, some substances can be explosive under certain conditions. Solvents and alcohols should never be poured down the sink since to do this constitutes a fire hazard, and some local authorities forbid their disposal into the main drainage systems. Inflammable waste should be collected into metal drums which should be stored in a cool place until their periodic disposal by a professional firm.

The following inflammable chemicals are those in common use in the cytogenetic laboratory:

Methanol

Methanol is the most commonly used alcohol in the cytogenetic laboratory, since the fixative made by adding it to glacial acetic acid is used for the processing of cultures. It is often used for destaining slides. Methanol is highly inflammable, and toxic both by ingestion and inhalation.

Ethanol

Ethanol is the other commonly used alcohol, both in absolute concentration, and 70% dilution (sometimes in association with hibitane, etc. to swab work-surfaces). This, like all alcohols, is highly inflammable. Excessive inhalation may produce intoxication and tolerance.

Fixative

The 3:1 methanol:acetic acid fixative (Carnoy's fixative) is used daily in cytogenetic laboratories. Like all fixatives, it is a poisonous chemical solution which causes coagulation of the proteins which make tissues firm and solid, thus preventing natural liquefaction. Living skin may also be fixed if in contact with fixative for 15 minutes or more. Gloves should, therefore, always be worn when working with this fixative, and procedures carried out in a fume cupboard.

Xylene

Xylene is the most common solvent found in the cytogenetic laboratory as it is the component of many slide mountants such as DPX. It may also be used for cleaning microscope slides. Aromatic hydrocarbon solvents such as xylene are volatile and toxic by all portals of entry, and should, therefore, always be dealt with in a fume cupboard. Xylene fumes may build up during a session of slide mounting, so this should be done in a well-ventilated area or within a fume cupboard.

Toxic, cytotoxic and carcinogenic chemicals and reagents

An increasing number of toxic, cytotoxic and potentially carcinogenic chemicals are being used in the cytogenetic laboratory as techniques become more sophisticated. In addition to the precautions already outlined above, it is advisable to wear an effective face mask whenever this category of reagent is used. This prevents inhalation of dust from the powdered forms, and particular care should be taken when using balances to weigh out these chemicals.

Aerosol formation from solutions of these reagents is as dangerous to the operator as aerosols from high-risk samples. These chemicals should never be handled on the open bench.

Material should be reduced to a non-carcinogenic state prior to disposal into a sewer or waste collection system. For instance, quinacrine mustard should be treated with hypochlorite solution. Controls for the use of carcinogens in hospitals are very strict, and staff should be familiar with their local code of conduct. Only experienced workers should handle such reagents. Particularly hazardous reagents used in the cytogenetic laboratory include:

1. *Colchicine*. Inhibitor of microtubules by specific binding to tubulin. Used routinely for producing metaphase spreads. This is a highly toxic irritant. The analogue Colcemid is less toxic.
2. *Vinblastine*. Another spindle inhibitor, less frequently used in cytogenetics. This is a highly toxic teratogen.
3. *Ethidium bromide*. A frameshift mutagen which intercalates double-stranded DNA and RNA. Used as an anti-condensing agent for high resolution banding. This is a mutagen irritant.
4. *Actinomycin D*. Also used as an anti-condensing agent. This is a cancer suspect agent.
5. *Methotrexate (l-Amethopterin dihydrate)*. Potent inhibitor of dihydrofolate reductase used to synchronize cell cultures for prometaphase banding. This is a highly toxic teratogen.
6. *5-Bromo-2-deoxyuridine (BudR)*. This is used in several techniques such as sister chromatid exchange, differential replication staining, etc. It is a teratogen mutagen.
7. *5-Fluorodeoxyuridine (FudR)*. Used for synchronizing cell cultures for prometaphase banding. It is highly toxic since it is an inhibitor of DNA synthesis.
8. *Mitomycin-C*. This reagent is used in tests for Fanconi's anaemia. It is a bioreductive alkylating agent and inhibits DNA synthesis. It is a highly toxic cancer suspect agent.
9. *Quinacrine mustard*. This is used for Q-banding. It is a powerful alkylating agent and is highly toxic and carcinogenic. Quinacrine dihydrochloride is a less toxic alternative for Q-banding techniques.

228

10. *12.0-tetradecanoylyphorbol-13 acetate (TPA)*. Used in B-cell disorders as a promoter of malignant cell growth. It is very toxic and a cancer suspect agent.

11. *Chromic acid (Chromium VI oxide)*. Sometimes used for cleaning slides and coverslips for tissue culture. is highly toxic and a cancer suspect agent.

Many of the remaining chemicals and reagents used in the cytogenetic laboratory are harmful on ingestion or inhalation, or are irritants. Care should be taken not to introduce them into the mouth by nail-biting, sucking of fingers, etc. other reagents which should be handled with caution include: *Distamycin A, DAPI(4,6-Diamidino-2-phenylindole), Hoechst 33258 (bisBenzimide), deoxycytidine, phytohaemagglutinin, pokeweed mitogen, DMSO (dimethylsulphoxide), copper sulphate, silver nitrate, immersion oil, hydrogen peroxide.*

Antibiotics and fungicides

The use of antibiotics and fungicides should be restricted to a minimum since resistant strains of pathogenic organisms can be established in the laboratory environment by excessive use. Those commonly used in the cytogenetic laboratory are penicillin (or derivatives) streptomycin, gentamicin, polymyxin, mycostatin, amphoteracin B.

ENZYMES

Trypsin is commonly used in the cytogenetic laboratory. Collagenase may be used for some tissue cultures. Enzymes may cause allergic reactions in some people, and gloves should be worn for handling.

It should be remembered that even the most innocuous reagents such as salts, amino acids and enzymes may be harmful if ingested, and care should be taken even when dealing with these. Absence of a warning sign should not be regarded as a guarantee of safety. If any substance is new or unfamiliar, and the hazards are not displayed on the items, safety data sheets should be made available from the customer services departments of the companies supplying these reagents.

Compressed and liquefied gases

CO_2 gas cylinders

These are used to produce a 0.5% CO_2 level inside incubators used for tissue culture. These cylinders should be placed outside the premises and protected from extremes of temperature. Warning notices should be displayed where the cylinders are stored and used, and trolleys should always be used to transport them. They must be securely supported during use and placed in a position such that they can be easily removed in an emergency. Water should always be used when testing valve sockets for leakages.

When operating the cylinder, the valve should be opened slowly at first, and then no more than is necessary to obtain the gas flow required. Cylinder valves, gauge, regulators or other fittings must not be oiled or greased at any time and white lead or paint must never be applied to them.

Liquid nitrogen

This is used in equipment for the freezing and storage of cells. It is important that proper protective clothing should be worn when handling liquid nitrogen, this consisting of a laboratory coat, asbestos gloves with long arms, and a transparent face shield. Sandals or open shoes should not be worn in case of splashes to the feet. The room must be well ventilated when pouring liquefied gases, and they must not be poured near flames. Metal objects which have been immersed in liquid nitrogen must not be touched with the bare hands since they can cause severe burns to the skin. Care should be taken over the storage of ampoules in liquid nitrogen. If nitrogen is trapped in a badly sealed ampoule, the ampoule will explode when it is withdrawn. Surrounding the ampoule with cotton wool or cloth will lessen the risk.

SAFETY PRECAUTIONS TO BE TAKEN WITH EQUIPMENT

Centrifuges

Precautions relating to the treatment of specimens to be centrifuged, and the action to be taken in case of accidents involving specimens in the centrifuge, have already been discussed. The following safety measures are, therefore, concerned solely with the prevention of risk from use of the machine itself.

The entire centrifuge and accessories should be cleaned regularly, and the bowl, head and accessories should be disinfected. All items should be autoclaved where possible. Centrifuges can be very dangerous if not operated correctly, and must be properly maintained and serviced at regular intervals. Only the heads and accessories recommended by the manufacturer must be used as replacement parts. Because corrosion is the main cause of centrifuge failure, all heads and accessories should be inspected frequently for signs of corrosion and hair cracks. Accessories and contents must be carefully balanced, and the load distributed symmetrically around the head, before starting the centrifuge. The containers must be of a size correct for the swing-out heads to ensure that there is an adequate clearance when the horizontal position is reached.

All centrifuges used in the cytogenetic laboratory must have sealed buckets, and there must be a few minutes' pause after the rotor has come to rest, during which the lid cannot be opened. The centrifuge should be of a type which will not operate unless the lid is securely fastened. The centrifuge must never be stopped by turning it off at the mains, neither should the head be stopped by hand. All changes in speed must be made slowly.

Safety cabinets

These are discussed in Chapter 9.

Microscopes

These should be properly adjusted and cleaned regularly to minimize straining the eyes. Good quality microscopes should be used for the analysis of banded preparations since this, in particular, can cause severe eyestrain if an unsuitable microscope is continually used. It is advisable to site microscopes to be used for banding analysis in a room with daylight and a fairly long-distance view so that the eyes can be relaxed on this periodically during a long session of such analysis.

CO_2 Incubators

These should not be situated in a small, sealed room unless there is an adequate ventilation system since the CO_2 level in the atmosphere may reach too high a level. Care should be taken to avoid condensation from humidified incubators reaching electrical components of the machine. Incubators should be cleaned at least once a week with non-hypochlorite disinfectant. All spillage of pathological material must be cleaned with swabs and cotton wool and non-hypochlorite disinfectant.

Cell banks

Cell banks containing liquid nitrogen must not be situated in a small, sealed room unless there is adequate ventilation, since the level of nitrogen may build up and cause suffocation.

Water baths

These should not be used at temperatures in excess of 80 °C. Some R-banding methods necessitate the use of waterbaths at 88 °C for about 10 minutes, if this is to be done, the work should be carried out as quickly and carefully as possible, and the temperature of the water reduced as soon as this treatment has been completed. This should, however, be avoided if possible since the danger of scalding is considerable.

12 Safety Measures to be Taken in a Botany Laboratory

M. P. Ramanujam

1. INTRODUCTION

Many wonder that specific precautions have to be taken in a Botany laboratory – a place dealing essentially with plant specimens. Developments since the nineteen fifties have rendered Botany an inter-disciplinary subject depending on Physics, Chemistry, Mathematics, Electronics etc. In fact, only after the adoption of analytical methods and induction of sophisticated instruments as investigatory tools, have the flood-gates of information been opened. Conventional botany has successfully adopted the experimental approach and, consequently, the botanical worker has to work in a milieu of instruments. With an increased risk in laboratory environment the need for adopting safety precautions has been increasingly appreciated. In the following pages an attempt has been made to present a comprehensive set of guidelines which would contribute to the safety of men and materials.

2. GENERAL CONSIDERATIONS

2.1 Designing the laboratory

An ideal Botany laboratory should have the following components: one or more working halls; a museum of plant specimens, a herbarium and a well-laid out garden with a greenhouse. With the increasing importance of microbiology and biotechnology, a culture-cum-growth chamber and an instrumentation centre are the desired additions.

A number of factors have to be borne in mind at the planning stage to avoid future complications:

(i)   space requirements for the present and future work.
(ii)   proximity to lecture halls, garden and museum to minimise movement and save time.
(iii) a calm and serene environment - away from the din and dust of playgrounds, auditoria etc.
(iv) an extensive electrical supply system and provisions for heat, water, ventilation and light.

These factors, though not falling under safety measures, indirectly influence them.

Experience has shown that top storeys are ideal locations for the biology laboratory. Such an attic location ensures adequate sunlight, ventilation and freedom from noise and dust. If the museum and herbarium are also located on the same floor, movement of men and materials up and down the stairs can be avoided. Large windows may be fixed in the walls of the laboratory hall to improve natural lighting and ventilation.

The chances of fire are rare; however, it is necessary to install fire-fighting devices at vulnerable points as part of the general precautions. Exits and emergency escape routes must be provided and indicated prominently.

2.2 Cleanliness and tidiness

The old adage "Cleanliness is next to Godliness" fits the laboratory most aptly. Sanitation and sterility of the laboratory environment are two aspects that have top priority in its maintenance since air, water and dust facilitate microbial contamination. An orderly display of furniture and equipment ensures clear passages enabling free movement without being jostled.

The floor must be kept clean and free from oil and water spills and dust. Such refuse can be the cause of fire hazards and makes footing unsure causing tripping.

Air is not an ideal environment in which the contaminant micro-organisms can thrive; yet their spores survive as aerosols, sticking to floating particles of dust, saliva, carbon etc.; yeasts, moulds (*Aspergillus; Mucor, Penicillium, Rhizopus* etc,) and bacilli bacteria are common. The number of contaminants is higher in an active room. Air-conditioned rooms are generally free from this menace.

It has been well established that air contains micro-organisms capable of causing respiratory infections. Virulent streptococci occur in the floor sweepings of hospitals and colleges. Diseases like brucellosis, tuberculosis, tularemia, pneumonia, influenza, mumps, diphtheria, scarlet-fever and chickenpox may be contracted from unclean environments (Salle, 1983).

Thorough dilution of contaminated air by ventilation is a very effective way of controlling air-borne infections. Application of oil-emulsions to the floors will attract and retain the microbes. Dust can be removed using dry vacuum pick-up followed by the application of disinfectants or detergent solutions (see Salle, 1983). Inactivation of air-borne microbes by chemical mists and vapours is also effective. Hypochloric acid or a hypochlorite and Propylene glycol suppress many bacteria and viruses. Spray-fogging with quaternary ammonium disinfectants is another effective method. Ultra-violet (uv) irradiation also checks micro-organisms but it is most efficacious in a smaller area like an inoculation/transfer chamber.

2.3 Personal protection and precautions

While safety of personnel and material is of equal importance, admittedly, human life is more precious. Therefore, adopt a "Safety First" norm at all times.

Before beginning work for the day be sure of what is to be done and how to proceed. If necessary, consent to a brief from experts who understand the principles and methodology underlying the experiment.

On entering the laboratory clean the work area using both dry and wet cloths and arrange things neatly. Assemble all the requirements on the work bench or at least ensure that you need not scramble for them during the experiments. Put away the apparatus not required for immediate use. Prepare a flow-chart of the experimental steps. Do not leave anything of consequence to chance or memory. The consequences of misplacements or wrong usages could be dangerous.

Follow the instructions very meticulously. One is not at liberty to proceed differently unless and until thoroughly convinced that the nature of the experiment demands a digression and that no danger is involved in so doing.

Even if something goes wrong, keep cool and retain your composure. Under no circumstances should one panic. Common sense, presence of mind and responsible behaviour could save an uncertain situation. Tension grips beginners at the slightest indication of some abnormality. Anxiety only adds to the confusion predisposing the worker to dangers. Imagine the plight of young students at times of practical examinations when they inflict cuts and burns on themselves because of their hurried behaviour. Avoid any thoughtless and hurried movements inside the laboratory. Concentrate fully on the job and don't allow distractions. Running, mass movements, and jostling are indications of irresponsible behaviour. Similarly, eating, drinking and smoking are to be strictly prohibited. Food and drink should not be stored in the laboratory refrigerator as they may be contaminated by chemicals stored therein, possibly leading to ingestion of chemicals and poisoning. Likewise, smoking may lead to fire hazards.

Wearing an apron or coat, spectacles or goggles and gloves have become routine steps. In addition, one must be familiar with the escape routes and exits, especially when working inside closed areas like instrumentation rooms and inoculation chambers. It is also good to know about the locations and handling of fire-fighting equipment. An additional qualification is to have received training in first-aid techniques and procedures.

Personal hygiene is a very important factor in any aseptic experiment. Hands must be washed thoroughly with soap and hot water before and after the experiments and also before treating any casualty of burns, cuts or eye injury. Strong detergents or disinfectants would affect the skin. Hexachlorophene which was employed as a disinfectant until recently was shown to penetrate the skin and cause rashes. It also has the potential to cause brain lesion and other serious human disorders. This has resulted in the banning of such chemicals being components of any cosmetic preparation.

2.4 Preservation and storage of specimens

It is always desirable to supply fresh specimens for study; the greenhouse and garden are intended for this purpose. However, the diversity of the plant kingdom is such that a number of plants must be preserved in the museum and a plant such as dried excicata in the herbarium. For the sake of convenience all plant specimens must be clearly labelled and arranged in an orderly fashion according to an accepted system of classification.

While preparing the plant specimens, cutting instruments like razor blades, scissors and cutters are used. It requires patience not to get injured either from the hooks and spines of plants or while handling the instruments.

Herbarium specimens are usually covered successively, with folders for species, genus, class etc. Paper of a cheaper quality is used during the drying and pressing stages. Invariably, the paper is retained for future use and very rarely discarded. This increases the risk of fire hazard in the herbarium. Fire has a devastating effect as highly combustible materials like paper, plants and wood are concentrated there. Nowadays, wooden cabinets have given way to steelware; the latter affords additional protection against insects and fire.

The use of chemicals is limited to the poisoning stage where copper sulphate or a dilute mercuric chloride solution (0.01%) is used. The latter is deadly poisonous and requires careful handling. Do not use bare hands. Lift the specimens with tongs for dipping into chemicals and use forceps to arrange them for pressing.

Contrary to the techniques practised in the herbarium, large volumes of preservative chemicals and different types of glassware are in common use in a museum. Many of the chemicals used like formalin and alcohol are slow in vaporizing and inflammable too. If the museum is kept closed for long periods of time, a concentration of such vapours builds up thus endangering the health of the workers.

In short, the herbarium and the museum should be spacious, well ventilated with exhausts and be provided with fire extinguishers. Frequently, the constraints of space results in a crowded display of materials thus aggravating the situation in times of fire.

2.5 Handling of glassware

Glassware of different designs and dimensions are used in the botany laboratory such as Ehrlenmeyer flasks, petri-plate pairs, boiling and test-tubes, pipettes and separation flasks. Storage tanks of various sizes are indispensable in a museum.

It is essential to make sure that no cracked glassware is used. Whatever is selected should be clean and dry. To avoid unnecessary breakages during jostling or collision, they should be carried in trays. Generally, test-tubes are used in large numbers and carrying them becomes problematic. Use wire-mesh-cages or multi-holed tube-trays.

Sometimes, the contents of the glassware may have to be boiled. Extra care is required in such cases as any spillage could damage the body.

Store glassware at about ground-level, preferably below the work benches. Categorize and display them neatly according to their size so that they are easy to choose from. Put away the used ones separately and wash them as soon as possible to minimize contamination. In doing so the waste is prevented from drying and sticking to the bottom of the glass vessel.

Cleaning of glassware: Chances of breakages and the resultant cuts and injuries are more frequent during washing since the detergent solution minimises friction. Disposable and pre-sterilized plasticware has already eliminated the problems of washing and also saves time; yet, most laboratories rely on glassware as the cost is not so prohibitive.

Any commercial cleaning powder containing an abrasive is suitable for washing glassware. If a substance is sticky, addition of some acetone will easily remove it. The old practice of heating the residue with acids is extremely dangerous and may lead to explosions. Again, attempts to use a mixture of nitric acid and ethanol should also be discarded as it results in violent explosions. In most laboratories chromic acid is found to be a very efficient cleaning solution. It is essentially a mixture of chromium trioxide and concentrated sulphuric acid, and is a highly corrosive chemical.

2.6 Disposal of waste

Collection and disposal of waste is a necessary adjunct to the maintenance of the laboratory. In fact, waste should be disposed of as often as necessary without waiting for the experiments to be concluded. The waste may be plant specimens, solids and liquids and each require a separate mode of disposal.

Hence, separate bins must be provided for broken glassware, solid waste, liquid waste etc. Disposal of radioactive waste is a technical exercise and is discussed elsewhere.

Liquid waste may be poured into the sink provided it does not contain any radioactive or highly reactive chemical. Solids should never be thrown into the sinks or waterways. Water insoluble organic substances and solid particles accumulate and choke the water system in the long run. Whenever chemicals are poured into the waterway they must be washed down the drain with an excess of water. Ensure that these chemicals do not stagnate or reach alarming levels affecting aquatic organisms and thereby endangering them.

Dry plant material may be collected in heaps outside the laboratory and can be utilised for making compost. Alternatively, it may be burnt periodically along with other materials. Burning of waste must be carried out outside office hours, in a distant place and after ascertaining that the direction and speed of the wind will not carry the sparks into the laboratory.

Waste from the microbiology and tissue-culture laboratory require special handling. In most cases the cultures are discarded before the nutrients are exhausted, but this facilitates uncontrolled growth of test-organisms. The unused medium also becomes a veritable nursery for many saprophytic organisms. Besides contaminating the atmosphere, many of them also pose health problems. *Mucor, Rhizopus, Aspergilli, Fusarium* are some such fungi of nuisance value. Fungal spores are known to cause allergic rhinitis and asthma in humans. The microbial cultures should be autoclaved before being discarded and should never be disposed of in the open.

3. INSIDE THE LABORATORY

3.1 Electrical and electronic installations

Most of the modern instruments are based on electronics and run on electricity. As a rule, these instruments must be installed in dust-free rooms, serviced periodically and maintained by trained personnel. If possible, a technically qualified person should be in charge of the instrumentation centre. It is advisable that the technician should receive training in first-aid techniques from a competent source. It is not desirable for a student or teacher with very little understanding of the principles of construction and function to meddle with these instruments.

Electrical safety considerations have often been overlooked. Malfunctioning of electrical appliances and their thoughtless handling often result in accidents. To insulate the workers against possible mishaps the following guidelines may be followed:

(a)   Have as many power points as possible. This precludes lengthy wires being laid on the floor and consequent risk of tripping. The risk is even greater when experiments have to be conducted in darkness. Display a warning on the door as a caution to visitors.

(b) Plugs of correct strength protected by a fuse of correct rating must be used. The fuse may be removed at the end of the experiment. Or install a switch-lock in each area of the power equipment if they are run simultaneously.

(c) An essential step is to ensure proper earthing which guards against electric shocks, especially in damp conditions.

(d) Use wires of standard quality. The international colour code for wires may be of some use to electricians. Live, neutral and earth wires are indicated respectively by brown, blue and green/yellow in the UK, white, black and green in the USA and by red, black and green in India.

(e) If the instruments are run continuously for long periods, the fuse-switch assembly may get heated up, leading to short-circuiting. Keep a watchful eye on the entire electrical system on these occasions.

(f) Don't move or carry any instrument when it is running.

(g) When high voltage equipment (like an electrophoresis apparatus) is used, take special care to wear rubber gloves.

(h) In damp weather moisture may collect within the switches which gives the user an electric shock. Be careful to wear gloves and not to go bare-footed.

3.2 Compressed gas cylinders

Compressed liquefied petroleum gas, which is the common substitute for an electrical burner, is highly objectionable, irritating to the eyes and nose, and causes pulmonary oedema. It is violently explosive despite the strong container. Hence, the tubing must be checked at regular intervals for any sign of leakage, and changed periodically. The pressure is extremely high and even a minor leakage may prove fatal if it catches fire. A very efficient and simple method for detecting gas leakages is to apply a dilute detergent solution and to look for gas bubbles. Keep the regulator and the main valve closed when not in use and check them frequently. Preferably, the cylinder should be tied to another firm support to prevent a lethal "jet-propelled missile-like" discharge. Always place the cylinder vertically and ensure moderate temperature and adequate ventilation.

3.3 Sterilization and inoculation procedures

Several techniques involving dry heat, wet heat, ultra-violet irradiation, ultra-filtration and chemicals have been perfected for the purpose of sterilization.

The word sterilization brings to mind an autoclave or a pressure-cooker. The former is used in large research laboratories while the latter serves the purpose in smaller institutions. In both, the articles, mostly media and materials, are heated by steam under pressure. At a pressure of 1.05 kg/cm² the temperature of the steam goes up to 115–120 °C. An explosion in such situations could be most damaging to men and materials. Hence, a close watch should be maintained on the thermometer and pressure-gauge of the autoclave, simultaneously. If necessary, the safety valve should be judiciously manipulated to keep the pressure under check. With the introduction of the gasket release system the risk of explosion is reduced to a minimum. However, the following additional points may be borne in mind to ensure safety:

(a) Do not overload the container; arrange the material in an orderly fashion to allow free passage of steam.
(b) Close the lid tightly to prevent leakage of steam
(c) Maintain the correct level of water
(d) Before closing the system ensure that all the air in the chamber has been completely expelled by steam
(e) Do not open the lid immediately after the sterilization is over. Allow the pressure to subside by leaving the cooker or autoclave undisturbed for a while. Otherwise, the steam will gush out and burn the skin and tissues causing blisters. In addition, the super-heated fluids may spill over from the containers, aggravating the injuries.

Glassware, mostly petri-plate pairs, flasks etc. are sterilized in hot-air ovens. This method of dry heat sterilization stretches over long periods (about 2 hours) at 165–170 °C. As with autoclaves, the oven should be opened only after allowing the temperature to subside. The great differences in temperature between the inner and outer sides of the oven will cause breakage of the glass screen if this is not done.

Chemical sterilization involves the use of a hypochlorite, ethanol or isopropanol for surface sterilization, mercuric chloride and copper sulphate for poisoning plant specimens and specific chemicals for fumigation exercises. Acidified alcohol (70%. v/v pH 2.0), used until recently for surface sterilization, has now been discarded because of its corrosive nature. The use of hypochlorite as a substitute is also beset with problems (see 5.2). Mercuric chloride is extremely poisonous leading to mental depression, and requires careful handling.

A very common exercise during inoculation is flaming the instruments dipped in alcohol. Being highly inflammable, the spilling of alcohol near a flame would lead to accidents. An element of personal risk is also involved when working inside a laminar air-flow system as the direction of the air would direct the flame towards the work. It is safer to use alcohol in metal containers since glassware will easily break, splashing the burning alcohol. Another undesirable practice is flaming the mouth of the flasks and tubes for a long time. Possibly, albeit unknowingly, one is introducing ethylene into the glassware and into the atmosphere.

Transfer of microbial propagules, cells, tissues and calluses is a delicate exercise which requires synchronization of mind and body. One may have to handle a lot of glassware at a time; to complicate matters, all the transfer procedures have to be carried out near the flame. Many people burn their fingers; the glassware breaks up due to excessive heating; the alcohol spills, and the cotton plugs catch fire. If the worker is not alert and cautious, not only does the entire inoculation go haywire, but the chances of accidents increase.

3.4 Ultra-violet irradiation

Ultra-violet (uv) light consists of a spectrum of irradiation with wavelengths ranging from 2000 Å to 4000 Å. Those wavelengths between 2300 Å and 2800 Å, and especially 2537 Å, are biologically most useful. The latter wavelength is microbicidal and kills even endospores of bacteria. Because of this property it is employed for sterilizing inoculation chambers. Some chemicals reflect uv light due to their structural design and the above attribute is exploited to detect the presence of these chemicals under uv-lamps. However, there are some inherent dangers in dealing with uv light although it is non-ionizing.

Short term effects of exposure to uv are skin disorders like sunburn and suntan. When uv light strikes the eyes it causes a painful burn called actinic keratitis. Prolonged exposure may lead to cancer as uv is also known to be mutagenic.

Arc lamps, uv lamps and other high intensity light sources should not be looked at directly. Even the uv light reflected from chromatographic columns or plates should be prevented from reaching the eyes. The insidious effects can be overcome by wearing close-fitting and uv-opaque goggles for the eyes, and gloves on the hands. If necessary, a larger glass barrier can be erected between the uv lamps and the worker.

Another important fall-out is the photochemical change prompted by uv light. Oxygen is converted to ozone in the presence of light of shorter wavelengths. If ozone accumulates in higher concentrations it becomes hazardous, causing irritation to the eyes and to the respiratory tract.

3.5 Laboratory procedures and practices

Every practical session should commence with a brief introduction by competent staff. The aim of the experiment, the principles involved and the procedural details should be outlined, enabling the worker to get to the crux of the problems with ease and confidence.

Plant specimens should be trimmed to size before sections are cut for microscopic study. Specimens may be as soft as a leaf or young stem or very hard like the wood of pine, oak, walnut, teak etc. Since trimming such specimens is a manual job, using knives and cutters, chances of physical injury are not uncommon. Sections may be cut, using a razor or blade. The material may be held between the index finger and thumb, or it may be placed between the split halves of pith or carrot root. When the material is held between the fingers, care must be taken not to run the sharp cutting edges into the fingers causing injuries. If the material is bulky, make a shallow groove on the support to accommodate its mass.

Fine sections can be obtained in a rotary or sliding microtome. However, since the knife moves across the specimen when this is done, fingers must be kept off its path. If the material is too hard for sectioning, soften it by treating with hydrofluoric acid.

Stains used in microtechnique, both basic as well as acidic dyes, are not known to cause any health hazards. Nevertheless, they are likely to leave clothes discoloured permanently. Persons suffering from colour blindness are at a distinct disadvantage during the staining process as they are unable to discern the colour variations. They should not hesitate to seek help from others.

Microscopes are very common instruments in any biology laboratory. Since they are costly and heavy they must be kept in special cabinets and should be carried to laboratory benches only when required. The acceptable mode of moving them is to grip the microscope arm firmly with the right hand, and the base with the left. The microscope should be lifted carefully from the cabinet, held close to the body and placed gently on the working bench. This will prevent collision against furniture or co-workers and protect the person and the instrument against damage.

It has been claimed that operations like pipetting, pouring and vigorous shaking of solutions often contaminate the environment. Dispensing aids like pipettes may be plugged with a piece of non-abosrobent cotton as a "stopper". This serves dual purposes; it prevents contamination of the contents and avoids back flow of the solutions into the mouth. Again, the pipettes should not be blown to get rid of the last drop of solution, as the scattering droplets form aerosols in the air to which other contaminants adhere.

A few other hints on some normal practices in the laboratory may not be out of place. Cork-boring is a patient and time-consuming exercise. To make it easy, lubricate the borer with a little glycerol or alcohol (too much would

242

make it slippery) and rotate steadily using gentle pressure. Excessive pressure would result in a narrow hole.

Broken glass rods and tubes piercing the skin are not an uncommon sight while inserting rubber tubing. Moisten the rubber tubes with a little alcohol before pushing them on. If the tubes are made of semisynthetic polymers, they may not be very flexible. In that case, immerse the ends of the tubes in boiling water before thrusting them on the glass tube.

For cutting rods or tubes to definite lengths, make a clear scratch with a triangular file, a glass-knife or a diamond pencil. Holding the rod with thumbs on either side of the scratch, bend it gently. The rod will break at the scratch mark. If necessary, smoothen the cut edges by fire-polishing them.

4. HANDLING OF PLANTS

4.1 Handling of micro-organisms

Bacteria and microscopic fungi dominate the discussion in this Section; mushrooms are discussed separately. Viruses pose few problems to the worker since no plant virus is known to cause any disease in human beings. The same is true for mycoplasma whose plant pathogenic capabilities were reported in the late sixties. Only very few fungi incite diseases in humans, e.g. *Cercospora apii, Aspergillus* sp., *Chlamydia* spp.

Many bacteria have exhibited dual pathogenicity to plants, animals and human beings; hence, strict regulations are imposed on their handling. Since the advent of genetic manipulation techniques an embargo has been clamped on tinkering with the genes of bacteria for fear of creating monsters and their accidental release.

Workers handling micro-organisms should be wary of bacteria and fungi, if they are also potential human pathogens. Records show that infection by *Brucella abortus, B. melitensis, Pasteurella aularensis, Salmonella typhosa*, are not uncommon in persons employed in a microbiology laboratory although the source of infection cannot be named with certainty. At any event, the fate of *Howard Taylor Ricketts*, the famous microbiologist who discovered the RLOs is worth recalling. So absorbed was he in his research on typhus infection that he accidentally contracted the bacterium and died.

The fungal diseases known to man are either *mycoses* caused by true infection, or *toxicoses* caused by the ingestion of toxic fungal metabolites. Some subcutaneous fungal pathogens are introduced beneath the skin by thorns or hooks or as contaminants of wood. But this rarely occurs in the laboratory.

Nevertheless, every aspect of microbial culture procedures needs careful scrutiny as best exemplified by the following incident. According to Barbeito *et al.*, petri-dishes containing the cultures of *Pasteurella aularensis* fell accidently in the hallway of a laboratory. An estimated fourteen persons passed that way during and after the incident. Five of them, including the two who stayed 20 metres away from the accident site, were affected by the bacterium (see Salle, 1983).

Therefore, not only the micro-organisms, but also their cultures, need careful handling. Wear gloves or at least apply spirit to the palms of hands before and after the experiments. Alternatively, the organisms can be killed before examination unless required alive. A simple way of ascertaining whether the bacteria are dead or not is to stain them. Generally, only killed cells retain colouring dyes.

Many fungi produce poisonous substances called mycotoxins which cause serious health disorders if ingested. Aflatoxins produced by Aspergilli and trichothecines produced by *Fusarium* spp. are mycotoxins of importance. The former are known to inhibit RNA synthesis; they are also potent carcinogens and are implicated in human liver cancer.

4.2 Handling of mushrooms

A different kind of problem, that of "mistaken identity", is commonly encountered while handling mushrooms. The student might have heard about the tastiness of the mushroom and its nutritive value.

It is true that mushrooms are considered table delicacies; but many are poisonous, yet attractive and enticing to look at. The student should be well advised in handling them since there is no general rule to differentiate between the poisonous and non-poisonous ones. The belief is that brightly coloured mushrooms are poisonous and that the creamy ones are edible, but the "Chanterelle" (*Cantherellus cibarius*) and the "Wood blewits" (*Tricholoma nudans*) are brightly coloured but are not poisonous. On the other hand, the "Death Cap" (*Amanita phalloides*), the "Fool's mushroom" (*A. verna*) and the "Destroying Angel" (*A. verosa*) are completely white, yet deadly poisonous. The agaricus group is an ideal example where some species are toxic and others are not. *A. arvensis, A. campestris, A. bispora* are eaten by people but *A. xanthoderma* is not. As the name indicates, the fungus changes its colour from white to yellow on touch or when damaged. It was pointed out earlier that many species of *Amanita* are banished from the table, but *A. rubescens* is edible. In the genus *Lepiota*, the green coloured *L. margoni* is poisonous and *L. rachodes* is edible. Though the foregoing would deter any student from experimenting with mushrooms, one should remember that only a critical microscopic examination would reveal the identification at species level. At collegiate level this is seldom attempted. Precautions should be made mandatory even in the field and at home, lest it should prove fatal. It may be relevant to mention here that *Gyromitra esculenta*, commonly known as the "saddle fungus", was sold as a favourite in America and Europe

244

Table 12.1 Defence structure of some plants

	Plant	Part modified
THORNS:	*Aegle marmelos*	Prophyll/axillary bud
	Bougainvillaea spp.	Axillary bud/stem
	Cassia sp.	Axillary bud/stem
	Duranta repens	Prophyll
	Flacourtia sp.	Axillary bud/stem
	Hygrophila auriculata	Axillary bud/stem
	Prunus sp.	Axillary bud/stem
	Ulex europaeus	Bigger thorns: axillary bud smaller thorns:- leaves
SPINES:	*Acanthorhiza* sp.	Roots
	Argemone mexicana	Leaf apices/segments
	Asparagus racemosus	Leaves
	Berberis vulgaris	Leaves
	Opuntia spp.	Leaves
	Phoenix dactylifera	Leaf apices
	Pothos armatus	Roots
	Prosopis juliflora	Axillary bud
	Punica granatum	Leaf petiole
	Quisqualis indica	Leaf petiole
	Spinifix squarrosus	Bracts
PRICKLES:	*Balanites roxburghii*	Superficial excrescences
	Mezoneurum cucullatum	Superficial excrescences
	Mimosa pudica	Superficial excrescences
	Opuntia spp.	Superficial excrescences
	Rosa spp.	Superficial excrescences
	Rubus spp.	Superficial excrescences
	Toddalia asiatica	Superficial excrescences
	Zanthoxylum limonella	Superficial excrescences

but was banned subsequently when its toxicity was discovered. Even the so-called edible mushrooms are not without undesirable effects. They cause indigestion when consumed in excess; some may cause an allergy in certain people; the "Ink Cap" mushroom, *Coprinus atramentarius* is known to cause transient purplish coloration of the skin when consumed with alcohol. The poisonous varieties leave temporary or permanent effects on the consumers. *Amanita phalloides* causes impairment of the nervous system; *A. muscaria* causes gastric disturbances followed by paralysis. *A. rubescens* is responsible for haemolytic anomalies. Gastric enteritis is the disorder caused by *Gyromitra esculentes*.

Whatever the source of poison, cases of mushroom poisoning must be attended to immediately. Vomiting may be induced to flush out the poison if medical attention is delayed.

4.3 Handling of higher plants

Commensurate with the extensive elaboration in their morphology, the seeded plants viz, Gymnosperms and Angiosperms have evolved various structural adaptations. Many plants have developed hooks, spines or thorns as part of their defence (Table 12.1) while some have developed stinging hairs, a bitter taste or a bad odour to deter pilferage (Table 12.2).

Table 12.2 Some important poisonous plants

Sl. No	Botanical name	Source of poison
1.	*Abroma angusta* Linn.f.	Irritant hairs
2.	*Anacardium occidentale* Linn	Juice from pericarp and trunk
3.	*Arisaema speciosum* (Wall) Mart	Juice, especially from tubers
4.	*Euphorbia antiquorum* Linn	Milky juice
5.	*Excoecaria agallocha* Linn	Milky juice
6.	*Fleurya interrupta* Gaundich	Stinging hairs on plant
7.	*Girardinia heterophylla* Decne	Stinging hairs on plant
8.	*Holigarna arnottiana* Hook.f.	Juice
9.	*Laportea crenulata* Gaudich	Stinging hairs on plant
10.	*Laportea terminalis* Wight	Stinging hairs on plant
11.	*Mucuna atropurpurea* DC.	Irritating bristles on pods
12.	*Mucuna gigantea* DC.	Irritating bristles on pods
13.	*Mucuna hirsuta* Wight & Arn	Irritating bristles on pods
14.	*Mucuna monosperma* DC.	Irritating bristles on pods
15.	*Mucuna nigricans* (Lour) Steud	Irritating bristles on pods
16.	*Mucuna prurita* Hook	Irritating bristles on pods
17.	*Rhus insignis* Hook.f.	Leaves, bark, fruit
18.	*Rhus punjabensis* Stew ex Brand	Leaves, bark, fruit
19.	*Rhus succedanea* Linn	Leaves, bark, fruit
20.	*Rhus wallichii* Hook.F.	Leaves, bark, fruit
21.	*Sachima wallichi* Choisy	Bark
22.	*Semecarpus anacardium* Linn.f.	Juice from pericap and bark
23.	*Semecarpus travancoricus* Bedd	Juice
24.	*Tragia bicolor* Mig.	Stinging hairs on plant
25.	*Tragia involucrata* Linn.	Stinging hairs on plant
26.	*Urtica dioica* Linn	Stinging hairs on plant
27.	*Urtica hyperborea* Jacquem ex Wedd	Stinging hairs on plant
28.	*Urtica parviflora* Roxb.	Stinging hairs on plant
29.	*Urtica pilulifera* Linn.	Stinging hairs on plant

After Chopra, Badhwar and Ghosh, 1974

The minute seeds of certain grasses like *Aristida, Stipa* and *Heteropogon* may pierce the skin and cause abcesses. The brown hairs of the cowhage plant, *Mucuna prurita* are rigid and pointed. On touching them, they enter the skin and cause irritation. Most of the xerophytes and many others have developed sharp and pointed protective outgrowths. At the family level this is best exemplified by the members of Cactaceae. As specimens for morphology and taxonomy students will have to handle spinous plants. Such specimens need careful handling as pricks from some of them will cause suffering for days.

Members of the genus *Urtica* are called "Stinging nettles". True to the name, they cause an itching sensation and swelling called "urticaria" in medical terms. The itching is caused while handling plants like *Tragia, Laportea* etc. Physical contact with *Laportea* leads to inflammation and blisters at the point of contact.

Species of *Rhus* of Anacardiaceae produce severe dermatitis associated with watery blisters. These blisters burst and spread quickly on the skin. *R. toxicodendron* (poison oak), *R. diversiloba* (Pacific poison oak) and *R. vernix* (poison elder) are important species containing allergens in the plant sap.

As with mushrooms, fruits of belladonna and cotoneaster are misleadingly attractive. Seeds of the laburnum plant are mistaken for green peas, and roots of hemlock for parsnips. Some of the poisonous plants are listed in Table 12.2. The reader should be prudent enough not to handle such specimens indiscriminately.

Avoid chewing or tasting any part of the plant as it may contain objectionable or poisonous substances as given below:

(a)   Latex from *Calotropis, Opuntia, Nerium, Euphorbia, Ficus* etc, may be disagreeable to taste and that of *Thevietia* is a well known poison.

(b)   Alkaloids which are medicinally useful in low dosages occur in concentrated form in plants and, hence, are strong poisons. e.g.:

        Nicotine (*Nicotiana* – leaves)
        Morphine (*Poppy* – fruit)
        Quinine (*Cinchona* – bark)
        Strychnine (*Strychnos* – fruits)
        Atropine (*Atropa* – leaves)
        The same is true of the glycoside digitoxin from the foxglove plant (*Digitalis* sp.)

(c)   Ergastic substances deposited as raphides and spheroraphides in *Amorphophallus* and many aroids are persistently irritating.

(d)   Unripe fruits such as guava (*Psidium*), banana (*Musa*) and tea leaves are rich in tannins; they are astringents and taste bitter.

Do not bring plants or twigs close to the face and avoid smelling them as you are increasing the chances of contracting pollens; sometimes the smell may be offensive as in *Poederia, Blumea, Balanophora, Rafflesia* etc.

4.4 Natural allergens

A number of plant materials like pollens and fungal spores elicit allergic reactions in sensitive individuals in whom histamines or histamine-like compounds are released due to antigen–antibody reactions. As a result, the person suffers from fever, asthma, dermatitis etc.

Pollen allergy which manifests itself as hay-fever may lead to asthma. A study in London has shown that pollen of timothy grass (*Phleum pratensis*) cocksfoot (*Dactylis glomerata*) and perennial rye (*Lolium perenne*) produce respiratory discomfort in sensitive individuals. In the United States, the pollens of rag weed (*Ambrosia* spp.) have been identified as the chief allergens. The allergic capabilities of the *Parthenium hysterophorus* have become legend by now, and some people have been driven to commit suicide in South India as a result of their suffering. Utmost caution is required when handling such specimens. As a general precaution, facial masks can be used and palynological studies may be conducted in a room with very little air-current.

Table 12.3 Chemicals commonly used in a botany laboratory

Chemicals	Uses	Properties	Parts affected
Acetic acid	killing, fixation	—	lungs, skin, mouth
Acetone	dehydration, solvent	inflammable, vaporizing	—
Ammonia solution	bleaching	corrosive	eyes, lungs, skin, mouth
Benzene	solvent	vaporizing	lungs, skin, mouth
Butyl alcohol	dehydration, clearing	inflammable	lungs, mouth
Chloral hydrate	clearing	vaporizing, poisonous	lungs, mouth
Chloroform	clearing	vaporizing, poisonous	lungs, mouth
Chromic acid	killing, fixation maceration	corrosive	lungs, skin, mouth
Copper sulphate	preservation, poisoning	poisonous	lungs, skin
Dichromates	killing, fixation	—	lungs, skin, mouth
Dioxan (diethylene oxide)	dehydration	inflammable, poisonous	lungs, mouth
Ethyl alcohol	dehydration	inflammable, intoxicating	—
Formaldehyde	dehydration, killing, fixing	irritating, poisonous	lungs, skin, mouth
Formalin	preservation	vaporizing, irritating	lungs, skin, mouth
Hydrochloric acid	maceration	corrosive	lungs, skin, mouth
Hydrogen peroxide	bleaching	corrosive	skin, mouth
Hypochlorites	sterilization, bleaching	corrosive	skin, mouth
Isopropyl alcohol	dehydration, clearing	inflammable	—
Mercuric chloride	preservation, poisoning	poisonous	lungs, skin, mouth
Methyl alcohol	dehydration	inflammable	—

248

Nitric acid	maceration	corrosive	lungs, skin, mouth
Nitrocelluloses:		explosive	
Celloidin	embedding		
Colloidin	embedding		
Parlidion	embedding		
Osmic acid	killing, fixation	corrosive, irritating	—
Perchloric acid	softening	reactive	skin, mouth
Phenol	clearing, solvent	corrosive	lungs, skin, mouth
Picric acid	killing, fixation	corrosive	skin, mouth
Sulphuric acid	maceration	corrosive	skin, mouth
Sodium sulphate	maceration	corrosive	skin
Trichloroethylene	clearing	—	lungs, skin, mouth

5 HANDLING OF CHEMICALS

5.1 General precautions

Table 12.3 will show the range of chemicals which a botanist has to handle very commonly. More complex chemicals are used in investigations of a sophisticated nature in research laboratories. There is a need for precaution in handling them due to their explosive, inflammable, volatile and poisonous nature.

Chemicals should be classified and stored according to their respective risks, volatile ones in fume cupboards and inflammable solvents in special cabinets. Every container should have a label detailing the name of the chemical, date of purchase, date of expiry and a note of caution on the dangerous aspects, if any.

As a general rule try to substitute a dangerous chemical with an innocuous or less dangerous one. Reactions generating heat (exothermic) or evolution of gases should be performed carefully and supported by cooling or trapping systems. The author has seen the curious spectacle of a container ballooning out and threatening to burst when an ignorant student used a plastic carboy for the preparation of chromic acid. Timely intervention by pouring ice-cold water on the carboy prevented an accident, the defect in this case being the choice of the wrong container. A heat-resistant, non-corrosive porcelain pot would have been ideal. In exothermic reactions the reagents should be added dropwise or in small quantities with rapid stirring. Always add acid to water and not vice-versa.

Many chemicals are highly corrosive. When some powerful oxidants are added to easily oxidised organic substances danger may ensue. Perchloric acid, which is often used as a softening agent in botanical microtechnique, reacts violently with organic materials like cork, rubber, cloth and wood. These materials absorb the chemical quickly and become susceptible to fire hazard. Hydrofluoric acid can be substituted for perchloric acid but it also has its own demerits. Both are vaporizing, highly corrosive health hazards. It was to avoid an explosion that the use of a mixture of alcohol and nitric acid for cleaning was discouraged earlier.

Never heat chemicals without knowing what the consequences might be. In attempts to remove tarry residues from glassware a little chromic acid or nitric acid is added and heated. The glassware may explode throwing splinters around. Such attempts should be made in exclusive locations only.

Fire hazards: Many chemicals, especially the organic solvents, are highly inflammable. That they are also highly vaporizing renders them doubly dangerous as the vapours might reach the sources of ignition. These vapours may also severely affect the nasal and pulmonary tracts. Store such chemicals inside the fume cupboards. Keep the containers away from naked flames and faulty electrical circuits. Sparks from electrical devices like thermostats, vacuum pumps and hot-air ovens could also be the cause of fire, as well as refrigerators, since the chemicals are stored in them. Nowadays, special types of refrigerators for the laboratory, with added safety features, are being marketed.

5.2 Reactive agents

Certain chemicals are highly reactive. Oxidising substances like alkalies and acids, belong to this category, and some, like nitric and sulphuric acids, are also vaporizing. Therefore, it is necessary to protect the eyes and exposed skin from these hazards. Care must be taken not to inhale the vapours, dust and mists as this would also spell a health hazard.

Improper handling of chemical substances may lead to permanent damage. On one occasion, an attendant, trying to open a sealed ammonia bottle carelessly, was soon writhing in pain, his vision severely affected by the ammonia vapour gushing out. He had to be hospitalized and had his sight restored after one month only. Cases of permanent loss of vision following ammonia splashing are not uncommon (Gopalan *et al.*, 1986). Wear full protective clothing including a respirator while handling such chemicals or keep them in the cold for some time before opening. In all cases of the skin, eye or mouth making contact with any injurious chemical substance, thorough rinsing with water should be the first treatment.

Nitric acid, perchloric acid, hydrofluoric acid, sulphuric acid and chromic acid are some of the acids which are strong and reactive. Some, like hydrofluoric acid, readily react with glass and quickly destroy organic materials.

Strong bases like ammonia, chromates and dichromates react violently with acids, generate heat on contact with water and affect eyes and skin. The dust of chromates dissolves nasal fluid and leads to perspiration. On continued exposure, ulcers or cancer may develop.

Toxic chemicals reach the inner tissues through ingestion, inhalation or direct absorption. Smoking, itself is dangerous to health. When smoking in the laboratory, other toxic chemical vapours also find their way into the lungs. To prevent ingestion of chemicals while pipetting, a "stopper" would do the trick. Avoid storing food, milk and drinks in the laboratory as they may become contaminated by chemicals. Some workers use their "sniffing" capacity to identify chemicals; this must be discouraged.

When chemicals are directly absorbed by the skin, dermatitis, an unsightly and irritating disease, may develop. The vapours may reach the internal body systems. The insidious effects include distressing physical and mental derangements. For this reason, herbarium workers are warned not to use their bare hands for poisoning the plants with mercuric chloride. An aqueous solution of sodium or calcium hypochlorite has been in use for a long time now to surface sterilize the specimens. The plant material is immersed in the chemical solution for about 10 minutes and thoroughly rinsed with several changes of sterile distilled water. Because of the corrosive nature of hypochlorite, the solution and the rinsewater must be discarded immediately. Furthermore, inhalation of hypochlorite can produce severe bronchial irritation and contact with the skin can be harmful (Dodds and Roberts, 1985, Salle, 1983). As for any other chemical, one should not use the mouth to pipette a hypochlorite solution. Keeping the chloride preparations under uv irradiation should be avoided as it releases free chlorine gas which is a serious health hazard (Hamilton, 1973, as quoted in Salle, 1983). Osmic acid which is used in preparing specimens for electron microscopy is not only expensive but its vapours are highly irritating; it also blackens the tissues. Vapour from methyl alcohol, chloral hydrate, could cause dizziness. Such chemicals should always be stored in closed containers, and spills, if any, should be washed. In cases of uncontrollable spillage of mercury, the area should be dusted with sulphur and washed later. It is emphasised that vomiting should never be induced in cases where the casualty is unconscious or has ingested corrosive poisons such as strong acids or alkalies or phenols.

5.3 Radioactive chemicals

Chemicals with radioactivity have become excellent investigatory tools in probes into the functional aspects of plants. They rank among the most dreaded substances as they emit ionizing radiation which may lead to cancer.

Very small quantities are used in biological experiments in contrast to the large amounts of labelled compounds used in research laboratories. Even then, they are to be handled with utmost caution as the deleterious effects are irreparable. In research institutions, work with these compounds is supervised by a technician with 'on-the-job' experience. In advanced institutions, the entire gamut of operations - purchase, storage, use and disposal - come under the "Radiation Control Officer".

While the general precautions for storage and handling of chemicals can be unreservedly extended to this type of chemical also, the following special precautions are to be scrupulously observed.

(a) Radioactive chemicals should be stored in a separate cupboard and in special containers - with labels marked "CARE RADIOACTIVE MATERIAL" on them.
(b) Radioactive solutions, however dilute, should not be pipetted by mouth as it may lead to accidental ingestion.
(c) Do not look into the mouth of the vessel containing the radioactive material as the radiation could be damaging to the eyes.
(d) Trim the finger nails closely and avoid handling the radioactive material with an open or even bandaged wound so as to exclude chances of the material entering the bloodstream.
(e) Despite all precautions traces of radioactive material coming into contact with the skin are not uncommon. Hence, it is safer to apply a barrier cream as a pre-treatment. If contamination is suspected wash the affected area with soap, scrub with a brush and pour water copiously.
(f) Place the containers with active material in trays and cover the working area with polythene sheets. A polished surface permits easy recovery of the spilled material. Using a finely drawn-out pasteur pipette fitted with a rubber teat most of the substance can be recovered.
(g) Do not throw radioactive waste into the sink or bins. It should be collected in a separate bin bearing a warning notice and disposed of scientifically. Generally it is buried deeply in concrete containers (see Bournsnell, 1958).

6 FIRST AID: TECHNIQUES AND PROCEDURES

6.1 First-aid box

A first-aid box must be kept in an easily accessible place and must contain the following items with clear labels.
- Bandages of different sizes, sterilized gauze, absorbent cotton, adhesive plaster of assorted sizes, unmedicated, sterile wound dressings.
- Delicate forceps, scissors, razor blades, safety pins
- Eye-bath, irrigation bottles, eye droppers, sterilized eye pads in sealed packets
- Aerosol sprays for various types of injuries, burnol, antiseptic ointments etc.

- – Disinfectants like Dettol, rectified spirit
- – A manual of first-aid procedures

It is also desirable to display prominentaly the name, address and location of the nearest available medical care source and fire service station. Providing their telephone number would be an added advantage.

6.2 Personal/psychological approach

Any affected person would be in a state of shock, the intensity of which would depend on the severity of the suffering. Therefore, our first attempt should be to comfort the victim. Make the casualty lie down and rest. Then proceed as indicated below and according to the nature of the suffering.

6.3 Cuts and injuries

Cuts and injuries are common during microtechnique and anatomy sessions. Abrasions are caused while handling carboys, packing-cases etc. If the cuts are minor ones, allow them to bleed for a few seconds. Remove any foreign material using clean forceps and apply antiseptic cream and bandage. If the bleeding is severe, press a gauze or a clean cotton swab firmly on the wound and hold it there until the blood clots. Then, wash the cut with alcohol and remove all foreign material. Apply a dilute solution of tincture of iodine, allow it to dry and, finally, put on a bandage. Do not apply tourniquets straight away in cases of bleeding injuries. Raising the injured part may also control the loss of blood. Any injury, slight or severe, must receive prompt treatment. Delay may result in a minor injury becoming a major one due to infection. In many cases stitching the wound may be necessary. Should an injury become in-flamed or painful, medical attention must be obtained.

6.4 Burns

Burns may be caused by heat or chemicals. If the burns are judged minor, apply boric acid, sterile vaseline or burnol. Put a loose bandage on if necess-ary. In cases of severe burns the affected area must be cooled immediately by plunging it into a bowl or sink of water or by continuously dousing it with water for at least ten minutes. Ice-cold water would also quickly absorb the heat from internal tissues.

If the burns are caused by chemicals, a different kind of treatment is required. Dilute solutions of sodium bicarbonate and acetic acid are used against acids and alkalies, respectively, for washing the burnt area. When corrosive chemicals like phenol spill over, wash off the material from the skin with copious amounts of water, swab gently with a pad of cotton soaked in ethanol, wash again with soap and water and, finally, apply boric acid or sterile vaseline. Do not lance or puncture the blisters, nor remove any piece of clothing sticking to a burn.

As an additional precaution, remove ornaments, dresses and other close-fitting appendages (rings, watches, belts, socks etc.) as the burnt area is likely to get inflamed. As a rule, do not use adhesive dressings and apply ointments indiscriminately.

6.5 Poisoning

Poisoning may result from ingestion or contact with chemicals, plant parts or plant products. When the poison has been in contact with the external surface of the body, proceed as described for phenol burns in the previous section. If the material has not been swallowed, spit it out at once and wash the mouth immediately with water. In cases of ingestion, induce vomiting, which is an effective step for poisons of plant origin. For chemical poisoning, inducing vomiting is not the panacea and, in certain cases, not desirable either. In such cases seek medical attention immediately.

6.6 Electrical shocks

First of all, disconnect the power supply and carefully remove the affected person from electrical contact. Never use a wet stick or towel as by doing so those assisting will themselves become hapless victims. Either use a dry stick or wear shock-proof gloves. Take the affected person into the open air and allow him to breathe freely. If necessary seek medical care.

6.7 Fires

In case of persons on fire, remove the burning clothing and roll the victims over. Smother the flames with a fire blanket or any other piece of thick cloth.

Turn off all other vulnerable fire sources like gas burners and electrical implements. Remove all inflammable chemicals.

Sometimes, the chemicals in a flask or beaker may catch fire. When this happens, cover the mouth of the vessel with a damp cloth. Dry sand will also put out the fire. If organic chemicals catch fire, add a mixture of sand and sodium carbonate or hydroxide. Desist from using water; it will only spread the fire.

The fire extinguisher can be used to quench fire in a certain spot, on a bench, in a heap of paper or in plant wastes. If the fire looks uncontrollable, call the fire-service immediately.

ACKNOWLEDGEMENTS

I am grateful to Professor S.B. Pal, the editor, for giving me an opportunity to contribute this chapter to this volume. I also acknowledge the useful suggestions of Dr B. Ambalanathan and the secretarial assistance of Mr G. Mohan.

REFERENCES

1. *Handbook of Mushrooms*, Nita Bahl (1984), Oxford and IBH Publishing Co., New Delhi
2. *Microbiology*, Pelczar, M J Jr., Reid, R D, and Chan, E C S (1977). Tata McGraw Hill Publishing Company Ltd., New Delhi
3. *Fundamental Principles of Bacteriology*, Salle, A. J. (1983). Tata McGraw Hill Publishing Co. Ltd., New Delhi
4. *Text Book of Microbiology*, Burrows, W. (1968), W. B. Saunders Company, London
5. *Poisonous Plants of India*, Chopra, R.N. Badhwar, R.L and Ghosh, S. (1984). Academic Publications, Jaipur
6. *The Medical and Poisonous Plants of India*, Caisus, J. F. (1986). Scientific Publications, Jodhpur
7. *Experiments in Plant Tissue Culture*, Dodds, J. H. and Roberts, L. W. (1985). Cambridge University Press, London, New York
8. *Pharmacognosy*, Trease, G. E. and Evans, W. C. (1978). Bailliere Tindall, London.
9. *Experimental Biology*, Van Norman, R. W. (1971). Prentice Hall, Inc. Englewood Cliffs, New Jersey.
10. *Safety Techniques for Radioactive Tracers*, Boursnell, J. C. (1958). Cambridge University Press, London.
11. *Botanical Microtechnique*, Sass, J. E. (1958). Oxford, IBH Publishing Co., Calcutta.
12. *Plant Microtechnique*, Johansen, D. A. (1940). McGraw Hill Book Company, New York.
13. *Methods in Plant Histochemistry*, Krishnamurthy, K. V. (1988). Viswanathan, S. (Printers & Publishers) Private Ltd., Madras.
14. *Vogel's Text Book of Organic Chemistry*, Furniss, B. S., Hannaford, A. J., Rogers, V., Smith, P. W. G., and Tatchell, A. R. (1978). English Language Book Society.
15. *Elements of Analytical Chemistry*, Gopalan, R., Subrahmaniam, P. S. and Rengarajan, K. (1986). Sultan Chand and Sons, New Delhi.

13 Safety Measures to be Taken in a Zoology Laboratory

C.M. Chaturvedi

INTRODUCTION

Most laboratory animals can induce diseases in man by laboratory-acquired infection such as zoonoses. Animals can also inflict physical injuries by biting or scratching. In addition to these possible dangers from animal contact, various laboratory work involving experimental techniques and the use of specific equipment and chemicals may also pose a hazard to the worker unless correct animal handling techniques and good laboratory practice are emphasized. The laboratory safety depends on the worker and cannot be replaced by sophisticated laboratory design and specialized equipment which can only supplement it. Moreover, good laboratory practice is the prime requirement for the safety of laboratory personnel.

This chapter will discuss the possible hazards involved while working in a zoological laboratory and safety measures that may be taken by laboratory workers to avoid infections and risks.

THE HANDLING OF LABORATORY ANIMALS

The handling of animals, their care and husbandry, involves a number of different practices and procedures depending upon the species. The maintenance of stock animals and their experimental use in zoological teaching as well as in research work, requires the handling of the animals. Although satisfactory procedures are described for the handling of animals, confidence and efficiency can only be developed with practice. In order to protect itself while being handled, the animal may struggle to escape, bite or scratch. Therefore, both fear and anger should be avoided and handling should be gentle but firm. Those who are new to handling must spend some time in merely picking the animals up and transferring them from one cage to another until confidence has been gained about the ability to control the animal. Different animal species require different handling techniques and the restraining techniques used should confirm acceptable practices, care being taken that neither handler nor animal is injured. It is not possible to describe a technique for each species, therefore, only those species which are more frequently used in Zoology laboratories are described in this chapter. In general, pregnant animals should be handled with great care, giving support to the posterior region and avoiding constriction on the abdomen.

Small Mammals

Mice

These animals are initially caught and lifted by the tail for transfer to another cage or scale, identification or sexing (Figure 13.1). But, for any treatment

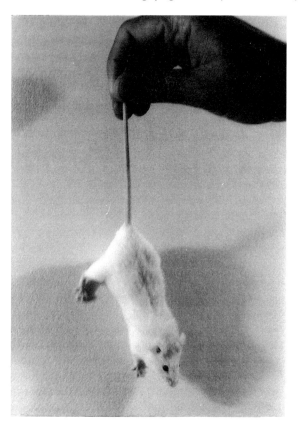

Figure 13.1   Grasping the tail of mice when lifting

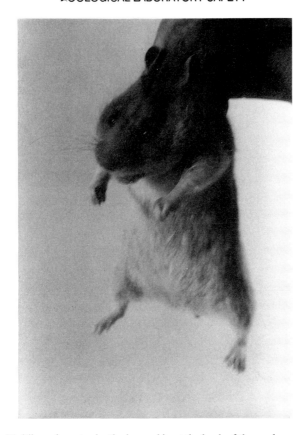

Figure 13.2   Holding a hamster by the loose skin at the back of the neck

and close examination, they may be held by grasping the loose skin at the back of the neck.

Hamster

Grasping the loose skin at the back of the neck and shoulders is effective for holding the animal with one hand (Figure 13.2). Restraint can also be accomplished by tightly grasping the loose skin across the back (Figure 13.3). The grip should not be so tight that the animal is unable to breathe. It may also be picked up by grasping the whole body (with palm over the back and side and thumb and index finger around the lower jaw).

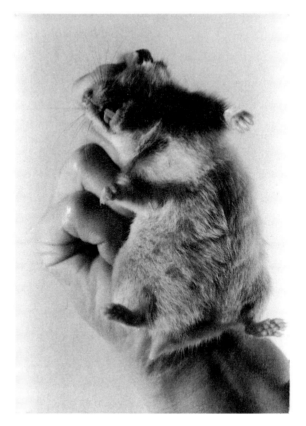

Figure 13.3   Restraint grip on the hamster across the back

Rats

They are normally lifted by grasping the whole body as described for the hamster. One hand hold is sufficient for control and treatment. Young rats may be handled similarly to mice.

Guinea pig

The docile nature of this animal makes its handling easier than for most laboratory animals. It should be held with the palm over the back and thumb and forefinger around the neck. When lifting, the other hand should support the lower part of the body.

Rabbits

Rabbits scratch effectively but rarely bite. They can be held by the loose skin at the back of the shoulders and the lower part of the body must be supported by the other hand. They should never be lifted by the ears.

Birds

Only four orders of class Aves are commonly used in zoological and biomedical research. These are Galliformes (chicken, turkeys, quails), Columbiformes (pigeons, doves), Passeriformes (crows, sparrows, finches) and Psittaciformes (Parrot family). Because of their unique anatomy, fragile nature, physiology and behaviour, development of special handling techniques and skills are required for birds. Most birds tend to be easily frightened or alarmed, so sudden noise should be avoided which may upset an entire flock. Generally, the stock of birds or experimental birds (to be exposed to natural day length) are maintained in an outdoor aviary which permits free access to the air and natural photoperiod. The area and height of the aviary should be sufficient for the normal maintenance of the stock, and twigs and branches of the trees (or bamboo sticks) should hang horizontally as perches for the birds. A net is used to capture the swifter birds from the aviary, the hoop of which must be made of a lightweight material to prevent injuries to the bird in case of an accidental blow.

While working with birds in the laboratory, the doors should always be closed to avoid the birds escaping out of the room in the event of uncontrollable release from the investigator's hands or, unexpectedly, from the cage during manipulation. The unwilling release of a bird is a common happening while handling these creatures and may create problems in case the bird is an active flyer (unlike galliformes). In such cases, dimming of room lights may be helpful for capture. The bird may also be forced to fly/exercise continuously until it is tired and slows down; it is then easy to catch by adopting a quiet method of approach. A traditional method generally used in India is also very helpful. A strong glue-like substance of plant origin (semi-liquid form) is fixed on the tip of a long thin bamboo stick, and even when the bird is at a great height or long distance from the worker, just a touch of the glued end of the bamboo stick makes the bird helpless as the feathers get stuck to the glue, thus making capture easy.

Galliformes – These birds are easy to handle and are not as fragile (except quails) as other species of birds. Although these birds are usually docile, they can peck or scratch. The flocking tendency of galliformes can be used to advantage while capturing a single bird from the flock because the bird often fails to suspect that it is the object of capture. While holding, the wings must

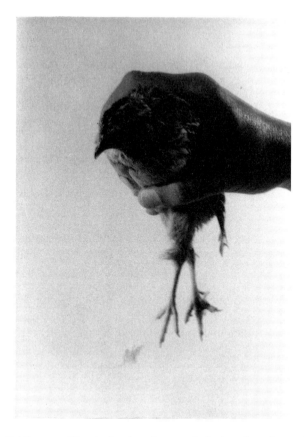

Figure 13.4 Holding a quail by placing the palm over the body and gently pressing the wings

be restrained, chickens can be carried by the legs but to calm them, gentle pressure on the wings helps. Turkeys are relatively easy to handle, but precautions should be taken as a large turkey, being stronger, can inflict injury with its powerful wings. Quails can be held or restrained by a palm over the body and by pressing the wings gently , with thumb and finger around the neck/body (Figure 13.4). For some treatment (injection, close observation, etc.) they may be held fully with the thumb and index finger on the ventral side and other fingers supporting it from the back (Figure 13.5). They may also be carried by their legs (Figure 13.6).

Columbiformes and Passeriformes – Due to their smaller size and flying capacity, these birds are swifter and more difficult to capture. However, capturing from the cage is easy. The door of the cage should be opened minimally (preferably a vertically operating door) just enough to allow the hand to enter, which minimizes the chance of the birds' escape out of the cage. Then they are held gently with the palm above the body and thumb and finger around the head (Figure 13.7). Later on, these birds can also be carried by the legs for close examination, etc. (see Figure 13.6). Restraining may be done in a similar way to that used for the quail (see Figure 13.5).

Psittaciformes – The same general technique as that described above may be used for the handling of these birds, but one has to be more careful while restraining the head due to their tendency to bite. To release the birds from restraint, they should be placed gently on the floor of the cage and the hand then withdrawn.

Reptiles

Because of their remote relationship with man and domestic animals these creatures are less used in medical and veterinary science, except in venom

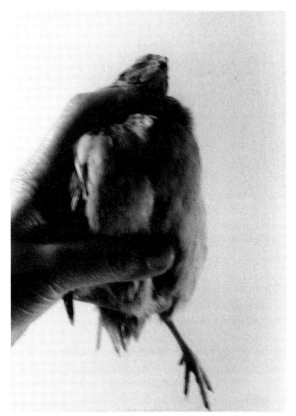

Figure 13.5   Restraint grip on the quail

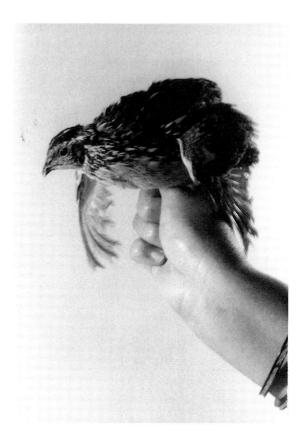

Figure 13.6   Carrying a quail by the legs

research. However, they are suitable for certain types of experimental work on the nervous system, vision research, tissue (tail) regeneration and embryonic studies.

Lizards – Small lizards are restrained by grasping their head with thumb and fingers, but they should not be held by their easily detachable tail, especially in the case of the wall lizard, etc.

Snakes – It should be emphasised that, in general, there is no easy way of distinguishing poisonous from non-poisonous snakes until examined closely (scales, teeth, etc) therefore, all unidentified snakes should be treated with caution. The use of live poisonous snakes is inadvisable unless necessary (as in venom research), but the best rule is to handle them as little as possible.

In the case of non-poisonous snakes, they should be grasped rapidly, firmly and confidently; after seizing the head, the snake's body must be supported comfortably with the other hand or by another person, to prevent the body and tail from thrashing about (Figure 13.8). Leather gloves may be useful protection from bites and scratches but are not easy to work in. Tongs or other instruments, such as snake rods or pole loops, used for restraining snakes should be used carefully, otherwise, they increase the risk of causing superficial damage to the creature.

Amphibians

Frogs – These are the most common animal models for zoological teaching at the preliminary level, and for the demonstration of certain physiological

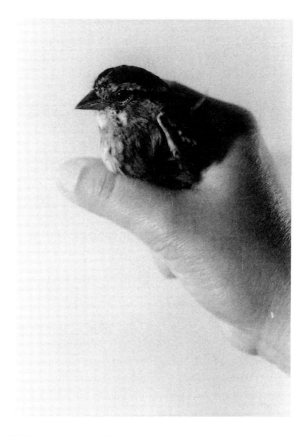

Figure 13.7 Holding a sparrow with the palm placed over the body and the fingers around the head

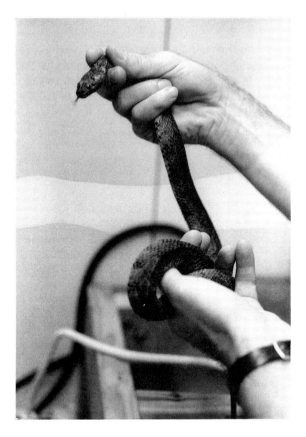

Figure 13 8   Grasping a snake's head with one hand and supporting the body with the other

experiments. The slippery secretion of their bodies makes handling difficult. They are picked up by placing fingers on each side and between the legs.

Fish

They require careful handling. Fish caught wild should not have mud on their gills and the protective mucus coat should not be removed. They are easy to catch with a small net from the aquarium and should not be taken out of the water for a lengthy period of time. The nature (temperature, oxygen content, etc.) of the home and transport water should not vary significantly.

USE OF RADIATION TECHNIQUES AND SAFETY MEASURES

With the ushering in of the atomic age, the number and variety of applications of radiation sources have increased enormously in scientific research, medicine and industry. Radio-autography, radioiodine uptake, tracer technique, radioimmunoassay, etc. are some of the techniques now commonly used in zoological research and teaching. There are a number of important factors that one has to bear in mind while handling the radiation sources. One is that these sources are completely safe to handle *provided* all necessary precautions are taken. However, careless handling could easily give rise to excessive exposures which, in turn, could result in undesirable physiological (somatic as well as genetic) effects, not only to the users, but also to other laboratory workers and members of the public. In assessing radiation hazards, it is important to bear in mind that its ill-effects are not immediately apparent (except in cases of high exposures) and there may be no general indication of the danger to which a person may be unwillingly exposed. The users, however, should be fully aware of all the potential hazards involved and the limits on the use of such materials. Since these radioactive materials could have detrimental effects on users as well as on the public if not handled responsibly, most countries have applied special regulations for their use. These legislations are based upon the recommendations of the International Commission on Radiological Protection (ICRP) and International Atomic Energy Agency (IAEA).

Laboratory design and handling procedure for radioisotopes

Laboratory

Frequently, a radioisotope laboratory has been set-up by converting an existing laboratory, but, there are a number of guiding principles which may be helpful in the interest of safe working.

1. There should be a gradient of activity so that higher activities can be confined to areas remote from inactive work.
2. Hoods are necessary for controlling possible airborne contamination arising from work with unsealed radioactive materials.
3. Near the entrance there should be some provision for washing and for contamination monitoring. One thin wall contamination monitor, preferably with aural indication, is suitable for day to day monitoring of possible contamination.
4. The top surfaces of work benches or tables should be covered with sunmica, formica or stainless steel and walls and doors painted with oil paint or plastic emulsion paint to facilitate decontamination.

5.   Elbow or foot operated water taps should be used.
6.   Foot operated dustbins are a 'must' in the laboratories using radiation.
7.   Appropriate radiation signs should be used.

The following procedures should be observed while handling radioactive substances or doing any kind of radiation work.

Protective clothing – suitable clothing and disposable gloves should always be worn while handling radioactive substances, and touching switches, door handles, taps, etc. should be avoided. Gloves should be cleaned while still on the hands and then disposed of. Laboratory coats and shoe covers should be worn. This clothing must not be taken out of the radioactive areas.

Protective equipment – preventing contamination is easier than decontaminating furniture and equipment. Radioactive work should be performed in trays that contain a protective lining with absorbent material and water repellent backing. Always use tweezers, tongs, forceps or other suitable devices to handle radioactive sources. Never pipette by mouth. If inhalation of vapour is possible use the fume hood.

General – eating, drinking, storing food, smoking, chewing gum or use of cosmetics should not be allowed in areas where radioactive materials are being used. Washing of hands with soap and water is a 'must' following the work, even though gloves are worn while working. An appropriate detection instrument must be used to monitor hands, clothing etc. for possible contamination, before leaving the work.

Working with animals – in the majority of experiments, only small quantities of radioactive substances are injected into animals ($< 50 \mu$Ci), so there is generally little risk of external irradiation, but internal contamination may result from inhalation of radioactive substances (absorbed on bedding materials, hair, feathers) and through skin contamination (by bites or scratches). Injection of radioactive materials into animals should be performed in trays lined with absorbent material, syringe shields may be used while injecting large quantities of beta and low energy gamma emitters. Animals' cages should be labelled properly, and should be segregated from those housing other animals. Adequate ventilation must be provided in places where animals are kept after an injection of a radioactive substance. The animal's handler must be aware of dose levels incorporated in the animals, time limitations in the area, and the handling requirements of the animals and excreta. For easy cleaning, the cages should be made of plastic, stainless steel or some such material and dust-proof bedding should be used.

Handling procedure for radioiodine

With the advancement of research, radioimmunoassay (RIA) has become a widely used technique for the sensitive and accurate assay of hormones in biological samples. Due to ease of labelling and many other characteristics, radioiodine is most widely used for this purpose. However, the use of radioiodine must be recommended with great caution because of its volatility and very low permissible concentrations. The following handling procedures are recommended when radioiodine is used.

1.   Work with radioiodine should be performed in well-ventilated fume hoods. Always open the vial in the hood because the pressure of radioiodine vapour builds up in the vial during storage. The vial should not be left open any longer than necessary and should be capped tightly when not in use.
2.   Two pairs of gloves should be used because radioiodine can diffuse through rubber or plastic.
3.   Contaminated vials/containers should be handled with forceps or other such devices and not directly. Forceps fitted with rubber gloves ensure a secure grip and can easily be replaced when contaminated.
4.   At low pH the volatility of I^{125} is enhanced significantly so acid should not be added to radioiodine solution.
5.   All contaminated materials should be kept in a double bag. Any spill may be decontaminated by using a solution of 100 mmol/l NaI, 100 mmol/l $Na_2S_2O_3$ and 100 mmol/l NaOH. This mixture helps to stabilize the material and minimize the evolution of volatile radioiodine. Cleaning should be completed with a detergent.
6.   A sodium-iodide detector should be used to monitor I^{125} contamination, it has an efficiency of about 20% at contact, compared with less than 0.5% from a G.M. counter.

Disposal of radioactive waste

During work with radioisotopes a certain amount of radioactive and inactive solid and liquid wastes are generated. Active and inactive wastes should be collected separately. Different disposal methods are used for different categories of waste.

1.   *Long-acting radioactive waste* – The waste containing significant amounts of long-acting radioisotopes (half-life in years) should be sent for safe disposal to the appropriate Radiological Protection Division. Carboys or Winchesters for liquids and bins with foot–operated lids for solids, should be used for the storage of the above mentioned wastes;

if needed prior to disposal, they may be stored, but proper shielding must be provided for high activities. Double containers or trays should be used for protection against breakage and all the vessels must be labelled with appropriate radiation signs.

2. *Short-acting solid radioactive waste* – This waste with a half-life of a few weeks to a few months may be stored in the laboratory, prior to general disposal, in a suitably shielded receptacle for a period of 7–10 half-lives. The waste may also be buried locally in a pit. An exclusive burial ground for solid radioactive waste should be located in an isolated area, duly fenced off. However, the site of such a burial ground should take into account the nature of the environment, topographical, geological, hydrological and meteorological characteristics, uses of ground and surface water in the general areas and affected facilities. For useful details for pits and radioactive disposal, a pamphlet is available from the Radiological Protection Division, Bhabha Atomic Research Centre (BARC), Bombay, India. After the period of a few half-lives (7–10) the waste in the pits may be disposed of as normal waste and the aforesaid pit may be reused. The radioactive foliage (paper, polythene sheets, aluminium foils etc.) after reduction in size (if possible by mechanical pressure), should be wrapped carefully in polythene bags. These bags may be stored in the laboratory or buried in pits as described above and then disposed of after a certain period.

3. *Short-acting liquid radioactive waste* – It is permitted to dispose of this waste in the sanitary sewage system provided the quantity is quite small. It should be soluble or dispersible in water and must be discharged into the sanitary sewer with a quantity of water such that its concentration is diluted by a factor of about one hundred in the main sewage.

4. *Animal carcasses, etc.* – Wrap animals in polythene bags ensuring that the claws are duly covered to avoid puncturing the bag. These bags may be buried in pits. Small animal carcasses/organs containing low activity may be incinerated. If the animal excreta is not mixed with sawdust or wood shavings, it may be disposed of via the sewer if the concentration is in accordance with the limits applicable to the liquid waste, otherwise, it may be placed in plastic bags and disposed of as solid waste. Each country has its own legislation with regard to the disposal of radioactive waste and the quantity it is permitted to dispose of by various routes per year. These rules should be strictly followed by laboratory workers in order to control and minimize radioactive contamination.

Contamination control/decontamination

Radioactive contamination is a hazard to health, may ruin experiments, and must be avoided. Much can be done by careful techniques and laboratory discipline. Some points to remember are cited below:

1. To reduce the risk of spillage, radioactive solutions should be handled in double containers. Volatile and high activity sources will almost certainly introduce contamination into the atmosphere so they must be used in a fume hood.
2. Sources should not be touched by hand and appropriate tools should be used.
3. For β-rays, protection of the eyes, face and body can be provided by shielding with transparent plates of moderate thickness.
4. Loose contamination should not be allowed on exposed surfaces such as work bench tops and floors. While working, bench tops should be covered with absorbent sheets and floors should be of a non-porous material to avoid contamination.
5. Work areas and personnel should be monitored after work with radioactive substances. It is useful to have contamination monitors with aural signals.

Preventing contamination is easier than decontamination. However, in the event of decontamination being necessary, the following methods must be used.

1. When hands, body and clothing, etc. become contaminated this should be prevented from spreading or from getting into any wound. Washing with soap and water is generally the best initial approach. While monitoring the hands, if the tips of the fingers show contamination, washing and clipping the fingernails may remove most of the radioactivity.
2. Ceramic tiles, painted surfaces, concrete, wood, etc. should be washed thoroughly with detergent and hot water, and, except for wood, may also be washed with a mild acid.
3. Laboratory taps and drains should be scoured with scouring powder or rust remover and flushed with a large volume of water.

Radiation hazards: evaluation and control

The increasing laboratory use of isotopes and radioactive substances in recent years has led to a heightened awareness of the hazards involved with radiation work. Radiation hazards may be broadly divided into two categories, i.e. external radiation hazards and internal radiation hazards.

1. *External radiation hazards* – The magnitude of this hazard depends upon the nature of the radiation, the strength of the radiation sources

and the exposure time. However, external radiation can be controlled by such factors as shielding and distance.

2. *Internal radiation hazards* – This occurs when radioactive substances are likely to get into the body system. The seriousness of this mainly depends upon the uptake and localization of the element in question and on the method and rate of elimination from the body. Control involves laboratory discipline, cleanliness and ventilation. It is emphasized that no radiation work should be carried out if there is any cut or wound to the hands, especially below the wrist. Eating and drinking should be strictly prohibited in radioactive laboratories.

To ensure safe working conditions for all radiation workers it is necessary that:

(a) Personnel are monitored regularly;
(b) The doses received by users are well within the prescribed limit; and,
(c) The cumulative dose records of the individual workers are maintained for the entire period during which they work with radiation sources.

Personal monitoring

External

This is the evaluation of radiation doses received by personnel working with radiation sources. There are two devices normally used for this purpose.

1. *Film badge* – This consists of personnel monitoring film along with a set of filters. Such a combination, worn on the chest or wrist, is used for the detection and evaluation of radiation doses. By selecting films of suitable sensitivity and proper thicknesses of filters one can easily cover a range of doses from 10 rem to 1000 rem. Although this requires processing, it is suitable for record keeping; it is useful to those exposed to X-rays, gamma rays, beta rays and slow neutrons.
2. *Thermoluminescent badges* – These are also being used for determining the external dose. The method used for dosimetry is the excitation of thermoluminescent materials, these also require processing, but this method is good for record keeping.

Internal

For internal radiation hazards, personnel dosimetry must be biological. Two methods are widely used for this purpose.

1. *Biological monitoring* – This involves the measurement of activity in the excreta, i.e. urine and faeces, analysis of exhaled air, or level of radioactivity in the blood.
2. *Body radioactivity measurement* – This is done with instruments (counters) and is useful in the case of gamma-emitting isotopes (I^{131} and I^{125} monitoring). It is also possible to do thyroid counting and to estimate body burden.

LABORATORY HAZARDS AND CONTROL

A hazard can be identified as anything that can cause injury, illness or deterioration in the health of the worker or the general public. A variety of hazards are associated with laboratory work, for example: biological, chemical, radiation, physical and mechanical hazards.

Biological hazards

The most common safety risks associated with workers in a zoological laboratory are the biological hazards, causing infections, etc. The risks associated with animal work may be grouped into four categories.

The zoonoses

Diseases which can be transmitted from animals to humans or from humans to animals are known as zoonoses. More than 200 zoonoses are reported in man; these may be caused by microbes (viruses, bacteria or protozoans), and some non-microbial zoonoses caused by helminths and arthropods. In the animal kingdom, some of these diseases are limited to certain species, while many have no such limitations. All laboratory animals can be unsymptomatic carriers of micro-organisms highly dangerous to man.

The modes of spreading these diseases are through contacts with infected animals, contaminated wool, hair fur, feathers, hides, air, food, water, etc. Inhalation of contaminated matter, dust, etc. and animal bites (flea, tick, mosquito, mammal, etc.) are the source of passive carriers of pathogens that infect man. Some of the notable diseases are smallpox, typhoid, plague, anthrax, tuberculosis, dysentery, whooping cough, measles, pneumonia, encephalitis, malaria, etc. With the above diseases in mind, it becomes obvious that great care is necessary in the purchase, maintenance and handling of animals. The obvious precautions of practising good personal hygiene will preclude most of the dangers in this area, and the use of antiseptic and sterilization procedures will prevent the infection of animal workers to a large extent. High standards of hygiene are essential, not only to protect the health of the workers, but also as an added protection for the animals themselves. On leaving the animal work area, hands should be washed thoroughly with a germicidal soap. All those in regular contact with laboratory animals should have an active immunization for tetanus.

Allergies

A number of people show severe allergic reactions to close contact with animals. Feathers, hair, fur and dust may not only cause minor respiratory troubles, but may also sometimes produce violent asthmatic attacks. The only permanent solution in acute cases is the cessation of contact with the allergy producing animals/materials. Diverting the attention of zoologists to another group of animals because of such allergies is not uncommon.

Problems associated with the handling of animals

If animals are not accustomed to being handled they become frightened and aggressive when approached. Mishandling of animals causes bites, scratches and abrasions to the handler which must be treated seriously, especially if inflicted by species which harbour pathogens. Appropriate medication such as anti-tetanus treatment should be available for personal safety, and recommended handling methods, as described in the first section of this chapter, should be practised.

Some exotic amphibians produce highly dangerous skin reactions and some produce irritating secretions. Such animals should be handled with protective gloves, and careful washing is specifically encouraged.

Problems of work environment

These are common even in well-equipped and suitably designed working facilities. The specific hazards in animal houses are generally noticed after they have occurred and caused an injury. Some of the hazards and steps which can be taken to prevent them are listed below.

Injuries by cuts – Caution should be exercised when putting arms into cages or when lifting them, as the edges may be sharp. Care should be taken when using sharp knives for cutting or scraping the cage trays. Glass tubes should be pushed carefully into rubber corks and broken glass should always be put into a special container and never into the sinks or dustbins. Sharp objects like scalpel blades, hypodermic needles and blood lancets should be carried, handled and used in a safe manner. Disposable sharp and pointed items should be placed in red-coloured sharps disposable boxes and when full, should be emptied into appropriate containers, sealed and discarded as solid hazardous waste.

Burns – Gloves should be used when handling hot items near autoclaves, ovens and incinerators. All exposed steam and hot water pipes should be kept covered with an insulating material.

Damage to clothing – Comfortable overalls without lengthy projections that can be trapped, should be worn.

Gas inhalation or explosion – Any gas leakage should be observed carefully. Gas cylinders must be stored safely and away from heat. Anaesthetics should only be used in a well-ventilated room, away from any heat source, and one should be careful and never smoke.

Electrical shocks – Check all electrical insulation and switches regularly.

Storage danger – Chemicals should be stored safely for easy access and inflammable ones should be kept in an appropriate manner. Animal bedding and other combustibles must be stored away from heat or fire.

General risks – Do not overreach to load or unload the cage racks. Care should be taken on ladders and on slippery floors in the wash area and on wet floors. The incidence of physical injury in the laboratory may be reduced by the provision of well-lit rooms, corridors and staircases, and by the use of non-slip floor surfaces.

Chemical hazards

Toxicity, corrosiveness, carcinogenicity, etc. are some of the hazards associated with laboratory chemicals. A safety shower and eye-wash facilities are the prime requirements to guard against chemical hazards. However, good laboratory practice and a knowledge in the use of chemicals to be handled are essential for personal safety. Dangerous chemicals should be stored in an area from which the fumes can be removed by an exhaust fan.

Radiation hazards

Radiological safety is of paramount importance to all persons working with radioactive substances. All radiochemical containers, storage cabinets and

275

doors to rooms where radiochemicals are used must be posted with appropriate signs, e.g. 'Caution Radioactive Area', 'Caution Radioactive Material', etc. The official Nuclear Regulatory Commission warning sign is the three–sided radioactive caution symbol (red or magenta on a yellow background). Additional precautions such as adequate shielding and detection equipment must be used. No food or drink is allowed in the radioactive area and storage and disposal of radioactive waste must follow the procedures outlined by the Radiation Protection Division. For details, see the section dealing with radiation techniques and safety measures.

Physical hazards

Electrical

One of the hazards of any working area is the possibility of electrical currents causing shocks to the workers. To prevent this, there should be red indicator lights to warn of the presence of high voltage, followed by electrical checks, at regular intervals. The ground wire must be intact, and power cord insulation must not be faulty or frayed. Minimum tension and correct voltage must be applied to all electrical outlets.

Among the relatively few hazards in an amphibian and fish facility, generally the greatest danger is posed by the extensive use of water and electrical appliances in the same work areas. Electrical insulation must be carried out by professionals who are aware of the nature of the facility and of this hazard.

Explosion

Explosive gases and those at high pressure should be so located that they are not in the immediate neighbourhood of the person working with them.

Fire

Adequate precautions must be taken to avoid fire, and the appropriate fire-fighting equipment must be readily available where these dangers are expected.

Mechanical hazards

Although a zoology laboratory does not have heavy machinery associated with mechanical hazards, dangerous conditions are always present with some instruments. One should remember the fact that accidents are generally caused by carelessness and rarely by a fault in the equipment or the existing facilities.

Centrifuge – This is the most frequently used instrument in almost all zoology laboratories. When in use it is necessary to ensure that the centrifuge tubes and buckets are accurately balanced. Precautions should be taken to see that the centrifuge is guarded by very strong side walls and heavy locking covers, otherwise, accidents might occur which could be very serious, if not fatal. An accident may be far more serious when the heads have been weakened or the safe speed or load has been exceeded.

Gas cylinders – Compressed gas cylinders must be handled with the appropriate control heads or pressure regulators. They must have screw caps on at all times when not in use. Cylinders must be firmly fixed or supported by chains and must not be used in areas near radiators, in those exposed to direct sunlight or in hot rooms.

Microtome – This is the basic instrument used in a zoology laboratory for cutting microscopic sections of tissues and organs, and requires a very sharp razor for the purpose. One has to be very careful while handling the microtome, especially during manipulation of the tissue block which should always be done in the locked position. When not in use, the razor should be kept covered and greasy. During sharpening of the razor, the handler should be very careful to avoid any cut due to its sharpness.

Surgical instruments – For dissecting or operating on laboratory animals, surgical instruments are used. These pointed devices must be handled carefully to avoid any cut or pricking. After use, these should be immediately and thoroughly washed with detergent and water to remove any biological material (tissue/blood clots, etc.) and sterilized to avoid infection and also for the maintenance of the instruments.

Glassware – Broken glass is one of the worst offenders as far as accidental cuts are concerned. For this reason, broken glass should be placed in specially marked containers and not with the ordinary solid waste, prior to safe disposal.

Other miscellaneous hazards

Cryogenic substances – Many laboratories use liquid, gases or cryogenic mixtures (solid CO_2 and ethyl alcohol) for low temperature work. Liquid nitrogen is widely used in the storage and preservation of biological material. If allowed to come into contact with the body, these liquids and mixtures may cause very painful and severe burns and tissue destruction. Therefore, suitable protective devices must always be used while handling them.

Aerosol production – Any operation or activity tending to generate airborne contamination should be avoided. Animals too are responsible for aerosol production either from their fur, hair, or via urine and faeces allowed to dry in bedding, and this may be inhaled by handlers, causing respiratory distress. Drop pans placed too far from the bottom of the cage could create aerosol through the splashing of urine and faeces and must be avoided, especially with infected animals. Sweeping dry floors and dry dusting of cages and other animal room equipment may also produce aerosol and should be avoided.

USE OF PROTECTIVE CLOTHING AND OTHER DEVICES

The risk of an infection/hazard can be minimized by the use of safety equipment/devices, practices and facilities. Some are as follows:

1. Laboratory coats, aprons, etc. should be worn while working in the laboratory or animal house. These over-garments protect the wearer's street clothing. Contaminated clothing should be changed and disinfected by appropriate means, and laboratory clothing should not be worn in non-laboratory areas.
2. Gloves should be worn for all those procedures which may involve direct contact with blood, infectious material or infected animals, etc.
3. Whether in the laboratory or animal areas, the chance of a foot injury is always present. Wearing street shoes in the animal rooms is generally the source of infection in the animal colony and should be avoided. Rubber shoes, boots/overboots are ideal in areas of chemical spills and wet areas. Shoe covers can be worn as a barrier between the wearer's shoe and the hazard (especially in the case of radiation hazard)
4. Eye Protectors/Safety Glasses should be used where operations present hazards of flying objects (dust, fur, etc.), glare, radiation, intense light etc. Care should be taken to protect eyes from ultraviolet light. Sufficient washing facilities (eye washes, deluge shower) should be available when handling liquids that may burn or irritate, etc.
5. Biological safety cabinets may be used to provide physical containment of specimen cultures and for the protection of personnel, where procedures creating hazardous aerosols are conducted. These cabinets are of different kinds depending upon the protection needed, the environment and the particular experiment.
6. Fume hoods should be used when handling hazardous fumes, gas or toxic solvents, etc.

7. Pipetting aids are available to replace mouth pipetting which should be prohibited.
8. Autoclaves should be available to sterilize contaminated materials.
9. Incinerators should be used to reduce aerosol production.
10. Screw-cap tubes and bottles provide positive specimen containment.

SUMMARY

The following basic laboratory practices look very simple, but require special attention by laboratory personnel for their safety and hygiene.

1. Eating, drinking, smoking, storing food and applying cosmetics should not be permitted in the laboratory work area.
2. Laboratory coats, gloves, etc. should not be worn out of the laboratory.
3. Hands should be washed after handling the animals and before leaving the laboratory.
4. Sharp objects like needles, broken glass, etc. should be disposed of properly in special containers.
5. Mouth pipetting should not be allowed.
6. All animals need to be handled carefully using prescribed handling and restraining techniques.
7. All inflammable and toxic chemicals should be used and stored properly.
8. If radioactive isotopes are used the area should be properly marked, radiation exposure monitored and proper shielding provided. To avoid contamination, the use of gloves, pipetting devices, a careful technique, approved radioactive disposal methods, and containment, should be observed.
9. Safety systems should cover fire and electrical emergencies, first aid, safety showers and eye wash facilities.

Human error and poor laboratory practice can compromise the best of laboratory safeguards and protective devices/equipment. Thus, laboratory safety requires not only the worker's awareness about the recognition and control of laboratory hazards, but also commonsense and good laboratory practice, which are key elements in the prevention of laboratory accidents, hazards and acquired infections. In general, it is perfectly safe to work in a laboratory when proper techniques, necessary precautions and good laboratory practice are being used.

LITERATURE CONSULTED

1. *Code of Practice for the Protection of Persons Exposed to Ionizing Radiation in Research and Teaching.* Department of Employment. (1968). (London: HMSO)
2. Fuscaldo, A.A. (ed.). (1980). *Laboratory Safety, Theory and Practice.* (New York: Academic Press)
3. *Laboratory Organization and Management.* (1979). Grover, F. and Wallace, P. (eds.) (London: Butterworths)
4. Inglis, J.K. (ed.) (1980). *Introduction to Laboratory Animal Science and Technology. (London: Pergamon Press Ltd)*
5. Krishan, D., Venkateswaran, T.V. and Ahmad, M. (1980). *Radiation protection in Radioimmunoassay Work. Publication of Isotope group, Babha Atomic Research Centre. (Bombay, India)*
6. National Institutes of Health. (1974). *Biohazards Safety Guide.* (Washington, DC: US Department of Health and Human Services)
7. Report (1980). *General Guidelines for the Disposal of Solid and Liquid Radioactive Waste to the Users Handling Small Quantities of Radioisotopes.* Division of Radiological Protection, Bhabha Atomic Research Centre (BARC) (Bombay, India)
8. Shapiro, J. (ed.). (1981). *Radiation Protection: A Guide for Scientists and Physicians.* 2nd Edn. (Cambridge, Massachusetts and London, England: Harvard University Press)
9. Spanski Jr, W.B. and Harkness, J.E. (eds.). (1984). *Manual for Assistant Laboratory Animal Technicians.* (USA: The American Association for Laboratory Animal Science)
10. World Health Organization. (1983). *Laboratory Biosafety Manual.* (Printed in England)

14 X-ray Hazards – Diagnostic and Therapeutic

R.G. Putney and N.W. Garvie

INTRODUCTION

This chapter deals with the hazards associated with the clinical use of X-rays, particularly for members of staff working within radiology and radiotherapy departments, who necessarily, during the course of their employment, suffer a level of occupational exposure.

Wilhelm Roentgen, a German physicist, is generally regarded as the founding father of the science of radiology, although the phenomena, of whose clinical significance he became aware, were brought to scientific attention through the development of cathode ray tubes in the earlier part of the nineteenth century. The first radiograph was obtained by Roentgen in 1895, using an exposure time of 30 minutes, and by the subsequent year X-ray apparatus began to be installed in hospitals. At the same time the adverse effects of X-rays began to be suspected. In 1896 Dr Daniel of Vanderbilt University reported depilation as a direct result of X-ray exposure. The risks were not, however, fully appreciated, and many X-ray pioneers eventually fell fatal victims to the side effects of their work. A growing awareness of these risks gave rise to the development of the science of radiation protection.

All life on earth has been exposed, since inception, to continuous low-level X-ray irradiation from a variety of sources, including cosmic rays from space, and naturally occurring radioactive minerals, and to this extent X-rays must be considered as part of man's natural environment. In the twentieth century these factors have been supplemented by the increasing use of artificially produced radiation, from such diverse sources as the development of the television set and the atmospheric testing of nuclear weapons, but the most significant contribution to the population dose in developed countries is from medical applications. In particular the diagnostic use of X-rays applies to people of all ages and it is important to minimize the quantity of radiation required to produce a satisfactory clinical result. There is a range of background radiation to which people are subjected which depends upon geographical location. Such variations can be considered a part of nature. These natural variations can be used as a guide as to what levels of radiation are acceptable. Thus the mean medical annual dose per head of population added to the mean annual background radiation level should be kept within the natural variation of background. Currently, diagnostic radiological procedures in developed countries add a dose of between one-fifth and two-thirds to that of natural background.

NATURE OF X-RAYS

X-radiation is electromagnetic in nature and forms part of the electromagnetic spectrum occupying the higher energy end. X-radiation behaves both as a particle and a wave; it has a dual nature. The X-ray particle is called a photon, and the photon also carries wave information in terms of having features which can be related to wavelengths. Photon energy is in direct proportion to its frequency, frequency and wavelength being uniquely related via the velocity of electromagnetic radiation which is 3×10^8 m/s. Photon energy is generally expressed in electron-volts (eV). Diagnostic X-ray photons have energies between 10 and 150 keV while for therapy they may reach several tens of MeV. X-rays have wavelengths of 10^{-9} metre or less and frequencies greater than 10^{17} Hz. The higher the photon energy the greater its penetrating ability, and consequently the thickness of protective devices has to increase with increasing photon energy in order to significantly attenuate the photon flux. X-radiation travels in straight lines and its intensity is reduced in proportion to the inverse square of the distance between the X-ray source and object. The total energy deposited by the X-radiation is directly related to the length of time of exposure; this also applies to biological material. These factors form the basis of radiation protection, i.e. the distance between radiation source and subject should be the maximum possible, an adequate thickness of protective material should be placed between the subject and the radiation source, where required, and the time spent in the vicinity of the radiation source should be kept to a minimum.

X-rays are produced when electrons having been accelerated by an electric field are rapidly decelerated by placing a high atomic number target in their path. This is practically achieved by the use of a specialized diode in which the potential difference between cathode and anode is of the order of 100 kV and the anode is made of tungsten or a tungsten alloy. The point of impact between electrons and anode is the source of the X-radiation, the X-radiation is more accurately termed *bremsstrahlung* (braking radiation). The kinetic energy of the electrons in keV is equivalent to the kilovoltage applied to the diode (X-ray tube). Thus the electron's kinetic energy is converted into heat and X-radiation when the electron is stopped by the anode. The maximum photon energy which can be achieved is equal to the peak kilovoltage applied, thus an X-ray tube operating at $100\,kV_p$ can produce maximum energy photons of 100 keV. The majority of the photons will have energies less than this and, therefore, a continuous X-ray spectrum will be produced from a few keV up to the maximum. The low-energy photons generally have little chance of influencing the clinical result and are, therefore, reduced by placing metal filters between the X-ray tube and the patient. These filters are a permanent fixture and a minimum thickness of material is specified for each range of kilovoltages. For diagnostic X-ray tubes a peak in the spectrum is obtained at about one-half to two-thirds the maximum energy, thus most X-ray photons are produced at this energy. Altering the kilovoltage shifts the spectrum up or down according to the direction of the kilovoltage change and this can be used to select the penetration to match the attenuator, i.e. an extremity X-ray kilovoltage will be lower than that for an abdomen. The intensity of the X-radiation is proportional to the square of the kilovoltage and directly proportional to the tube current. The kilovoltage, therefore, controls both the intensity and the penetrating ability of the X-ray beam.

X-RAYS – EFFECT ON BIOLOGICAL MATERIAL

When X-rays are absorbed by living cells the transfer of energy produces effects which are potentially harmful to biological material. The extent of the damage depends upon the level of exposure, and upon the amount of energy absorbed by the recipient tissue. The energy contained in the X-ray photon is transferred to the cell by heat production, excitation of ions and molecules, and by ionization. In particular, radiolysis of water leads to the appearance of highly reactive uncharged hydrogen and hydroxyl free radicals which react with organic molecules within tissue. This process may produce a variety of effects, including enzyme destruction and alteration in DNA, and may ultimately lead to inhibition of cell division, premature cell death, or the production of transmissible or inheritable changes, particularly within germ cells, which may be propagated by subsequent cell multiplication. Although the chemical changes induced by X-rays within the environment of the cell occur instantaneously, the biological effects of X-irradiation may manifest over a widely varying time-scale, from a few hours to many years.

A radiation dose in excess of 10 Gy (1000 rads) to the human body will cause death within a week, and a dose of 5 Gy (500 rads) will prove fatal to 50% of the exposed population within 2–3 weeks. There is considerably more uncertainty, however, about the effect of low-level exposure to radiation, such as experienced by occupationally exposed workers. Accurate data are difficult to provide, because of the long latent period that may elapse before effects manifest. There is continuing debate concerning whether or not, for example, the risk of cancer formation is linearly proportional to radiation dose at all dose levels, or whether a 'safe threshold' dose exists below which cancer does not develop. It is known, however, that long term effects of exposure to radiation include the development of certain tumours of the thyroid, lung and bone, leukaemia, and cataract formation. Other effects, such as dermatitis and skin cancer, are seen at higher sustained dose levels. Tissues with a high inherent cell multiplication rate, such as bone marrow and intestinal mucosa, are particularly liable to radiation damage. In addition, it has been shown that exposure of pregnant females to ionizing radiation may result in damage to the developing embryo. These risks are believed to be greatest if exposure occurs during the first 2 months of pregnancy.

Table 14.1 Dose limits for occupationally exposed workers aged 18 years or over

	Annual limit	*Other limit*
Whole body	50 mSv (5 rem)	
Effective dose (from partial body exposure)	50 mSv (5 rem)	
Abdomen of woman of reproductive capacity		13 mSv (1.3 rem) in a quarter
Abdomen of a pregnant woman		10 mSv (1 rem) between declaration of pregnancy and delivery
Lens of the eye	150 mSv (15 rem)	
Skin (averaged over any area of 100 cm^2)*	500 mSv (50 rem)	
Hands, forearms, feet and ankles	500 mSv (50 rem)	
Any other organ or tissue (average in organ)	500 mSv (50 rem)	

* 100 cm^2 applies to doses from radioactive contamination; a smaller averaging area should be used for radiation beams.
It must be noted that the dose shown for any other organ or tissue may be less than the limit shown by an amount which depends on a factor which relates to a particular organ's radiosensitivity (ICRP 26).

Because of concern over the possible effects of radiation on occupationally exposed workers, most countries have developed regulations or recommendations specifying the dose limits for exposed staff, which should not be exceeded (Table 14.1). These limits, which are necessarily arbitrary, although founded so far as possible upon scientific facts, are under continuous review. It is interesting to note that the safe dose recommended by the International Commission on Radiation Protection has been revised downwards over the past 50 years. For example, the 'tolerable dose' in 1934 was 1.0 rads per week, whereas in 1956 the 'maximum permissible dose' was designated as 0.1 rads per week. For the general population, however, X-irradiation from medical and industrial sources forms only a small part of the total exposure level, which remains largely due to cosmic radiation, and localized gamma radiation. Whatever the prescribed safety levels for absorbed dose, it remains a fundamental feature of radiation protection that, within these levels, all reasonable steps should be taken to minimize unnecessary staff exposure to keep the absorbed dose 'as low as reasonably achievable'. In response to continuing public and scientific concern it is likely that further downward revision of the recommended safety levels will occur.

X-RAY MEASUREMENT

The energy contained in a beam of X-radiation is specified as the radiation exposure. This quantity is measured by collecting the electrical charge released from a known mass of air contained within the X-ray beam. The quantity associated with the energy absorbed from the X-ray beam by the medium through which it passes is called the dose. Thus radiation exposure is the dose in air. Finally, the quantity which takes account of the relative biological damage inflicted by different types of ionizing radiation is called the dose equivalent. The units of dose and dose equivalent are the Gray (Gy) and the Sievert (Sv), respectively. These units are in accordance with the SI system. The units of dose and dose equivalent used prior to these were the rad and the rem respectively. The unit of exposure was the Roentgen, but the SI system has not specified a particular unit in this case and so exposure is quoted as coulombs per kilogram of air or dose in air. Table 14.2 lists the units and their interrelationship.

Table 14.2

Quantity	Pre-SI unit	SI unit	Base units
Radiation exposure	Roentgen		$C\,kg^{-1}$
Dose	Rad	Gray	$J\,kg^{-1}$
Dose equivalent	Rem	Sievert	$J\,kg^{-1}$

1 Gy = 100 rads; 1 Sv = 100 rems

The most common practical method of measuring X-radiation is with an ionization chamber. Such chambers are air equivalent and are designed in a number of geometries, of which the cylindrical or thimble chamber type is most common. A knowledge of the mass absorption coefficients of air and the material being irradiated will, in principle, enable the reading of the ionization chamber dosimeter system to be converted to dose. Dose equivalent can be found by consideration of the density depositions of energy which is based on the type of radiation. For X-radiation the factor for converting Gray to Sievert is unity.

RADIATION DOSAGES TO EXPOSED GROUPS

The basis for safe working within such departments as diagnostic radiology and radiotherapy must be a knowledge of what levels of radiation are considered acceptable. The International Commission on Radiological Protection (ICRP) continually reviews, in the light of the latest information, all aspects of the use of such radiation and it is on the Commission's reports that methods of safe working practice can be instigated. The philosophy of the ICRP is that 'Radiation protection is concerned with the protection of individuals, their progeny and mankind as a whole, while still allowing necessary activities from which radiation exposure might result'. Additional information concerning the balance of risk to benefit of radiation is produced by the United Nations Scientific Committee on the Effects of Atomic Radiation (UNSCEAR), International Atomic Energy Agency (IAEA) and World Health Organisation (WHO).

In a department, there are four groups of persons to consider for radiation protection purposes:

1. members of the public whose visit to the department is temporary;
2. staff not directly concerned with the application of radiation, such as secretarial staff;
3. staff directly involved with the application of radiation, such as radiographers;
4. the patient.

For all these groups the ALARA principle (as low as reasonably achievable) holds: for the first three groups a dose equivalent limit (DEL) has been set, which must not be exceeded. The fourth group, the patient, can reasonably expect that the application of radiation for their diagnosis and treatment is controlled in order that damage to tissue not directly affected by the disease is kept as low as possible unless this jeopardizes the treatment.

The dose equivalent limits (DELs) are subject to continual review. Many requirements for safe working practice, however, are fundamental and are based on what are considered to be the best working methods to achieve the required result at the minimum dose to the staff. Such requirements may be generalized as follows:

1. *Correct room design*. The diagnostic and treatment rooms can be considered as radiation containers, and their layout and construction must be such as to reduce the level of radiation scattered or transmitted outside to within that which is currently acceptable.
2. *Radiation dose monitoring of areas and staff involved with radiation*. Personal monitoring relates to particular individuals carrying at all times during work a device which records the amount of radiation

286

received. Such a device is termed a personal dosemeter. It is mandatory for individuals to have personal dosemeters in situations where they are likely to receive doses in excess of 3/10 of a dose limit. In such cases the personal dosemeter must be supplied by an approved laboratory, where 'approved' means that the laboratory has demonstrated to a national radiation laboratory a certain precision in the results obtained with such dosemeters. Additionally, a good record keeping system for such results has also been proven by such laboratories. Personal do-semeters are usually either based on a small piece of photographic film (film badge) or on thermoluminescent effects the TLD badge. In each case the personal dosemeter requires careful calibration and sophisti-cated readout facilities. It should be noted that personal dosemeters merely record the radiation to which an individual has been exposed and does not in any way protect them from such radiation. All such devices are clearly retrospective, in situations where the radiation levels are required to be known immediately other devices are available and would be appropriate, however such devices should not replace the film or TLD badge.

3. Adequate training of staff and the provision of all relevant radiation protective devices and equipment necessary to carry out their duties with minimal dose to themselves.

4. To provide a logical and approachable responsible organization in order that staff at all levels know the procedure for ensuring that any comments or problems they have which have radiological protection implications may be impartially considered.

5. That rules relating to particular machines are written by suitably quali-fied persons in which any unusual aspects of the equipment are indi-cated, prepared working methods are described, persons immediately responsible for radiation protection of the equipment are listed and emergency procedures are described. These rules are known as local rules.

6. Every member of staff must understand the codes of practice which are drawn up by governmental bodies and are based on the reports of the international commissions. They describe the methods by which staff can pursue their function within the department while minimizing dose to themselves and others. Also any relevant local rules must be read and understood by staff. Staff should sign a statement saying that they have read and understood these rules.

7. Women of reproductive age are considered as a special group among radiation workers. The possibility of pregnancy is present which, when confirmed, may require additional protective measures. The quarterly DEL for these workers should not exceed one-quarter of the annual dose limit. These staff have a responsibility to inform their heads of departments when a pregnancy is confirmed in order that consideration

can be given to temporarily changing their work function in order to reduce dose. Currently following confirmation of pregnancy the dose limit should be set at 10 millisievert (mSv)/(1 rem) for the remaining term of the pregnancy.

ORGANIZATIONAL STRUCTURE OF RADIOLOGICAL PROTECTION

It is not possible to run a department which uses ionizing radiation safely without organizing a clearly defined structure of people who are responsible for the control and administration of procedures involving the use of such radiation and thereby the well-being of the people carrying out those procedures. A typical organizational structure is as follows.

The administrative organization of radiological protection

Controlling authority

The controlling authority (the employer) carries the ultimate responsibility for radiological protection and safety. In order to comply with this responsibility the controlling authority would need to appoint a number of qualified persons to advise and execute instructions.

Radiological protection adviser (RPA)

The RPA is a qualified and experienced physicist appointed by the controlling authority. The controlling authority is likely to have little or no understanding of radiation protection; the RPA is appointed to give that expert advice to the controlling authority. In order to carry out his duties the RPA will need to regularly visit the hospitals and departments to which he has been nominated, to review, in consultation with the heads of department the protection measures laid down. Such discussions would normally include input from any professional or safety representatives within each department. Any changes which are deemed necessary would be channelled through the controlling authority especially where equipment is required to be purchased or any structural alterations need to be effected. The RPA should meet regularly with the controlling authority in order that they may be kept informed as to the current state of radiological protection within their jurisdiction.

Head of department

Where radiation is used, the head of department, in collaboration with the radiological safety organization must ensure that any national codes of practice and all local rules are observed within his department. The head of department would be responsible for ensuring that any defective X-ray equipment or radiation protection devices were not used until repaired or replaced. It would be the responsibility of staff within the department to bring such situations to the immediate notice of the head of department. The head of department would also be responsible for the safe use of X-ray equipment used outside the confines of his department. An obvious example of this would be the use of mobile X-ray equipment. In such situations it is likely that arrangements would have to be made with the staff in the other department such that the authority of the radiographer or person in charge of the X-ray equipment was recognized. To this end collaboration between the heads of department would be necessary.

Appointed doctor

The appointed doctor is designated by the controlling authority to be responsible for the medical supervision of all appropriate staff. Staff designated as classified, that is staff likely to receive more than 3/10 of any dose limit would be subject to annual medicals and to have certain medical tests (such as blood count) as and when the appointed doctor sees fit. The appointed doctor would be expected to be familiar with the biological effects of radiation and to medically supervise any staff who have been significantly irradiated as the result of accidental exposure to ionizing radiation. Any planned special exposure to radiation would be subject to approval and control by the appointed doctor.

Radiological safety committee (RSC)

The controlling authority may set up a committee to advise on radiation protection matters. Membership of the committee would involve staff representatives from each group which had regular contact with radiation sources. Thus nurses, radiographers, radiologists and radiotherapists would be among those expected to be represented on such a committee. RPAs would naturally be part of any RSC. Although, currently advice is given by the RPA and there is no mention of RSCs in the latest legislation on the use of ionizing radiation in the UK, many hospitals feel that the multidisciplinary input of the RSC is valuable and will continue to use them. Thus, in the UK, while hospitals have a duty, by law, to appoint an RPA, the setting up of an RSC is at the discretion of the controlling authority.

Occupationally exposed persons – designation

For the purpose of monitoring and surveillance, a clear distinction is made between two categories of workers. A worker is designated as a 'classified' radiation worker if he receives or is likely to receive a dose in excess of 3/10 of any dose limit. With the current annual dose limit of 50 mSv the three-tenths limit corresponds to 15 mSv which as an approximate guide is 1.25 mSv per month. The other category is a worker who receives less than the three-tenths dose limit in a year. Areas in which the dose levels are such that persons remaining there for 40 hours per week would exceed the three–tenths limit are designated as controlled radiation areas. By definition, therefore, only classified radiation workers may enter a controlled area. In many instances, however, this would be an unnecessary burden, and so it is possible for non-classified persons to enter a controlled area, provided it is done by following a system of work. The system of work should be written into the local rules for that area and should clearly describe all precautions required to enter the controlled area safely. One obvious likely requirement under such a system of work would be for any person requiring to enter the room for the purpose of a work activity to be issued with a personal do-semeter. A classified worker does not have to enter a controlled area under a system of work.

Assessment of individual doses must be systematic for classified workers and be carried out by an approved dosimetry service. The dose results should be submitted to the worker, the RPA and the appointed doctor. Thus the RPA and the appointed doctor can fulfil their roles by (in the case of the RPA) checking that the radiation protection arrangements are satisfactory and (in the case of the appointed doctor) fulfilling his responsibility in relation to the health of the worker.

Medical supervision of classified persons must include a pre-employment medical examination, general medical surveillance and periodic reviews of health (at least annually). In accordance with this supervision, the medical state of a classified person with respect to his fitness for work must be defined by one of three classifications, namely fit, fit subject to certain conditions, or unfit. A medical record and a record of individual monitoring information must be opened and kept up to date for every classified person. Thereafter, the records must be retained in the archives for a period of at least 50 years. Only classified persons can be subjected to planned special exposures. Individual monitoring and special medical supervision of all other persons, i.e. non classified workers, is not required but can be implemented discretionally.

Radiation Protection Supervisor (RPS)

The RPS is a competent person of sufficient knowledge, experience and seniority to supervise the use of radiation within a defined area. The RPS is appointed in writing by the Controlling Authority and the letter of appointment should list the responsibilities of the RPS. It is usual to appoint a different RPS for every department in which radiation is used.

Duties of the RPS – General duties   The RPS has a duty to ensure that protection measures are carried out. Three fundamental aspects of this duty are to:

1. ensure that the code of practice and any local rules are observed in the department;
2. ensure that personnel monitoring devices are used where necessary and in the correct manner;
3. maintain safe working practices in the department by instruction, supervision and, not least, by example to other personnel. In this way, the RPS can strive to keep the occupational exposure of workers as low as is reasonably practicable.

The RPS, in consultation with the head of department, must report to the Radiological Protection Adviser in writing when:

1. it is suspected that a radiation hazard exists;
2. any maintenance or servicing has been carried out, or any new technique adopted, which may affect the protection of a machine or a protected area;
3. any member of staff has been repeatedly breaking protection rules, as specified by the code of practice or the local rules.

RADIOTHERAPY – INTRODUCTION

The following rules primarily relate to radiotherapy techniques, that is, in situations where a large enough radiation dose is delivered to a region within the patient causing an immediate change in the constitution of the tissues within the defined region. The equipment used in such situations has, in general, a significantly higher radiation output than in diagnostic equipment where great care is taken to minimize any alteration to the tissues subject to irradiation. Therefore, while many of the following points relating to safe working practice may be similar to the diagnostic situation there are major differences, the most obvious of which is that in diagnostic radiology it is common practice for some staff under clearly defined conditions (systems of work) to be present in the X-ray room while the equipment is producing radiation. This is never allowed in the radiotherapy situation. It is fundamental to both situations that only the specified tissues are subject to irradiation. In radiotherapy the aim is to uniformly irradiate the specified region to the prescribed dose while minimizing irradiation of all other tissues. In diagnostic radiology it is the aim to irradiate the specified region to the minimum doses consistent with obtaining a diagnostic image while minimizing irradiation of all other tissues.

In radiotherapy there are two distinct methods of treatment. Brachytherapy relates to the treatment of the diseased tissue using radioactive sealed sources (that is sources contained within a sealed metal container usually in the form of wire, rods or needles) which are placed in close proximity to or within the tissue to be treated. This method poses a different set of protection problems where control and care of the sources is paramount in contrast to the second general treatment method termed teletherapy. In this case an extremely active source is contained within a machine which is housed in a specially designed treatment room. The room is made from materials which absorb the radiation scattered within the room when the machine is on. Thus the operator is protected from the effects of the radiation. The patient lies on a couch beneath the unit and the head is aligned with the region to be treated using a light beam to simulate the radiation beam. The source is generally about 1 metre from the patient and treatment times last only a few minutes. The patient is left alone in the room, and the operator removes a shutter remotely from outside, the time the shutter is removed dictates the treatment time and hence the dose delivered. Radiation protection in this situation hinges around emergency procedures, for example if the shutter fails to close at the end of the treatment time, and specifying working procedures to ensure that inadvertent irradiation of staff members cannot occur. A further treatment method is becoming very common and is termed afterloading: it consists of loading dummy (non-active) substitutes into tubes within the patient. This ensures that positioning of the dummies radiographically is correct before the patient is taken to a protected room where the active sources may be remotely loaded. Nursing activities may be carried out with the sources withdrawn which minimizes any radiation protection problems. There are numerous devices and variations on this idea, but in all cases it has the radiation protection advantage that a large amount of the work in loading and checking position etc. can be done with dummy sources. Wherever possible afterloading techniques should be employed.

GENERAL MEASURES FOR RADIOLOGICAL PROTECTION

All activities in the department must be carried out within the requirements set out in the current code of practice for the protection of persons against ionizing radiation arising from medical use.

All members of staff must read, understand and follow the local safety rules for the department.

Following a fire in the department, the complete area around the department must be sealed off until the RPA and the appropriate radiological monitoring department have checked the area.

All barriers and doors to treatment rooms should remain open except when the unit is to be energized. Treatment keys must be removed at all times when staff are not present.

Emergency 'off' switches should be available at prominent positions within the treatment room.

PROTECTION OF STAFF

All members of staff must be aware of warning signs in the department, e.g. red lights by treatment doors, and must ensure that they do not enter any area where the warning sign indicates that it is unsafe to do so.

All members of staff who are occupationally exposed to ionizing radiation must wear a personal monitoring device, either a film badge or an alternative monitoring device as supplied by the radiological monitoring department. Staff must ensure that their personal monitoring device is used in the correct manner and that they are changed at the appropriate times.

Every member of staff is responsible for the use and safe-keeping of their personal monitoring device. If any problems arise, staff should not hesitate to contact the departmental RPS or the head of department, or the radiological monitoring department.

Any radiation incident involving staff must be reported to the head of department, to the RPA and to the RPS.

In gamma-ray units, the radionuclide radiates continuously and so, despite shielding, there will be an inevitable low level of transmitted radiation. Accordingly, the treatment room must remain unoccupied at all times except for the purposes of treating a patient, for maintenance of equipment or for any other essential activity.

When treating a patient, the most senior radiographer present must ensure that no member of staff is in the treatment room before irradiation begins. All staff must be very familiar with the location of the emergency 'off' switches on all the treatment machines.

PROTECTION OF PATIENTS

A patient's radiotherapy treatment must only be administered as prescribed on the patient's treatment sheet. Details of the irradiation must be recorded immediately on the treatment sheet.

Members of staff should consider themselves responsible for the radiation that they administer.

If a radiation incident occurs involving a patient, the radiographers or other staff members involved must report details both to the superintendent radiographer and to the doctor responsible for the patient.

For women of childbearing age there may be special treatment requirements which the radiotherapist will specify in order to minimise the dose to reproductive organs.

SAFETY MEASURES IN RADIOTHERAPY WORK: SEALED SOURCES LABORATORY – GENERAL SAFETY RULES

Introduction

Radiotherapy is concerned with the use of ionizing radiation (most commonly X- or γ-radiation) for the treatment of disease. This form of treatment requires a dose of radiation to be delivered to the prescribed region, which must be large enough to ensure that within the treatment volume all of the affected tissue is sterilized. Methods of delivering such a dose can be divided into external beam machines (teletherapy), of which an X-ray machine is an obvious example, and the use of radioactive materials which are placed in close proximity to the treatment region (brachytherapy). The use of radiation in this way is generally restricted to large hospitals and the building and organization of such a radiotherapy department must be arranged according to internationally accepted methods.

All procedures carried out must conform with the relevant codes of practice for the protection of persons against ionizing radiations arising from medical use.

Persons to be designated responsible for the safety of the laboratory:

1. custodian of radioactive sealed sources;
2. deputy custodian;
3. radiation protection supervisor (RPS);
4. radiation protection adviser (RPA).

The custodian may also serve as RPS if appropriate.

Preparation of radioactive sources must be carried out behind shielding of adequate thickness to protect the operator and any other persons in the vicinity of the handling area.

The storage of radioactive sources (temporary or permanent) must be such as to minimize exposure to radiation (during transfer to and from the storage units). Individual storage compartments should not contain more than 20 sources or be of higher γ-ray activity than 100 milligrams of radium-226 or 10 GB$_q$ (270 mCi) of caesium-137.

A sealed source register must be maintained giving details of all radioactive sources held in stock. This register must show the initial date of receipt of the source, the type of source, its activity, physical dimensions and serial number. Record dates of examinations, leak and wipe testing and, when appropriate, the disposal date and destination of the source.

A quarterly audit must be carried out by the custodian to account for all registered sources. A yearly audit and tests in accordance with the current 'codes of practice' must be carried out by the responsible radiological protection department.

Detailed records must be kept of all radioactive sources issued or returned recording the following:

1.   the name of the patient or person using the source;
2.   the method of loading if appropriate;
3.   the type of applicator;
4.   the initials of issuing officer and recipient if a staff member.

A record sheet must accompany all sources issued for treatment purposes giving details of:

1.   the sources and the applicator used;
2.   the date and time required in the ward or operating theatre;
3.   the date and time of insertion and removal, with the signature of staff responsible for insertion and removal;
4.   the prescribed dose and duration of treatment.

A wall chart should be maintained in the sealed sources laboratory giving:

1.   the location of sources in use;
2.   the number and type of sources;
3.   the date of issue and approximate date and time of return.

Radioactive sources must be transported in protective containers specified for this purpose. The container must give adequate protection to all persons in the vicinity of the container. All containers must be marked with radiation warnings and show the name of the patient and the ward.

Sterilization procedures must be in accordance with recommended methods as prescribed for the type of material in use.

Wards having patients undergoing treatment with radioactive sources must be checked frequently and regularly by the radiological monitoring department to ensure correct functioning of the incinerator monitors. Such radiation monitors give clear warning if any material to be disposed of by incineration is contaminated with radioactive substances. Similarly, all material for disposal from the radioactive sealed sources laboratory must first be monitored before being cleared for disposal.

Patients being treated with radioactive sources must not be transferred from one ward to another without prior notification to the custodian, to enable adequate checks to be made on ward incinerator monitors and any necessary radiation protection measurements to be made in the vicinity of the patient undergoing treatment.

RADIOTHERAPY – DUTIES OF THE RADIATION PROTECTION SUPERVISOR (RPS)

Sealed sources

If it is suspected that a sealed source has been lost or damaged, the RPS must set the appropriate emergency procedure in motion. In the particular event of the loss or suspected loss of a sealed source, the RPS must arrange for an immediate search for the lost source to be made by a competent person. During the search it is vitally important to cover the possibility that the source may have located itself in protective material where its presence may not be readily detectable using monitoring instruments.

The RPS must ensure that all entrances to wards or other areas in which patients are liable to be undergoing sealed source therapy, carry the standard symbol denoting the possible presence of ionizing radiation. The RPS must also ensure that all beds occupied by such patients carry a notice to indicate the fact that radiation is present. The notice must also include the standard hazard symbol. Details which should be included on the notice are the number and nature of sources, the total activity of the radioactive substances, the time and date of application and removal, and all relevant nursing instructions.

On wards or in other locations where patients undergoing therapy reside, the RPS of the relevant ward or department must measure or otherwise estimate the dose rate around the patient, paying particular attention to gaps between mobile protective screens where 'hot spots' may occur. Care should be taken to ensure the dose rates are low, i.e. less than $0.75\,\mu$Sv h^{-1} in areas occupied by other persons, either staff, patients or visitors, etc. Standard radiation notices should be fitted to the beds and the entrance to the room if appropriate. There should be a suitable source container and handling tools in close vicinity to the patient in order that safe storage for the source is readily to hand if required. The RPS must issue specific instructions regarding the daily time allowable for nursing procedures and visiting.

External beam therapy

The duties of the RPS are to:

1. see that all safety interlocks and warning lights on treatment room doors are operational;
2. see that all radiation monitors in the megavoltage therapy rooms are operational;
3. see that staff are aware of any special local rules, if applicable, to any individual treatment rooms;
4. ensure that the radiotherapy department provides training for newly appointed staff in emergency rules, particularly in γ-ray therapy;
5. see that newly appointed staff read and understand all the relevant sections of the Code of Practice.

THE CUSTODIAN OF SEALED SOURCES – DUTIES AND RELEVANT RADIOLOGICAL PROTECTION INFORMATION

The storage and movement of radioactive substances: definitions and fundamental duties

In each hospital where radioactive substances are used, a custodian must be appointed to be responsible, in consultation with the RPS, RPA/RSC, for organizing the security during storage and use of all sealed sources and for ensuring that all necessary records are kept.

A specific person, or persons, must be appointed to be directly responsible under the custodian for the receipt, storage, maintenance and issue of sealed sources.

Full records must be kept of all sealed sources received, stored and issued.

The stores must be maintained in an orderly fashion and must be inspected regularly either by the custodian or by another person who has been specifically appointed to accept this responsibility.

Issuing of sources

Sealed sources must be issued from a main store only by the custodian or by one of the individuals who has been specifically appointed to carry out this duty. Once issued, the use or storage of sealed sources and the basic, relevant radiological protection measures associated with their use or storage, must at all times be entrusted to the care of responsible individuals until the return or disposal of the sources. Ideally, all aspects of radiological care should be supervised by the RPS responsible for the ward or department in which the sealed sources are being used.

Whenever sealed sources are transferred from the care of one person to another, the recipient must sign a receipt on a form provided for this purpose. This receipt must state the radionuclide, the approximate activity, the type and number of sources and the person or department from which they were received.

Audits, registers and records

A sealed sources register must be kept showing full particulars of all sealed sources having a half-life greater than a few days. This register must include all relevant information concerning the radionuclide, its activity on a given date and the construction, dimensions and serial numbers (where appropriate) of each type of source. Records of examination, leakage tests and repairs must also be included in the register.

Records must be kept of all sealed sources received at or issued from the main store. These records must be signed, either by the custodian or by an individual with specifically allocated authority. The records must be of sufficient clarity and detail to enable the reader to immediately ascertain the precise whereabouts of any source and also to know its expected date of return. A record should also be made permanently available of all the sources of each type that are actually in the store and available for issue. At regular and frequent intervals the custodian, or an individual with specifically allocated authority, must undertake an audit to account for every source listed in the sealed sources register. All the sources in the store must be counted, although it is not necessary to check serial numbers. If a group of sources have remained in a sealed container since the last audit, then the previous count may be accepted. Sources which have left the store must be covered by a current receipt.

Damage to sealed sources

After use, all sealed sources must be inspected for evidence of damage before being returned to main store.

All sealed sources must be regularly examined by a specifically authorized person so as to permit the early detection of progressive damage to the protective encasement of a source. In some circumstances this will become the duty of the custodian. If not, the custodian should help ensure that this task is performed by requesting the service of the person who has been appointed the duty at the appropriate times. Examination of this type should be conducted using a lead glass window of suitable protective capacity together with a suitable magnifying lens.

All sealed sources must be tested for leakage and surface contamination when new, annually, and whenever damage to the source is suspected. The source must initially be considered leaking if the test indicates a free activity of more than 200 B_q (5 nCi). This decision can only be changed if the free activity can be positively identified as surface contamination. In this event it may be possible either to remove the surface contamination or to allow it to decay to an acceptably safe level. The custodian must not hesitate to seek expert advice if needed concerning any aspect of the treatment of surface contamination. Records of leakage tests must be entered into the sealed sources register.

If it is suspected that radioactive material is leaking, or is liable to leak, from a sealed source, the source must be placed immediately in an airtight container. If the source is radium, repairs can only be undertaken by an outside specialist agency.

Transport of sealed sources

If sealed sources are transported within the hospital they must be carried in containers that have been specifically provided for this purpose. All sealed source containers must bear the conventional symbol to denote the presence of substances which emit ionizing radiation and provide satisfactory radiation protection.

The sterilization and disinfection of small sealed sources

During procedures undertaken to sterilize or disinfect small sealed sources, the following basic precautions must always be observed:

1. the radiation exposure to the worker(s) involved and to any other staff who are liable to be in the vicinity at the time must be kept as low as is reasonably practicable through the adoption and conscientious execution of safe techniques;
2. damage to the sources must be avoided at all times;
3. at all stages during these procedures, the techniques adopted must help to minimize the possibility of losing a source.

If there are any doubts concerning the efficiency of the current techniques with reference to any of these points, the custodian must not hesitate to seek the advice of the RPA. Expert advice on the most effective methods of achieving a desired degree of sterilization or disinfection, should be sought from a consultant pathologist.

Radioactive source emergency – procedure in the event of loss or damage of a radioactive sealed source

The following persons must be informed in the event of suspected loss or damage to a radioactive sealed source:

1.   the radiation protection supervisor for sealed sources;
2.   the radiological protection adviser for sealed sources;
3.   the medical officer in charge;
4.   the duty administrator for the hospital;
5.   the nursing officer (if appropriate).

The following procedures *must* be followed immediately:

1.   if it is suspected that a source has been lost, ensure that no material or liquid is removed from the area concerned;
2.   if it is suspected that a source has been damaged, restrict the movements of all the personnel who have been involved in handling the source so that they remain in the affected area until they have been cleared through radiation monitoring;
3.   no attempt must be made to move any suspect material until experienced personnel have arrived;
4.   all the activities related to radioactive emergencies must be carried out by the custodian, the radiological monitoring department and the medical officer concerned.

EXTERNAL BEAM THERAPY – RADIONUCLIDE SOURCE UNIT – EMERGENCY PROCEDURE IN THE EVENT OF TECHNICAL FAILURE

Shutter failure

If, at the end of the treatment time, the source fails to return to the 'off' position, the following action should be taken. These facilities should always be present on this type of machine.

Press radiation off button

If this action fails to close shutter:

Press shutter emergency button

This action causes the collimator to be closed to the smallest field size by the motor. The shutter motor is turned on to move the shutter to the 'radiation off' position. The shutter emergency button lights up red when the collimator has reached the smallest field size. If, despite the action mentioned above, the beam has not been shut off, then immediately arrange for the patient to be removed from the room. Before entering the room the best and quickest way to assist the patient's removal from the room should be determined. Whilst in the treatment room, movement should be quick and avoidance of the path of the primary radiation beam is essential. Ensure the personal monitoring device is present and use a dose-rate monitor to measure the dose as it is received.

An accurate estimate of the prolongation of the patient's treatment should be made. If possible, a stop-watch should be used, which ought to be switched on the moment the shutter failure is noted.

Make sure the treatment room is unoccupied; lock the door; notify the Superintendent Radiographer and the RPS.

Action to be taken in case of technical failure other than shutter failure

If there is a technical failure other than shutter failure, i.e. gantry will not stop rotating during rotation treatment or patient is receiving an electric shock from table etc., the following action should be taken:

Press mains emergency button

These machines will have such a switch which should disconnect the mains supply to all parts of the machine and table, independent of the position of the source. If the source is in treatment position, it may be necessary to switch the mains back on to determine the position of the source, but care should be taken to ensure that if the faulty part has not been corrected, this will not endanger either the patient or the operator. It is advisable to remove the patient from the unit before switching mains on.

Action to be taken in case of mains failure

If the mains supply is interrupted during a treatment the source should automatically close. In this situation there may be no indication that the source is in a safe position. Proceed as above for 'press shutter emergency button' from 'the beam has not been shut off'; in case the source has remained in the open position. Note the reading on the timer so that an assessment of the actual treatment delivered can be made.

SAFETY ASPECTS OF BRACHYTHERAPY IN THE PATIENT'S VICINITY

Treatment times for brachytherapy patients can be as long as 1 week. This poses radiological protection problems for the nursing and other staff who care for the patient during this period. It is advisable to restrict treatment of this type, wherever possible, to particular wards were staff will become more familiar with looking after such patients and some degree of training in radiation protection may be implemented. It is further advisable, wherever possible, to provide these patients with a separate room, this will simplify the application of control which will be required of persons visiting the patient during this time. The safest method of treating such patients while minimizing radiation protection problems is by the use of afterloading machines. Using such machines the patient is fitted with an applicator which will accept the radioactive sources; however, it is not necessary to load the applicator with the radioactive sources until the patient is situated in a room specially designed for the treatment. This removes the problem of moving the patient through the hospital with radioactive material present and eradicates the radiation dose received by the person who would normally have inserted the sources (radiotherapist). When the patient reaches the treatment room the applicator is connected to the machine which contains the source. The sources can then remotely, and for preset periods automatically, load and unload the applicator. Nurses can override the system and have the sources removed before entering the room. There are two types of unit of this type: one uses high-activity sources and treatment times are short (several minutes), the patient is treated similarly to someone receiving teletherapy in as much as they are taken to the room at specific times for their treatment. Safety aspects in respect of these rooms are, therefore, similar to those for teletherapy rooms and sources failing to retract are also considered in a similar way. A second type of machine uses lower activity sources and the treatment time is normally several days. In this case the treatment room is provided with the usual radiological protection and the patient stays in a bed in the room for the duration of treatment. When nursing care is required, or visitors allowed, the sources are retracted. The radiation dose to staff is very small and in cases where the sources fail to retract there is normally plenty of time to inform the custodian who will instigate the appropriate manual source retrieval sequence required for a particular machine.

In situations where patients are being treated with radioactive material which is required to be permanently attached for a fixed period the nursing and allied radiation protection problems are more difficult. There are three types of such treatment, termed intracavitary, interstitial and surface loading. With these methods the radioactive material is loaded (usually in an operating theatre) into a natural body cavity, into tissue or fitted on the body surface respectively. The sources are provided in a number of geometries, i.e. wires, needles, tubes, etc., the geometry having been tailored for a particular application. The following is a list of procedures required when an emergency occurs with such patients. As many of the staff involved with these patients will not be familiar with handling radioactive material a brief set of rules is included as an example of what would be required in the local rules. Nursing staff, etc., would be expected to read these rules and be encouraged to discuss any fears or problems with their immediate superiors who can arrange for the RPS or RPA to provide more detailed explanation.

Basic principles of radiation protection

Protection from ionizing radiation is based on:

Distance

The farther an individual is from the source of radiation, the lower the dose received. Doubling the distance will quarter the dose received. Nursing staff should not work close to the source of radiation, if it is practicable to do the work even slightly farther away.

Speed

The shorter the time spent near the source of radiation, the less dose is received. Nurses should carry out only essential nursing duties and should work as rapidly as is compatible with acceptable standards.

Shielding

Protective barriers containing several centimetres of lead or several inches of concrete are required to absorb a significant proportion of a beam of radiation. Lead aprons should *not* be worn as they are too thin to provide any protection and merely restrict mobility. Portable lead screens are used in certain rooms to reduce the dosage to critical areas.

Vulnerability

Young individuals are more at risk than the elderly. The developing fetus is particularly sensitive and can be damaged by quite small doses of radiation. Pregnant staff must not work on wards where radioactive sources are used. Visiting should be limited to those over 50 years of age, and pregnant visitors must not be allowed.

Emergency procedure for patients bearing radioactive materials

If a radioactive source becomes detached from the patient do *not* attempt to replace the source. It should be picked up with long-handled forceps and placed inside the lead pot or transport box (which must always be available in the room). If it is necessary to cut any attached thread, the cut should be made away from the source. The exact time of removal must be noted in the nursing record and the radiotherapy registrar must be informed.

Suspected loss or damage to a radioactive source

The following personnel must be informed immediately:

1. the radiotherapy registrar on call;
2. sealed sources custodian or deputy;
3. radiological protection adviser.

While awaiting expert assistance, *nothing* should be removed from the room and unnecessary traffic in and out of the room should be prohibited. If a source is thought to be damaged, all involved personnel should remain beside the patient's room so that they can be monitored for radioactive contamination (significant contamination is most unlikely).

The radiation alarm on the ward incinerator is activated

In wards a radiation monitor may be present on the ward incinerator to detect radioactive material in the refuse. Warning that this has occurred is given by a siren or light. Contact the relevant staff who can offer expert help. While awaiting expert assistance, nothing must be removed from the incinerator and the refuse must not be burned.

Fire

Patients should be evacuated with the sources *in situ* along with their yellow radiation notices. Once safe, they should be placed in a single room or in an area with 2.5 m of clear space around the bed.

Patient requires artificial respiration

An Ambu bag or Brooke airway must be available and should be used rather than mouth-to-mouth respiration. This is *absolutely* vital where there are radioactive needles in the lip or tongue.

Cardiac arrest

External cardiac massage should be carried out as usual if this is appropriate. Where there is a chest wall implant or chest plaque, no one individual should perform external cardiac massage for longer than 5 minutes.

Death of a patient

The radioactive sources must be removed in the normal fashion before the body is taken to the mortuary.

Safety requirement for patients with brachytherapy sources

The patient should be nursed in a single room identified by the radiation hazard symbol. A portable lead pot or lead safe must be available in the room.

The form which accompanies the patient from the operating theatre must be displayed outside the room. This will specify the number and types of sources and the time they were inserted. The date and time of removal will be added by the radiotherapist when the final treatment time has been calculated.

The patient(s) occupying the adjacent bed(s) should be over the age of 50 years and ideally should be ambulant so that part of the day can be spent away from the source of radiation. Exceptions to this rule are patients having radiotherapy.

Pregnant members of staff (including domestics) must not work on the ward.

The patient must not get out of bed for any reason.

No visitors less than 50 years of age for the duration of the treatment.

Pregnant women of any age must be prohibited. A total of 2 h visiting over the duration of the period of the treatment should be the maximum permitted for any one individual.

Essential nursing procedures only must be carried out prior to removal of the sources. The nurse should work as rapidly as possible and keep as far from the source of radiation as possible. When a portable lead screen has been provided, the nurse should work from behind the screen whenever possible. The nurse should plan precisely what he/she intends to do before entering the room.

Following removal of the sources, the above restrictions must not be relaxed and the patient must not be discharged until written authorization (clearance certificate) is received from the sealed sources custodian. This ensures that all sources have been accounted for.

DIAGNOSTIC RADIOLOGY

Staff working with X-ray equipment are exposed to risks from a number of potential sources. Although precautions should be taken at all times to prevent accidental and unnecessary exposure to radiation, it is a fact that, in general, these risks are well minimized, and the biggest potential cause of staff morbidity is related to other factors, such as electrocution due to faulty circuits, and trauma due to working with heavy equipment.

Safety measures in diagnostic radiology

Tube factors

Although X-rays are generally thought of as being confined to the beam emergent from the tube, in fact they radiate with approximately equal intensity in every direction from the target. In addition to the primary rays produced, secondary scattered radiation further increases the level of radiation intensity within the tube. This radiation, if allowed to escape, would result in unnecessary exposure of personnel. These risks are higher in an older tube, where deposition of metal on the lining of the tube produces a 'secondary anode' for electron bombardment.

For this reason all X-ray tubes should be contained within a shield of appropriate absorptive material, except in the region of the beam window. Occasionally cracks may develop within the shield, particularly due to excessive heating and subsequent cooling. The integrity of the shield housing the tube should be checked visually, but monitoring may be necessary to exclude all small defects.

Current recommendations are that leakage radiation should not exceed

306

0.87 mGy in air per hour under maximum conditions at 1 metre from the focus averaged over an area of 100 cm^2.

Filtration

Diagnostic X-ray beams are composed of a wide spectrum of photon energies. The lower energies are completely absorbed by soft tissue, and do not contribute to picture quality. They contribute significantly, however, to skin dose, and can be removed by interposition of an appropriate material between the tube window and the patient.

In choosing a filter material, it is important that the emission of soft 'characteristic' radiation from the filter material is not substituted, such as may occur when copper filters alone are used. For this reason filters can be complex multi-layer sheets of various absorptive materials, selected to produce a beam quality consistent with the physical requirements of the examination. Inevitably the use of absorptive filters increases exposure time and the 'wear and tear' on the X-ray tube. A material used commonly for filtration purposes is aluminium and a minimum thickness of this material of 2.5 mm is required for most X-ray equipment. Other materials are quoted in aluminium equivalence.

Beam restriction

The greatest potential source of unnecessary exposure to patients and staff alike occurs with the use of poorly confined beams, such that the radiation is not restricted purely to the area of the patient under examination. Beam restriction may be achieved in a variety of ways, but all techniques employ the use of attenuating materials to absorb stray photons at the periphery of the desired beam.

The simplest type of beam restrictor is an aperture diaphragm, which consists of a lead sheet with central hole, the dimensions of which are determined by the size and shape of the desired X-ray beam. Beyond this, beam restriction may be achieved by the use of cylindrical or conical metallic devices, or movable collimators.

The width of the beam can be observed using a light beam, from a bulb mounted in the collimator. It is important that, to avoid distortion, the light bulb filament and X-ray focus should be at exactly the same distance from the collimator.

To prevent unnecessary X-ray exposure the light beam should be used before each radiographic exposure, whenever possible. The use of automatic beam restriction, limited to the size of the X-ray cassette, is now widely available with the newer types of X-ray equipment.

Interlocks

All conventional X-ray machines incorporate interlocks, which are automatic devices designed to limit exposure times, particularly in order to protect and safeguard the tube. This may also prevent exposure when the door to the X-ray room is open or no cassette has been inserted.

Automatic exposure control

The use of ionization chambers for automatic exposure determination is now widespread. This device, inserted between the patient and the cassette, is aimed to result in a satisfactory and acceptable level of film blackening, so that repeat radiographs should not be necessary. An audible warning device should be used during fluoroscopy, to advise staff when a given interval has elapsed. Most modern fluoroscopic units incorporate an automatic exposure control thus ensuring that the equipment operates at the correct dose rate.

Controlled areas

The fundamental concept in designating areas in which radiation is present as controlled or not lies in whether an individual working in this area for 40 hours per week may receive a radiation dose in excess of 3/10 of any dose limit. Thus, at its simplest, if the mean hourly dose rate exceeds 7.5 μSv, then the area has to be designated as a controlled radiation area. Generally, all diagnostic X-ray rooms are controlled areas. The boundary of the controlled area must be clearly marked or delineated, as by the walls of an X-ray room, and prominent warning signs should be present stating that the room is controlled. It is normal for the entrances of X-ray rooms to be fitted with red warning lights which light up when X-rays are about to be produced by the machine. Staff should not generally be allowed to enter the room when the warning light is on. Only classified staff may enter a controlled area; however, non-classified staff may enter provided this is done under a system of work. Generally, anyone working in a controlled area regardless of their designation, should be issued with a personal dosemeter. For a complete explanation of controlled areas the current Code of Practice should be consulted.

Protective barriers

To contain the radiation within the controlled area and prevent accidental exposure of personnel outside it, a system of barriers is used. A primary barrier is required in all areas of a room which may be exposed to the incident primary beam from the tube. Secondary barriers are required, where necessary, to eliminate scattered radiation.

In designing a primary barrier, various factors have to be taken into account, including the workload, exposure, occupancy and use factors, and distance of the barrier from the X-ray tube. Lead or concrete is generally used and is incorporated in the construction of the individual X-ray suites.

Secondary barriers are used for areas not exposed to the primary beam, such as adjacent offices. The radiographer should be protected at the console by a suitable barrier, with lead glass to view the patient.

The cable from the hand switch should not be long enough to permit the radiographers to leave the barrier during an exposure.

Fluoroscopy

During fluoroscopy, the staff work in very close proximity to the primary beam. It may on occasion even be necessary for the operator to insert a hand into the beam, during screening, in order to manipulate the patient. On such occasions lead gloves should be worn.

Lead aprons of suitable thickness between 0.15 and 0.5 mm of lead should be worn by staff during fluoroscopy. The aprons should extend from the neck to the mid thigh, and cover the surface of the operator exposed to the scattered radiation. More recently there has been a tendency towards 'remote screening', using remote control of the image intensifier behind a console protected by lead glass.

During fluoroscopy, screening should not be continuous, but only used when necessary. For complex radiography involving both screening for long times and close proximity to the patient (as in cardiac catherization) the use of a thyroid protector and lead glass spectacles should be considered. Staff not immediately required in the region close to the patient should step back whenever possible, especially during serial radiography or cine runs etc. Automatic time-limiting switches should be used when screening. Movable lead flaps should be present on the base of image intensifiers, to reduce the scattered radiation to the operator.

Radiographic technique

Only staff essential to the individual investigations should be present in the X-ray room during exposure. If care is taken to ensure a satisfactory quality of films, unnecessary second exposures will be kept to a minimum. The examination should be carefully explained to the patient in advance, and a good level of patient co-operation obtained. Immobilizing devices may be required for children and adults.

It should be remembered that the patient, and the couch on which he may lie, are important sources of secondary scattered radiation, and that, even if staff are situated outside the primary beam, they may be getting a significant level of secondary irradiation from the patient.

X-rays, like other electromagnetic radiation, obey the inverse square law. In other words, the intensity of the radiation is in proportion to the distance between the source and the exposed person. For this reason staff should endeavour to keep as far as practical away from the primary beam, even when using a protective apron.

In the case of restless children, radiographic staff should never volunteer to hold the patient. This is better done, in any event, by a near relative, who is able to achieve a closer rapport with the patient, and who is not subject to occupational exposure. Such a relative should, of course, wear a lead apron. All lead aprons should be frequently checked, since they will tend to crack as they age.

Patient radiation exposure record

It is required in some countries to record the quantity of radiation adminis-tered for each examination carried out. This may be done in two ways. Firstly for simple apparatus and simple examinations, the radiation exposure is readily determinable by reference to the exposure conditions applied, thus a written record of the number of exposures and exposure condition is adequ-ate. A second method is required for more complex equipment or more involved examinations; this requires that the X-ray equipment is fitted with an ionization chamber which is designed in such a way that it can monitor the whole cross-section of the radiation beam. The data which this equipment records, therefore, is exposure area product μGy m^{-2} in air (R cm^{-2}). The final figure can be printed automatically at the end of the examination and a copy attached to the patient's record. This type of equipment is also a useful aid in training as the effects of radiation administered by increasing the field size, etc., can be readily demonstrated. For each examination a typical value of exposure area product will be established and this will encourage staff to try to keep within this figure. On X-ray units where no such equipment is present it is necessary that the radiation output is checked by a competent person at regular intervals and also following servicing or a breakdown of the equipment.

Electrical safety

The use of equipment which operates or produces voltages in excess of 50 volts will inevitably have an associated risk of imparting an electric shock to the operator or the subject of the equipment's function. This is important with X-ray equipment as very high voltages are generated and many of the external surfaces of the equipment are made of electrically conducting material. The risk of suffering a potentially lethal electric shock at work with such apparatus is much greater than the risk of receiving a lethal dose of radiation.

Electrical protection is provided by making apparatus comply with international regulations, for example, *IEC Publication 601-1* which deals with the safety of medical electrical equipment. It is important that regular checks are made on such equipment, to ensure that all external conducting parts are adequately earthed, any loose wires or connections, frayed cables, damaged insulation, overheating of equipment or any other indication of apparently defective equipment be reported to a competent engineer. The testing of the earth quality should be routinely carried out by suitably qualified staff. Similarly, mobile equipment should not be overlooked and identical care should be taken to ensure such apparatus is electrically safe. If there exists a doubt as to whether the equipment is safe then the equipment should not be used until it has been examined by an appropriate person. In the case of a fire starting in such apparatus, the equipment should be disconnected or isolated from the electrical supply and the patient should immediately be removed to a safe place. Notify the fire authority immediately and prepare to evacuate the area. The room should have a fire extinguisher of a suitable type which may be used on electrical equipment, water-based extinguishers should not be used, if the extinguisher fails to cope, seal the room or (in the case of mobile units) isolate the equipment and evacuate the building. Be ready to direct the fire-fighting service to the area of the fire. A fundamental rule of general safety is for the operator to know the equipment; familiarization with all controls, procedures and mains switches is absolutely vital. In the event of a patient or other person receiving an electric shock, always switch off the equipment before going to their aid. Failure to do this may mean that in touching the victim who may still be connected to the electrical source, the person coming to the victim's aid may himself become a victim of the same electrical fault.

Electrical equipment can be checked for electrical safety by competent engineers. Failure to have this regularly carried out may result in various aspects of legal action regardless of whether anyone is seriously injured or not. Likewise, equipment with substantial mechanical structures (like X-ray machines) should, for the same reasons, have their mechanical safety regularly checked.

Other hazards

Staff should always seek assistance when lifting heavy patients or objects.

X-ray suites should be designed so that these procedures are minimized and made easy.

Hazards such as floor cables and protruding objects should, as far as possible, be removed.

All movable heavy equipment should possess a braking system capable of immobilizing the device.

Particular precautions must be taken to avoid contamination with body fluids and excretion from patients suffering from hepatitis or similar body fluid borne diseases. Medical advice must be sought whenever any possible exposure may have occurred.

Patient protection – 10 day rule

Gonad shields must be used on all patients of reproductive age or less when this is practicable.

Special precautions must be adopted for the radiography of pregnant women. Only essential examinations should be performed, and every care taken to avoid irradiation of the pelvis. In women of reproductive age, in whom there is a possibility of pregnancy, non-urgent examinations of the lower abdomen and pelvis should be delayed until the possibility of pregnancy has been excluded. The use of the ten day rule has been applied for many years. This allows X-ray examinations to be made providing the timing is such that it is within 10 days following the onset of menstruation. This method (called the 10 day rule) is in the light of current research probably not achieving the desired results. The reason for this is that although the patient is not pregnant the ovum is ripening and is sensitive to radiation, paradoxically following conception (normally after the 10 day period) the zygote is not particularly sensitive to radiation. Sensitivity to radiation increases when the cells differentiate especially when the central nervous system forms. This normally occurs about 8 weeks after conception. Thus, the current use of the 10 day rule is questionable, but does give the radiographic staff an easy test to determine whether they should proceed with an examination. The alternative of questioning the patients as to whether or not they may be pregnant is obviously fraught with problems.

The dose to the patient should be kept to the minimum consistent with providing adequate clinical information when possible by the use of fast films, intensifying screens, correct use of diaphragms, and avoidance of unnecessary and repeated exposures.

Only the patient being examined should be present in the X-ray room unless satisfactory radiation protection using mobile screens or lead rubber ceiling suspended curtains is available to protect the other patients.

CONCLUSION

These rules relate to those which exist within one hospital situated in the UK. The rules have been applied and amended over many years and are based on the code of practice for ionizing radiation arising from medical and dental use, and on ICRP and other international bodies recommendations. It is not possible for all situations to be envisaged, and it is because of this that local rules which are in line with the current recommendations must be drawn up. The local rules are very important and it is essential that they are devised by a competent person with sufficient experience to consider and define the maximum number of possibilities. The dosimetric monitoring of staff is considered to be very important as it not only enables staff dose to be carefully monitored, but also by implication is a check on the quality of the radiation protection, both procedural and physical, which exists in a department. It also ensures that poor working practice is unlikely to become a significant problem. Good radiation protection cannot be expected if staff are inadequately trained. It is essential that staff directly involved with the use of ionizing radiation are well trained, and that staff whose contact with such radiation is infrequent are taught the basis of good working practice and are made aware of the channels through which they can contact the people responsible for their radiological safety.

15 Precautions to be Taken when Working in an X-ray Crystallography Laboratory

M.J. Minski and R.S. Osborn

INTRODUCTION

This chapter outlines the procedures necessary to provide protection from radiation for workers in the field of X-ray crystallography. The suggestions are based on the requirements currently in force in the UK as embodied in the *Approved Code of Practice, Ionising Radiations Regulations 1985* (IRR '85)[1]. Although the legal requirements in other countries may differ slightly from the above, the basic principles are relevant to all situations.

Before considering precautions in detail it is important to explain the nature of the radiation hazard in this work, particularly as it differs from that in the better known field of medical X-rays. The X-rays used in crystallography have much lower penetrating power than those used in medicine and are mainly absorbed within a few mm of the skin surface. The dose-rate close to the window of a typical crystallographic X-ray tube, operating at about 1 kW, is of the order of tens of Gy sec^{-1} (units will be defined later), so if the skin is exposed to the primary beam from the window, a considerable amount of energy is absorbed in a small depth of tissue, even in one second. The result is a serious burn which is very slow to heal, and for longer exposures or those involving more highly rated tubes, there is a danger of permanent damage to the skin. In addition to these superficial effects there may be other biological changes which are discussed in the next section.

BIOLOGICAL EFFECTS

The basic process when radiation interacts with matter is one of ionization.

In biological systems this process may result in molecular rearrangement which can subsequently affect the development of the organism. Radiation such as heat and light does not have sufficient energy to cause ionization but X-ray radiation does. The changes that occur in tissue or cells due to radiation can be described in a series of stages, and since these systems are 90% water, the processes can be related to the ionization of water. The initial physical stage allows energy deposition in the cell with subsequent ionization (e.g. $H_2O \rightarrow H_2O^+ + e^-$); this is followed by a physicochemical stage where ions interact with other water molecules to give further ions and free radicals ($H_2O^+ \rightarrow H^+ + OH^-$; $H_2O + e^- \rightarrow H_2O^-$; $H_2O^- \rightarrow H^0 + OH^-$). Free radicals are highly reactive and can produce oxidizing agents such as hydrogen peroxide ($OH^0 + OH^0 \rightarrow H_2O_2$). These reaction products react with organic molecules in the cell, in particular DNA and the complex molecules of chromosomes. The final stage, which can vary in length from minutes to years, results in early cell death, prevention or delay of cell division, permanent modification in sexual reproductive organs, and cancers. Biological effects of radiation can result from acute or chronic exposure; the former is usually a single dose at high level, whereas the latter is exposure over a long period at a fairly low level. The type of radiation will influence the resulting biological effects as will the nature of the irradiated tissue and the age, sex and health of the individual.

A single, acute dose of about 3 Gy is lethal to man if the whole body is irradiated, but higher doses can be tolerated if only part of the body is involved. Short-term effects resulting from an acute high level radiation dose manifest themselves within hours or weeks of exposure and are due to a major depletion of cell population in a number of body organs – in particular, bone marrow, the gastrointestinal tract and the central nervous system, all of which are particularly radiosensitive. Initial radiation sickness is due to damage to cells lining the intestine and, during the first 24–48 hours, lymphocytes in the peripheral blood are reduced. Haemorrhages occur within 4–5 days after exposure and risk of infection is increased.

Chronic exposure to radiation does not produce the short-term effects but can cause long-term or delayed effects leading to cancer induction. The increased risk of cancer is complicated by the long latent period between exposure and the appearance of the cancer, typical latent periods being 8–10 years for leukaemia, 15 years for bone cancer, 15–30 years for thyroid cancers, 10–20 years for lung cancer and 5–10 years for cataract formation.

Since it is not known whether there is a threshold for cancer induction by radiation, it is assumed for the purposes of radiological protection that any dose, however small, carries some risk. To assess this risk it is necessary to extrapolate from the high doses received by groups such as A-bomb casualties, radium dial painters, uranium mine workers and those receiving medical X-ray treatment, which are known to cause cancer, to the low doses as received by the majority of individuals. This requires a knowledge of the dose/response relationship and this is currently a topic of some controversy. In radiological protection a linear dose/effect relationship is assumed with no threshold, thus erring on the side of overcaution. International bodies, such as UNSCEAR (The United Nations Scientific Committee on the Effects of Atomic Radiation)[2], BEIR (The Committee on Biological Effects of Ionising Radiations)[3] and ICRP (The International Commission on Radiological Protection)[4], are currently reviewing the risks of radiation-induced cancers. From these findings the total cancers induced by radiation are 13 per 10^6 per milliSievert (mSv) compared with 2000 per 10^6 cancers produced spontaneously.

These radiation effects are somatic, affecting the individual irradiated, but future generations can be affected and these are hereditary or genetic effects of radiation. Although detectable in animal experiments there is no evidence of radiation-induced hereditary effects in man at any dose level. Attempts to predict the possible magnitude of hereditary disorders suggest a mean value of approximately 0.2 hereditary disorders per 10^6 per lifetime Sv. This compares with naturally occurring hereditary disorders of 30 000–100 000 per million live births, thus indicating the difficulty in detecting any excesses at the levels proposed for radiation.

In the context of X-ray crystallography the most likely biological effects are skin burns if a high level acute dose is received from the main beam or low level effects from secondary radiation.

Dose limits

To protect workers and the general public from unwanted exposure to radiation, certain dose limits have been proposed, based mainly on the recommendations of *ICRP Publication 26*[5]. These levels are recommendations and the individual countries produce their own legislation based on these levels.

The main requirements for radiation protection as expressed by *ICRP 26* are:

1. No practice shall be adopted unless it produces a positive net benefit;
2. All exposures shall be kept *as low as is reasonably achievable* (ALARA), economic and social factors being taken into account; and,
3. The dose to individuals shall not exceed the limits recommended for the appropriate circumstances.

For the whole body the dose limit is 50 mSv annually for a radiation worker, and for skin (averaged over any area of 100 cm^{-2}) it is 500 mSv annually, this latter figure applying to contamination and, therefore, a smaller averaging area should be used for a concentrated X-ray beam.

To ensure that these dose limits are not exceeded, personnel and area monitoring is carried out. To understand the readings of a monitor it is necessary to be familiar with the units used in radiation protection. X-rays were originally detected by their ionizing effects in air, and radiation exposure was defined in terms of the electrostatic charge produced by X-rays in 1 cc of air at NTP. This was the Roentgen. However, the measurement of interest is the dose to human tissue, so the concept of absorbed dose was introduced to allow for exposure to tissue rather than air. The SI unit of absorbed dose is the Gray (Gy), defined as the quantity of radiation which causes an energy absorption of 1 Joule kg^{-1} in irradiated material. The pre SI unit is the rad. 1 Gy = 100 rad.

Damage to tissue is also a function of the type of radiation, and varies widely between alpha particles, beta particles, neutrons, X-rays and gamma-rays. To allow for this a quality factor, Q is used and the unit is *dose equivalent* = absorbed dose x quality factor. It is measured in SI units by the Sievert (Sv) and the pre SI unit is the rem. (1 Sv = 100 rem). For X-rays the quality factor is 1.

Most monitoring instruments make use of an ionization chamber for measuring dose rates and are calibrated variously as Roentgen h^{-1}, rad h^{-1}, Gy h^{-1}, Sv h^{-1} depending on the age of the instrument. The latest UK legislation requires dose rates to be measured in Sv h^{-1}. In the case of X-rays it is difficult to convert the value measured by the ionization chamber to a dose equivalent but it can be done using the mass absorption coefficients of air and the material being irradiated.

PRINCIPLES OF RADIATION PROTECTION IN X-RAY CRYSTALLOGRAPHY

The principles and procedures described in this chapter apply equally well to industrial or academic situations, the most important differences being that industrial laboratories may handle a higher proportion of routine work than those in academic establishments, while the latter are likely to be used for teaching as well as research and so will need to cater for inexperienced workers on a regular basis.

Radiation protection in X-ray crystallography is based on the same principles as for any other ionizing radiation, namely,

1. *Time* – Minimization of the time spent near the source of radiation since the total dose received is proportional to the length of the exposure to radiation;
2. *Distance* – Maximization of the distance from the source, since X-rays obey the inverse square law, i.e. the dose-rate diminishes by a factor of four, if the distance from the source is doubled;

3.   *Shielding* – Provision of radiation-proof shielding to minimize the chances of workers receiving any dose at all.

Work in this field is also subject to the general requirement of the ALARA principle.

LOCATION OF WORK

If possible, an X-ray crystallography laboratory should not be used for any other work. Where exclusive use of a room is precluded, the part used for X-ray work must be partitioned off in such a way that the dose-rate outside the partition does not exceed that permitted for the general public. Ideally, even within the X-ray area, each X-ray generator and its equipment should be housed in an individual small room or cubicle, but if this is not feasible as much space as possible should be kept clear around each generator. If necessary, fixed barriers or shielding should be installed to ensure, as far as possible, that no worker would be at risk in the event of mistakes by other workers nearby. It is advisable to remember at all stages of planning and development that no safety device is totally infallible, and some can be deliberately disabled by irresponsible persons who may think 'it saves time' or 'it makes it easier ...'.

APPARATUS

Equipment for X-ray crystallography consists of two main categories:

1.   X-ray generators, and
2.   Cameras, diffractometers, etc, in which the samples are exposed to X-rays and the resulting diffraction patterns are recorded.

Generators

The X-ray tube is frequently mounted on a bench-top directly above the transformer, but if this is not convenient the HT cable connecting it to the transformer must be firmly supported so that it has no sharp bends, and is kept away from water and chemicals.

The hoses carrying cooling water to the tube must be firmly fixed to the inlet and outlet points. It is not unusual for water pressure to rise at night in urban areas and it has been known for water hoses to blow off after staff have left, causing costly damage.

An X-ray tube has one or more 'windows' through which the primary beam of X-rays can emerge. Each window in regular use should have an automatic shutter or other device to control the X-ray beam and all unused windows should be covered by fixed shielding.

Interlocks

Many safety features of the equipment used in this field depend on interlocks. An interlock is a device which automatically prevents X-rays being switched on or shutters being opened unless the apparatus is safe. Interlocks may operate electrically or mechanically or by a combination of both methods.

One example of a mechanical interlock is an automatic window shutter of the spring loaded type; the shutter is closed by a strong spring unless held open by apparatus mounted at the tube window.

Electrical interlocks consist of suitable switches (proximity type, etc) connected into circuits controlling production of X-rays or opening of shutters in such a way that the circuit is only complete when apparatus or essential shielding is correctly positioned.

A mechanical–electrical combination is used in the system wherein a pressure switch is mounted on the tube housing, near a window with an electrically operated shutter. Unless the switch is pressed in by a lever attached to apparatus to be used at the window, the shutter circuit is not completed and the shutter cannot be opened. The lever is designed so that it only operates the pressure switch when the apparatus is correctly assembled and mounted at the tube window.

In addition to the need to safeguard against the removal of an entire piece of equipment from the tube window, there are also many situations where sections of apparatus (film holders, sample chamber covers, etc) are regularly removed. Such items frequently form part of the essential radiation shielding, and must, therefore, be individually interlocked to an X-ray-generating or shutter-control circuit.

Enclosures

If it is not possible to achieve safety by the methods indicated above, the apparatus must be enclosed by shielding. This may consist of a fixed enclosure with interlocked doors or access panels, or it may be more convenient to use large hinged, sliding, or demountable interlocked panels. If it is necessary to provide entry openings for cables, the holes must be too small to allow persons to insert any part of themselves into an area of significant dose-rate. In some cases a simple one-piece removable cover may be used, the cover being interlocked to the base on which the apparatus stands.

Alternatively, it may be possible to make a close fitting interlocked cover for part of the apparatus, to prevent access to beam paths. Diagrams and instructions for making various types of enclosures, interlocks, etc are given in reference 6.

X-ray diffractometry

It is not possible to give detailed descriptions of all safety devices here because there is a great variety of equipment available, but there is one group of instruments in widespread use and having a number of features in common, namely X-ray diffractometers. They may be designed for work with single crystals or with crystalline powders; in either case the diffraction pattern is not recorded photographically but by an X-ray detector.

In powder diffractometers the detector rotates around the sample in one plane, and modern instruments are provided with flexible or overlapping shielding to accommodate the motion. However, older machines should be checked over the whole accessible range of Bragg angles (θ), since in some cases, dangerous gaps between parts of the shielding may occur at certain positions. This is particularly dangerous at values of θ near zero since the direct beam could escape in such cases.

In single crystal instruments the detector is usually fixed, but the crystal mount is capable of movement in three dimensions. However, most of the operations are computer controlled during normal use, so that the entire system of X-ray tube window, crystal mount and detector can be surrounded by a total enclosure with interlocked access panels.

Computer control is also increasingly used for powder diffractometers, and modern instruments are very well protected, with interlocked covers for all points where access to beam paths is needed. Older equipment, which may still be adequate for purposes of data-collection, is likely to have some covers which are not interlocked, e.g. caps over access points for slit-changing. In these cases some means of preventing removal or opening of such covers, while X-rays are on and the shutter is open, must be provided.

In upgrading old machines to present safety requirements some limitations on modes of use may have to be accepted, but this may well be preferable to scrapping the equipment completely.

X-ray fluorescence spectrometry

Although this is not strictly speaking a branch of X-ray crystallography, it frequently runs in parallel with crystallographic techniques, often in the same laboratory, so it seems appropriate to mention it. Modern equipment is very well protected, with all inspection panels interlocked so that in normal use there will be no radiation safety problems. With some older machines, however, there may be a small dose-rate at the bottom of the sample well, but this does not cause a hazard provided samples are loaded and unloaded using tongs. In fact, tongs should always be used for this purpose unless there are very strong reasons for not doing so.

Warning signs

Effective warning signs are an essential part of the necessary safety measures in all X-ray work. The international symbol for radiation hazards should be fixed at all entrances to areas where X-ray work is carried on. Metal or self-adhesive plastic labels carrying this symbol may be obtained from firms specializing in hazard warning signs.

Every X-ray tube must be provided with a sign which automatically indicates when X-rays are being produced. The sign should display the words 'X-rays ON', illuminated immediately when X-rays are switched on, but not legible when X-rays are off.

This sign must be close to the tube window, and clearly visible from all positions where persons could be at risk from X-rays.

Such signs must be 'fail-safe', that is, there must be no possibility of X-rays being on if the sign is not illuminated. If it is not possible to arrange for lamp-failure to cause X-rays to be switched off or the shutter to be closed, then it may be acceptable to use two lamps connected in parallel, since it is unlikely that both would fail simultaneously. However, if this method is used a rigorous system of checking and replacement of bulbs must be followed.

Where a tube window is provided with a shutter, there must be a sign indicating clearly whether the shutter is open or closed, and it should operate automatically if reasonably practicable.

MONITORING

Monitoring of equipment

It is essential to make regular checks to ensure that no radiation leaks have developed in any part of the equipment. One of the 'Mini-monitor' range of instruments has been designed for X-ray work, and it is particularly suitable for use with crystallographic apparatus, because the small physical size of the probe enables it to be used in confined spaces. The intensity of radiation detected is indicated by a meter reading and by an audible signal.

A monitor must be available in every X-ray laboratory, and must be used to make the following checks:

1. Test all shielding to make sure that it continues to provide adequate protection;

2.   Monitor junctions between covers that are regularly removed and the main body of the apparatus;
3.   Monitor the junction between the apparatus and the tube window;
4.   Monitor the part of the apparatus where the main beam is terminated, if accessible.

Clearly, tests 2, 3 and 4 will not be possible, or indeed necessary, if the equipment is protected by a total enclosure.

The monitor itself must be checked once a year against a standard source of radiation, or against an instrument which has been calibrated by a recognized laboratory. The state of the battery must be noted every time the monitor is used, the mini-monitor being provided with a testing device for this purpose.

The reading given by a simple test source should also be observed, so that self-consistency of readings can be checked. A suitable source for this purpose consists of a small piece of uranium foil encased in Perspex.

Monitoring of personnel

In normal use crystallographic equipment should be safe enough to make the wearing of personal monitoring devices unnecessary. For those involved with alignment or similar operations it is advisable to wear a thermoluminescent device (TLD) on a finger. The device usually takes the form of a small packet of thermoluminescent powder attached to a plastic finger-stall.

Badge-type personal monitors for wearing on the trunk are not generally suitable for this work, because even if a radiation leak does occur, it is likely to be in the form of a very narrow beam. The probability of such a beam striking the small area of a personal monitor is extremely low, so that a nil-dose indication would not necessarily mean that no dose had been received and this could obviously be dangerously misleading. In the UK, TLD personal monitors are supplied, processed, and dose-records notified to users by laboratories authorized to provide such a service.

Exceptions to normal practice

Occasionally, situations arise when a necessary procedure cannot be carried out with all safety devices operative. For example, some alignment procedures require access, with X-rays on and shutters open, to parts of the apparatus that would normally be enclosed by interlocked shielding. If possible, alternative safety measures should be devised, but if this is not reasonably practicable a permit-to-work system should be operated. A method must be worked out whereby the procedure can be carried out without exposing the worker to radiation, even though some safety devices may need to be overridden. There must be written instructions specifying which safety measures may be suspended and outlining the practical steps in the procedure.

For instance, in alignment procedures it is often possible to make preliminary settings visually without X-rays on, and some equipment is supplied with alignment templates to facilitate mounting with optimum values of distance and take-off angle from the tube window. The amount of adjustment needed with X-rays on can be substantially reduced if these initial settings are done carefully. It is also advisable to restrict adjustments to small increments while X-rays are on and the shutter open, since large alterations to the angle and/or position of a camera may cause gaps to open between the tube window and the collimator, with consequent danger of exposure to the primary beam.

A small piece of fluorescent screen material fixed to a thin wooden or Perspex handle about 20 cm long can be a useful aid to alignment as it enables the worker to observe the effects of adjustments from a safe distance or from behind shielding.

Permit-to-work systems should not be instituted for reasons of convenience; serious efforts must be made to provide safety devices which permit all necessary operations to be carried out. Only experienced workers should be allowed to override safety devices and carry out permit-to-work procedures, and their names must be entered in the permit-to-work instructions and in the local rules (see next section).

ADMINISTRATION

However small the number of X-ray workers in the laboratory or section, a certain amount of administrative work will be involved.

Some form of registration of the work being done and of the persons involved will be essential. The work registration should include details of equipment to be used, its location, a brief outline of the nature of the work and the names of those responsible for running the section. Registrations of personnel should contain details of age, sex and previous experience of work with X-rays, if any.

In establishments where there are large numbers of X-ray workers, it may be necessary to produce printed forms for registration of work and personnel, but whatever method is used, records must be kept. In laboratories where persons are frequently only working in X-ray crystallography for periods of 4 weeks or less (e.g. in a teaching situation), full registration procedures may not be necessary, but lists of names of such persons should be kept.

It is necessary to draw up a code of practice for the general running of the laboratory, covering such matters as access for persons who are not registered X-ray workers, emergency procedures, etc. Cleaning staff will regularly need

324

access to the laboratory, and occasionally maintenance or security personnel will need to enter it so arrangements enabling them to do this safely must be made. This is particularly important since crystallographic X-ray equipment often needs to be left running unattended for long periods, including overnight.

Certain basic rules of work must be defined, covering such matters as checks to be carried out before switching on X-rays, monitoring procedures, etc. Written statements of all such rules and instructions must be available; these constitute the Local Rules referred to in the *Approved Code of Practice IRR '85*.

It is often desirable to display sections of the local rules in the laboratory, and large establishments may find it helpful to produce their local rules in printed form for distribution to all workers[7].

SAFE WORKING PRACTICES

Of far greater importance than any safety devices, warning signs etc, are the working habits and attitude to safety of the workers themselves. It is essential that all workers fully understand the nature of the hazard involved, and the precautions necessary to avoid exposure to radiation.

Those in charge of X-ray crystallography laboratories must make sure that all workers receive a thorough training before starting work. In some cases it may be useful to preface individual training by a group lecture or video programme[8], but each worker must be given full practical instruction in the handling of the apparatus they intend to use.

Finally, it must be strongly emphasized that workers should not rely on safety devices but should maintain constant vigilance, and should develop a rigorous safety routine, including the following points:

1. Before switching on X-rays, or exposing beam paths, check that the tube window shutter is closed;
2. Make sure that *all* windows of a multi-window tube are safe before switching on X-rays;
3. Check that apparatus is correctly assembled and mounted at the tube window and that all shielding is fully in place before opening the shutter;
4. Check operation of warning signs when switching on X-rays and opening shutters. If illuminated signs contain two or more bulbs, note whether any have failed; if so replace them before continuing work.

References

1. Health and Safety Executive. (1985). *The Ionising Radiations Regulations*. (London:

HMSO)

2. United Nations Scientific Committee on the Effects of Atomic Radiation. (1982). *Ionising Radiation Sources and Biological Effects*. (United Nations)

3. Committee on the Biological Effects of Ionising Radiations (BEIR). (1980). *The Effects on Populations of Exposure to Low Levels of Ionising Radiations*. (National Academy Press)

4. Annals of the International Commission on Radiological Protection.

5. International Commission on Radiological Protection. (ICRP). (1977). *Recommendations of the ICRP Publication 26* (Oxford: Pergamon Press)

6. Occupational Hygiene Monograph No 15. (1986). *A Guide to Radiation Protection in the Use of X-ray Optics Equipment*. (Science Reviews Ltd)

7. Imperial College, London. (1986). *Rules for Safe Working Practices with X-rays*.

8. Imperial College, London. (1986). *X-ray Crystallography – Principles of Safety. (Imperial College Television Studio)*

16 Radiation Protection in Radionuclide Investigations

D.M. Taylor

Within a very few years of their discovery at the end of the last century, X-rays, radioactive materials and other types of radiation sources had found important applications in medicine and in research. During the past 40 years the use of radioactive materials and radiation sources in hospitals, industry and in research has mushroomed and today radiation must be added to the list of potential dangers to which laboratory personnel may be exposed.

Like electricity and most of the chemical substances commonly used in laboratories ionizing radiations arising from X-ray machines, charged particle generators or from radioactive materials, are a potential hazard to human health. However, if the nature of the danger is clearly understood and the appropriate techniques are employed in their manipulation, radiation sources probably represent a very much smaller hazard to the individual than, for example, many toxic chemicals.

In contrast to many chemicals whose dangers were only realized when a considerable number of people died or suffered severe ill-health, the ability of ionizing radiations to cause serious biological damage was recognized before they came into widespread use. Consequently, it has been possible to draw up guidelines, often called 'codes of practice', for the safe handling and use of radioactive materials and all other types of radiation sources. In recent years guidelines have been supported in many countries by statutory legislation for the conduct of all types of radiation work. As a result of the early recognition of the harmful effects of radiation and the introduction of recommended safety procedures, serious radiation injury has been a very rare occurrence, despite the many thousands of people throughout the world who now use radioactive materials or other radiation sources in their everyday work.

In order to appreciate the risks involved in handling any toxic agent, and to understand the principles on which the recommended safety procedures are based, it is necessary to know the properties of the agent and the nature of the injuries it may produce. The aim of this chapter is to describe the basic properties of ionizing radiations, the nature of biological damage they may induce, and the basic principles which must be applied for the safe use of radiation sources and radioactive materials.

RADIATION AND RADIOACTIVITY

All matter is made up from chemical elements and the smallest unit of any element which can exist is the atom. Atoms are composed of three fundamental particles: protons, neutrons and electrons. Protons carry a positive electrical charge; neutrons, which have almost the same size as protons, carry no electrical charge. Electrons, the smallest of the particles, carry a negative electrical charge of equal size to the positive charge of the proton. Atoms possess characteristic structures consisting of a nucleus, containing the protons and neutrons, surrounded by electrons. The numbers of protons and electrons in an atom are equal so that the atom is electrically neutral. For any given element the atoms contain a fixed number of protons and electrons, but the number of neutrons in the nucleus may vary. Atoms containing the same number of protons but different numbers of neutrons are called isotopes. Since the chemical properties of an atom are determined by the number of electrons, and thus by the number of protons in the nucleus, the isotopes of any element have identical chemical properties, and differ from each other only in their mass.

If some external influence causes an atom to lose or gain an electron, the atom is left with a net electrical charge; this process is called ionization, and the charged atom is known as an ion. If the neutron:proton ratio falls above or below certain limits the nucleus may be unstable and disintegrate with the release of a large amount of energy and, usually, one or more of the component particles of the atom; this process is called radioactive decay. The common types of particle or electromagnetic radiation which may arise from radioactive decay or which may be produced by X-ray and other machines, are described briefly below.

ALPHA PARTICLES

These are doubly charged helium nuclei which have little ability to penetrate matter. Due to their very short range, 30–60 μm, in biological tissue they give up all their great energy in a very small volume.

BETA PARTICLES

These are very high-speed electrons. Their energy may vary considerably according to their source of production, thus their ability to penetrate biological tissue may range from a fraction of a millimetre to a few centimetres. Nuclides with too few neutrons for stability may decay by the emission of a positively charged electron – a positron, or beta-plus particle. In this process a proton in the nucleus is converted to a neutron. The positron may have any energy up to a maximum of 0.63 MeV. When a positron is ejected from the nucleus it loses its energy by interaction with surrounding atoms; when it has lost its energy it is annihilated by combination with an electron to form two photons each with an energy of 0.51 MeV which are emitted at 180° to each other. This so-called annihilation radiation is identical to gamma radiation. Positron-emitting radionuclides such as ^{11}C or ^{18}F are becoming increasingly important in diagnostic nuclear medicine.

NEUTRONS

During some types of radioactive decay neutrons may be ejected with high energy; they may also be produced in nuclear reactors, cyclotrons or similar electrical machines. Being uncharged, neutrons are not repelled by charged nuclei but may enter them to form radionuclides which decay with the emission of alpha or beta particles, or gamma rays.

ELECTROMAGNETIC RADIATION

In addition to the ejection of particles, radioactive decay is often also associated with the emission of gamma-rays or X-rays. These two radiations are examples of the electromagnetic radiations which include radiowaves, microwaves, visible and ultraviolet light in addition to X- and gamma-rays. Electromagnetic radiation consists of 'packets' of energy, quanta, which are transmitted in the form of a wave motion. The wavelength of electromagnetic radiation covers a very broad spectrum ranging from radiowaves, with wavelengths of a few km to a few cm, to gamma-rays whose wavelengths are of the order of 10^{-12} m.

The energy of the quantum, or photon, of electromagnetic radiations is inversely proportional to the wavelength, thus the quanta of radiowaves carry little energy while the quanta of gamma-rays carry much energy. All electromagnetic radiation travels through space with the velocity of light and both gamma-rays and X-rays can have great penetrating power. The more energetic gamma-rays may pass through several centimetres of lead, or tens of centimetres of concrete, and may pass through the human body with relatively little deposition of energy.

Gamma-rays and X-rays are in most respects identical, the main difference being that gamma-rays are emitted as the result of a change in the atomic nucleus while X-rays arise from changes in the orbital electron shells either as a result of radioactive decay or by the application of electrical energy in machines such as those used for X-ray crystallography or for diagnostic or therapeutic purposes in human and veterinary medicine.

Charged particles, such as electrons, protons, deuterons or alpha particles with very high energies may be produced in machines such as cyclotrons, linear accelerators or van der Graaf machines.

UNITS OF RADIOACTIVITY AND RADIATION

The relatively new International System of Units (SI) has necessitated changes in many of the units which are commonly used in radiation work. However, the old units are still in widespread use and both the new and the old quantities will be described.

The energy of any radiation is generally expressed in terms of the electron-volt which may be defined as the energy gained by an electron when it is accelerated through a potential difference of 1 volt. This is a very small unit and the commonly used unit is a million-electron-volts, which is abbreviated to MeV.

The basic unit of radioactivity is the Becquerel (Bq) which is defined as the amount of a radioactive substance which decays at a rate of 1 disintegration per second. This is a very small unit and radioactivities are usually described in terms of kilobecquerels (kBq), Megabecquerels (MBq) or Gigabecquerels (GBq) which represent 10^3, 10^6 and 10^9 Bq respectively. The old unit of radioactivity, which is still very widely used, is the Curie (Ci) which is defined as the amount of radioactive substance which has an activity of 3.7 x 10^{10} disintegrations per second. In contrast to the Bq this is a very large unit and it is subdivided into smaller units, the millicurie (mCi), which is one thousandth of a Curie, and the microcurie (μCi), nanocurie (nCi) and picocurie (pCi) representing 10^{-6}, 10^{-9} and 10^{-12} of a Curie respectively. One Curie is equivalent to 37 GBq and 1 μCi is equivalent to 37 kBq. The units of radiation which are most important in relation to radiation protection are those which are based on the amount of energy deposited in matter by ionizing radiation. The unit dose is the Gray (Gy) which is defined as the absorption of 1 Joule of radiation energy per kilogramme of matter (1 Jkg^{-1}). The old unit of absorbed dose is the rad which was defined as the absorption of 100 ergs per gramme (0.01 Jkg^{-1}). Thus 1 Gray is equivalent to 100 rads.

The biological effects of radiation vary with the type of radiation to which the organism is exposed, as will be discussed later, and it is desirable for radiation protection purposes to have a unit which takes into account both the physical and biological characteristics of the radiation. Such a unit of 'dose equivalent' has therefore been introduced. This is defined as the absorbed dose (D) multiplied by a quality factor (Q), which is related to the physical properties of the radiation, and a modifying (N) factor which takes account of other factors, thus:

Dose equivalent $= D.Q.N.$

The absorbed dose D is given in Gy, the value of N is at present defined as 1 and the value of Q may range from 1 to 20. This unit of dose equivalent is called the Sievert (Sv). The old unit of dose equivalent is the rem, which is defined as the absorbed dose in rads multiplied by the quality factor Q. One Sievert is therefore equivalent to 100 rem.

BIOLOGICAL EFFECTS OF RADIATION

The passage of ionizing radiation through living tissue damages the cells in its path. However, the mechanism by which the damage is produced is not fully understood. It is assumed that the chemical reactions associated with the ionization which occurs along the track of the radiation cause deleterious changes in the complex molecular systems within the cell. Exposure of living tissue to large doses of radiation results in the death of a high proportion of its cells. This effect is utilized in the treatment of cancer by X-rays and other types of radiation. The response of cells or tissues to radiation varies greatly from cell type to cell type and depends on factors such as the type of radiation and the dose rate and frequency with which it is administered. For example, a rat will die within a few days if it is exposed to about 7 Gy of X-rays administered in a few minutes, but it will survive for months if exposed continuously to gamma radiation of equivalent energy at 0.5 Gy per day. Although they penetrate only a few micrometres into tissues, alpha particles cause very intense, localized areas of ionization which may cause much more severe damage to a cell than would be caused by the absorption of an equal amount of beta or gamma radiation in the same cell.

Much of our knowledge of the effects of radiation on mammalian systems comes from studies in experimental animals but some direct information on human response has been derived from the study of patients treated with X-rays or other radiation; from studies of the survivors of the atomic bomb explosions in Japan, from early workers with radium and from uranium ore miners. The effects of radiation on human beings can be placed in two classes; early, or acute, effects such as nausea, vomiting and anaemia which appear within hours or days of exposure to large doses of radiation (more than 1 Gy);

and late effects such as leukaemia, cancer, cataract, sterility and genetic damage which may appear many months or years after exposure to much lower doses of radiation.

In the use of radioactive materials in laboratories, accidents resulting in radiation doses high enough to produce acute radiation effects should never occur and the prevention, or minimization, of the risk of producing late effects is the major factor involved in the development of procedures for the 'safe' handling of radiation sources.

Many experimental studies have shown that the embryonic or juvenile mammal is more sensitive to irradiation than the adult. A large number of observations on children born to women who were exposed to X-rays, either for diagnosis or treatment during pregnancy, have shown that irradiation *in utero* can lead to serious abnormality in the offspring. The defects observed in these cases include mongolism (Down's Syndrome), hydrocephalus, micro-ophthalmia and limb malformation. This human experience, together with the information from animal studies, suggests that the risks of damage to the developing embryo are greatest during the first 2 months of pregnancy and decrease gradually at later times. This relatively high risk of radiation damage to the embryo during the early stages of pregnancy makes it extremely important that any unnecessary radiation exposure during this period is avoided.

It is important to recognize that human exposure to radiation is not limited to those persons working with radiation or receiving radiation for medical purposes. Throughout human existence mankind has been exposed to con-tinuous and inescapable irradiation from cosmic radiation and from the naturally radioactive elements, such as uranium and thorium, which occur in the rocks and soil. Some of these elements, or their decay products, enter the human body through food, water or air and become deposited in bone and other tissues, thus delivering a continuous internal irradiation of our tissues. The level of the natural external and internal radiation received by man varies considerably between various parts of the world, or even within the same country, due to changes in cosmic ray intensity with latitude and altitude and to variations in the composition of the rocks and soil. In Europe and much of North America the average annual radiation dose from natural internal and external radiation is about 2 mSv. To this dose must be added a further contribution of about 0.5 mSv derived from human technological activities, including occupational exposure to radiation, disposal of radioactive waste, fall-out from nuclear weapons and other sources; about 90% of this man-made dose is derived from medical use of radiation for diagnosis or treat-ment.

Radioactive material may enter the human body accidentally, by swallow-ing, by inhalation of gases, dusts or aerosols or by entry through the skin or through a wound. The ultimate fate of radionuclides which enter the body depends on their chemical properties and on their interactions with the natural components of cells and tissues. Some materials may become distributed widely within the body while others may deposit in specific organs, for example radioisotopes of iodine, as iodide, localize in the thyroid gland while the radioisotopes of calcium, strontium and radium are deposited predominantly in the skeleton. The fate of a radionuclide in the body may also be influenced by the chemical form in which it is administered. For instance, carbon-14 administered in the form of ^{14}C-labelled cortisol is rapidly eliminated from the body by excretion whereas ^{14}C-labelled glycine undergoes metabolic conversion in the body to enter proteins, fats, etc. where some of the ^{14}C may be retained for periods ranging up to many months. ^{14}C or ^{3}H labelled nucleosides, e.g. thymidine, are incorporated into the desoxyribonucleic acid of dividing cells and thus irradiate the cell nucleus directly, which may lead to severe damage to the genetic apparatus. The retention of radionuclides in the the body may vary very widely, some materials being completely eliminated from the body in a few hours, while others, especially those which deposit in the skeleton, may be retained for many years.

Table 16.1 Classification of radionuclide toxicity: some examples of the radionuclides in the different categories (International Atomic Energy Agency, 1963)

Class I high toxicity	Class II medium toxicity, upper sub-group A	Class III medium toxicity, lower sub-group B	Class IV low toxicity
Strontium-90	Calcium-45	Calcium-47	Hydrogen-3
Lead-210	Chlorine-36	Carbon-14	Zinc-69
Radium-226	Manganese-54	Fluorine-18	Technetium-99m
Thorium-228	Cobalt-60	Sodium-24	Indium-113m
Plutonium-239	Strontium-89	Phosphorus-32	Xenon-133
Californium-252	Iodine-131	Potassium-42	Platinum-193m
	Caesium-137	Chromium-51	Uranium-235
	Barium-140	Iron-55	Uranium-238
	Bismuth-210	Iron-59	
	Lead-212	Cobalt-57	
		Copper-64	
		Zinc-65	
		Strontium-85	
		Molybdenum-99	
		Cadmium-115	
		Gold-198	
		Mercury-203	

The radiotoxicity of a radionuclide depends not only on its biological behaviour but also on its physical half-life and the characteristics of its radiations. On the basis of these various factors radionuclides have been

333

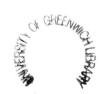

placed in four categories of toxicity. Some examples of the radionuclides in these various categories are listed in Table 16.1.

THE PHILOSOPHY OR RADIATION PROTECTION

The early recognition of the potentially harmful effects of radiation led to the creation in 1928 of the body now known as the International Commission on Radiological Protection (ICRP). This body keeps a watching brief on the fundamental principles upon which appropriate radiation protection measures can be based and makes recommendations concerning systems of dose limitation which it considers will permit ionizing radiations to be used without creating an unacceptable risk of damage to individuals, their children or to mankind as a whole. The Commission makes recommendations only, and it is the responsibility of the authorities in individual countries to implement those recommendations which they consider appropriate to their own particular circumstances. Revised recommendations were published in 1977 (International Commission on Radiological Protection, 1977) and the system of dose limitation now recommended is based on the following principles:

1. No radiation procedure should be adopted unless it can be shown to have a positive benefit.
2. All exposures should be kept as low as is reasonably achievable, taking account of both economic and social factors. This is often described as the ALARA principle.
3. The radiation dose equivalent should not exceed the limits recommended for different groups of people and particular circumstances.

The detrimental effects of radiation against which it is necessary to provide protection are called somatic and hereditary effects. Somatic effects are those which arise in the exposed person, while hereditary effects are those which affect his, or her, children and their descendants. In the recommended dose limits ICRP considers two classes of radiation effects, stochastic effects, which are those whose occurrence increases with increasing radiation dose without any 'threshold' below which the effects do not occur, and non-stochastic effects which are those that in the light of present knowledge are believed not to occur until a certain threshold dose of radiation has been exceeded.

Dose limits

The dose limits which ICRP believes will prevent non-stochastic effects and limit the occurrence of stochastic effects to an acceptable level are as follows:

(a) For non-stochastic effects in all tissues except the lens of the eye 0.5 Sv (50 rem) in a year. The dose equivalent limit for the lens of the eye was 0.3 Sv per year but this was reduced by ICRP in 1980 to 0.15 Sv (15 rem) in a year.

(b) For stochastic effects the recommended limits are based on the principle that the risk should be equal whether the whole body is uniformly irradiated or only part of the body is irradiated. For uniform whole-body irradiation the dose limit is 50 mSv (5 rem) per year. When only individual tissues or organs are irradiated the relevant individual organ dose limits are obtained by multiplying the whole body dose limit by an appropriate weighting factor. These weighting factors are listed in Table 16.2.

Recently, new analyses of the basic human biology database, derived to a very large extent from the study of the survivors of the two atomic bomb explosions in Japan, have suggested that the risks for the induction of, at least certain types of, cancer by radiation are greater than previously thought. In the light of this new information ICRP is currently revising its recommendations and the revised recommendations are expected to be published in late 1990 or 1991. It appears most likely that the new recommendations will propose new dose limits in the region of 20 mSv per year.

Table 16.2   Tissue weighting factors for the calculation of dose equivalent (International Commission on Radiological Protection, 1977)

Tissue	Weighting factors
Gonads	0.25
Breast	0.15
Red bone marrow	0.12
Lung	0.12
Thyroid	0.03
Bone surfaces	0.03
Remaining tissues (except the lens of the eye, skin, hands, forearms, feet, ankles)	0.30

For members of the general public lower dose limits, 1mSv per year, are recommended, and it is also recommended that pregnant women should be allowed to work only under conditions in which it is most unlikely that the radiation exposure will exceed three-tenths of the recommended dose limit.

The maximum amounts of different radionuclides which, if accumulated and retained in the body will deliver the dose limit to the organs and tissue, may be derived from the physical and biological characteristics of the individual nuclides. From these values it is possible to calculate the maximum amounts of specific radioactive materials which may be taken into the body in a year without exceeding the annual radiation dose limits. These quantities, the annual limits of intake (ALI), vary widely from radionuclide to radionuclide, thus for ^{3}H as tritiated water the ALI is 96 MBq ($2.6 \times 10^3 \mu$Ci per year, while for the long-lived alpha particle emitting nuclide ^{226}Ra which is deposited largely in the skeleton where it remains for many years, the ALI is only 3 kBq (0.08μCi) per year for soluble compounds.

PRACTICAL ASPECTS OF RADIATION PROTECTION

'Radiation work' nowadays covers a very wide range of activities. In hospitals X-rays are used for diagnosis and treatment, large sealed radionuclide sources (^{60}Co or ^{137}Cs) are also used for therapy and a wide variety of radionuclide compounds – radiopharmaceuticals – are administered to patients for diagnostic investigations and to a lesser extent for therapy. As well as these *in vivo* procedures, radionuclides are also used *in vitro* in radioimmunoassay and other analytical procedures. In other laboratories a wide range of radionuclide tracer studies may be carried out for research or other purposes. Such studies may also involve administration of radionuclides to experimental animals. Radiations from X-ray generators, linear accelerators, cyclotrons and sealed nuclide sources may be used for a variety of purposes including X-ray crystallography, radiation or radiochemistry and radiobiology. Although each type of work has its own specific requirements in terms of laboratory design, equipment and detailed working procedures, there are certain basic principles which are common to all work with radiation sources from X-ray generators to radionuclide solutions. The basic objectives of radiation protection are to minimize, or prevent, injury to individuals and to minimize the risk of genetic damage to the population. In order to achieve these aims it is necessary that all work involving radiation sources or radioactive materials is carried out carefully and with strict observance of these few basic principles.

In work with sources of penetrating radiation which may irradiate the body from outside there are three cardinal points to remember. The operations with the active source should be carried out in the minimum time necessary for the satisfactory and safe completion of the task, since the shorter the period of exposure the less the dose received by the operator. The operator should work at the largest practicable distance from the source, since radiation intensity decreases by the square of the distance from the source, i.e. the dose rate at 2 m is one-quarter of that at 1 m from the source. The operations should always be carried out behind an adequate amount of shielding. Shielding is required to reduce the intensity of the radiation to an acceptable working level. The amount and nature of the shielding material required will depend on the type and intensity of the source. For high-energy X-rays or gamma-rays several inches of lead may be required, whereas high-energy beta particles may be almost completely stopped by 1 cm of Perspex or similar material; low-energy beta particles or alpha particles have so little penetrating power that they are totally absorbed by the walls of their container.

These principles of time, distance and shielding apply to all work with radiation sources whether they are X-ray generators, radiation generators consisting of a radionuclide permanently mounted in a leakproof container (a so-called 'sealed' source), or solutions of radioactive compounds or other types of open or 'unsealed' source. Work with unsealed sources requires additional precautions of which the most important is the principle of containment. This requires the design of apparatus and procedures so that the escape of radioactive material from the container into the general laboratory environment is prevented, thus minimizing the risks of ingestion or inhalation of radioactive material by workers in the area. The type of shielding, containment and other facilities required for the use of radioactive materials will vary considerably according to the nature of the work and the activity, physico-chemical form and toxicity of the radionuclide concerned.

WORK WITH UNSEALED RADIATION SOURCES

The range of work now carried out using unsealed radionuclides is very large. At one end of the scale investigators may be working with only a few Bq of radioactivity while at the other radiochemists may be carrying out synthetic or preparative work with tens or hundreds of MBq. Work with unsealed, or open, radionuclides poses more potential radiation protection problems than that with X-rays or radiations from sealed sources. The main problems arise from the need to 'contain' the radionuclide within a defined area in order to prevent contamination of the laboratory, personnel or samples.

As mentioned earlier the exact type of facility required for radionuclide work will depend on the activity, radiotoxicity, radiation characteristics and physicochemical characteristics of the radionuclides to be used, as well as on the actual operations to be carried out. Radionuclide compounds may be used or produced as solids, liquids or gases; in addition, as a result of the manipulations to be carried out radioactive vapours or aerosols may be generated. All these factors must be taken into account in deciding on the exact facilities required for the proposed work. A detailed discussion of the facilities required for all types of radionuclide work is beyond the scope of this chapter but a few general comments may be made.

For simple operations involving simple mixing of solutions of radionuclides, containing less than 37 MBq of low-, or 3.7 MBq of medium-toxicity radionuclides, and when the possibility of aerosol or vapour formation can be excluded, no very elaborate facilities are needed. Preferably a separate laboratory should be set aside for such radioactive work and this should conform to requirements similar to those of a Class C laboratory (United

Kingdom, Committee of Vice-Chancellors and Principals, 1966), that is, it should be well ventilated and the walls and floor should be of non-absorbent, easily cleaned materials. All joints between flooring materials and between walls and floor should be sealed. The floor should be cleaned by wet mopping, not by dry sweeping. If the radionuclide is volatile, for example radionuclides of iodine, or if there is any chance that radioactive vapours or aerosols may be generated during the procedure, then a fume hood should be used. The addition of scintillant to samples for liquid scintillation counting may give rise to radioactive aerosols plus chemically toxic vapours and is best carried out in a fume hood. The design of fume hoods for radioactive work has been discussed by Hughes (1974). Basically fume hoods for radioactive work should be designed and constructed that they may be easily cleaned and that they should have an air flow (face velocity) of at least 0.5 metre per second through the working aperture of the hood. The extraction system must be carefully designed and the discharge arrangements outside the building must comply with local and national radiation safety requirements.

For work with large quantities of radioactivity or with highly radiotoxic nuclides more elaborate facilities are needed. These may range from the use of a 'glove box' in a suitably designed laboratory to special 'hot' cells constructed of high-density concrete, with special ventilation, in which all work is carried out using remote handling devices.

When work is being carried out on open benches or in fume hoods the bench surfaces should be lined with absorbent paper to facilitate easy decontamination in the event of a spillage of radioactive material, impervious, plastic-backed absorbent paper, such as Whatman 'Benchkote' (Whatman, England) is very convenient for this purpose, but polyethylene sheeting covered with any suitable absorbent paper is equally satisfactory. So far as it is practicable it is desirable to carry out work with radioactive materials in plastic or metal trays lined with absorbent paper. In the event of a spill the tray should retain the major part of the radioactivity thus making the task of decontamination easier. For work with gamma-ray emitting radionuclides appropriate shielding may be provided by walls built of lead bricks or by placing the radioactive solutions, etc. inside suitable lead 'pots'. In erecting appropriate shielding it must not be forgotten that the radiation is emitted in all directions and that adequate protection all round and above and below the source is needed. A clear Perspex or Plexiglas screen 1 to 2 cm thick will provide protection against the more energetic β-particles and also give valuable protection against facial or body contamination in case of a spillage of radioactive material.

For all work with radioactive material a carefully thought out experimental protocol should be prepared and tested with non-radioactive materials before work with radioactivity is commenced. In drawing up such protocols it is generally desirable to seek the advice of the local radiation safety officer (see later) or of some other person with experience in the requirements for radiation safety. Protocols should be kept as simple as is consistent with the satisfactory execution of the required procedure. When procedures involve the manipulation of relatively large amounts of gamma-ray-emitting radio-nuclides directly by hand the radiation dose to the fingers or whole hand may be quite large, thus in such circumstances thermoluminescent dosimeters should be worn on the hands or fingers.

The main stocks of radionuclides should be kept in a suitable shielded and locked store. For small quantities of radioactive materials a suitably shielded locked cupboard in the isotope laboratory may be authorized, but more usually a separate isotope store is required. It is important that adequate records of the receipt, use and disposal of all radioactive materials are kept at all times.

Radioactive contamination in the laboratory carries not only the risk that the worker or his or her colleagues may become contaminated externally or internally but also that experimental materials or samples may become contaminated, thus rendering work useless or of questionable validity. There-fore an important requirement in all laboratories where radioactive materials are used is the maintenance of high standards of personal and laboratory hygiene. At the personal level the following basic rules should be observed strictly in all work with radioactive materials:

1. Rubber or plastic gloves should be worn for all work with radioactive materials and in radioactive areas. It should always be remembered that anything touched with contaminated gloves will usually become con-taminated, consequently it is necessary to avoid touching switches, taps or apparatus outside the radioactive area. Gloves should be cleaned while still on the hands and the hands should be thoroughly washed immediately after leaving the radioactive area. Disposable gloves should be used whenever possible.
2. Separate overalls, or other protective clothing, should be kept, and must be worn to work in the radioactive area, these should not be worn outside the area.
3. For any work involving the risk of inhalation of dust, for example, cage cleaning in an experimental animal facility, a dust mask which com-pletely covers the nose and mouth should be worn.
4. An appropriate film, thermoluminescent or ionization chamber do-simeter should be worn at all times when working in, or near, radioac-tive areas.
5. No radioactive solution, or any inactive solution used in the radioactive area should be drawn into a pipette by mouth. Suitable pipetting devices must always be used.
6. Eating, drinking, smoking and the application of cosmetics are abso-lutely forbidden in radioactive areas. Obviously it is also forbidden to store foodstuffs or personal drinking vessels in such areas.

7. Since radioactive materials can enter the body through open wounds, work with radioactivity should not be undertaken if open scratches, cuts or sores are present on hands, face or other exposed areas of the body. If such work must be undertaken in these circumstances the wound should be well covered by a waterproof dressing.

In the radioactive area a regular programme of monitoring should be carried out under the supervision of the radiological safety officer. This should include bench tops, floors, walls, ceiling, sinks and waste traps as well as all equipment. Staff should monitor their hands and clothing at the end of each session of work in the radioactive area and appropriate beta-gamma monitoring equipment should be provided for this purpose. The type of monitoring equipment required will vary according to the radionuclides used and the amount of radioactive work carried out. In establishments using only small quantities of hard beta- or gamma-emitting radionuclides a simple, inexpensive, general-purpose, beta-gamma sensitive Geiger-Mueller type monitor will suffice, but laboratories making extensive use of radioactive isotope techniques involving a wide range of radionuclides will require more sophisticated instruments, with a variety of different types of alpha-, beta- or gamma-sensitive probes. Monitoring of hands and clothing following work with the isotopes ^{14}C and ^{3}H is impracticable, because of the difficulties of detecting the low-energy beta particles emitted by these nuclides; very high personal hygiene standards are therefore essential.

Benches, etc. can be monitored for ^{14}C and ^{3}H by wipe tests using a small piece of filter paper or paper tissue and subsequently assaying this for radioactivity in a liquid scintillation counter. Such monitoring should be carried out at frequent intervals.

RADIONUCLIDE STUDIES IN EXPERIMENTAL ANIMALS

The majority of experiments in which radioactive substances are administered to animals involve the use of only small quantities, 185 kBq (50 μCi) or less, of low or moderate toxicity radionuclides; thus, even when these emit gamma-rays, there is usually little risk of serious external irradiation of animal technicians by the treated animals. The major problems arise because of the risks of internal contamination of personnel by the radionuclide used. Internal contamination may result from inhalation or ingestion of radionuclides absorbed on to dust particles arising from bedding materials, by inhalation of gaseous radioactive compounds exhaled by the animals, through contamination of the skin by excreta, or from bites or scratches. All of these risks can be reduced to negligible proportions by the good design of facilities and operating procedures and the maintenance at all times of high standards of personal and animal house hygiene.

Animals should be housed in easily cleaned cages, constructed of plastic material, aluminium, stainless steel or glass. Bedding should be of a non-dusty type such as cellulose wadding, absorbent paper or coarse-grain vermiculite. When only very small amounts of activity are used and the excretion is expected to be low, a coarse sawdust may be used. The disposal of contaminated bedding, excreta, etc. will be discussed later. If the work involves the use of large animals, such as dogs or sheep, the pens in which the animals are kept should be so designed that they may be easily cleaned and decontaminated by hosing down or mopping out. It may be necessary for the drains from these pens to lead into delay tanks so that effluent can be decontaminated before it is pumped into the main drainage system. If, as is often the case, it is desired to collect excreta for analysis, the animals will need to be housed in metabolism cages. These may be of any convenient design but they should be so constructed that they may easily be dismantled for cleaning and decontamination. All cages used for radioactive work should be kept separate from those used for other animal work.

If it is necessary to work with high-toxicity radionuclides, or greater amounts than about 40 MBq of low or moderate toxicity nuclides, or to administer radioactive materials continuously in the diet, more elaborate facilities will be needed. The additional facilities are required to ensure containment of the radioactive materials within a well-defined area and to permit the discharge of radioactive gases or vapours through suitable trunking and filters to the outside of the building.

The problems of radiation, and general safety in the animal house, have been discussed extensively, but with special reference to British practice, by Seamer and Wood (1981).

RADIATION SAFETY DURING CLINICAL INVESTIGATIONS

The use of radionuclides in clinical diagnosis or therapy often involves larger amounts of radioactivity or radiation than are encountered in most laboratory situations, thus the radiation safety measures necessary to keep radiation doses to staff well within the ICRP dose limits may have to be rather more extensive than those required in other laboratories.

In laboratories where radiopharmaceuticals are prepared for administration to patients, usually by intravenous injection, the requirements for good radiation safety must be combined with those required for the safe preparation of pharmaceuticals for human use. This may involve more elaborate facilities such as 'clean rooms' and additional working rules. The preparation of radiopharmaceuticals has been discussed in several recent publications (BIR, 1979; Kristensen, 1979). The radiation exposure of the patient during medical treatment or investigations should be governed by the ALARA principle, that is the radiation dose should be kept to the minimum required to ensure that the investigation or treatment is likely to yield a satisfactory result. This involves the balancing of the possible risks from radiation against the direct benefits likely to accrue to the patient from the investigation or treatment; this is principally a matter for the patient's physician to decide. However, all persons responsible for the conduct of such investigations or treatments have an obligation to ensure that the procedure is properly designed and executed in order to avoid unnecessary further irradiation because the investigation was technically unsatisfactory.

In view of the sensitivity of the developing embryo, it has been recommended that radiographic investigations in women of childbearing age should be limited to the 10-day period following menstruation since during this period there is no risk of an unrecognized pregnancy (ICRP, 1982); there is no general agreement about whether this rule should also apply to radionuclide investigations.

A special situation arises with the use of human volunteers for investigations involving the administration of radioactive substances for research purposes when the exposure is unrelated to any illness in the subject. Such investigations may only be carried out on persons who have given their consent, usually in writing, after the exact nature of the procedure and its risks have been fully explained to them. Such investigations should only be undertaken with the consent of the authorities in the institution concerned and after the advice of an expert advisory group has been obtained; they must also comply with any national and local rules concerning such investigations. In general such investigations should not be performed on children or other persons who may not legally give their informed consent to the procedure.

The protection of the patient in radionuclide investigations has been discussed in several specialist monographs (ICRP, 1969, 1982; Langmead, 1983).

LEGISLATIVE CONTROL OF RADIATION WORK

In most of the developed countries of the world the use of radiation sources and radioactive materials is governed by some form of legislation (WHO, 1972). In the past this legislation, and any associated regulations, has normally followed closely the philosophy and dose limitations recommended by the ICRP. The ICRP Recommendations, which were discussed in a previous section, involved both a change in the basic philosophy and in the numerical values of the dose limits and as a result some alterations have been or should be expected to be made to most legislative regulations. Further changes will be needed to take account of the new ICRP Recommendations which are in preparation.

Within the European Community all member states are subject to the provision of the Treaty which established the European Atomic Energy

Community (Euratom). Article 30 of this Treaty states that basic standards must be formulated for the protection of the health of the general public and of workers against the dangers of ionizing radiations. Under Article 33 of the Treaty member states are required to enact the appropriate legislation and regulations to enable them to comply with the standards which have been laid down (Euratom Directive, 1976, 1980). Thus radiation protection standards and regulations should be broadly similar throughout most countries of Western Europe. The different member states of the European Community have their own national laws controlling the use of radiation and radioactive substances and these laws must be brought into harmony with the Euratom Directive. For example, in the United Kingdom the relevant legislation is contained in the 'Radioactive Substances Acts of 1948 and 1960' and in the 'Health and Safety at Work, etc. Act, 1974'; in France the principal provisions are contained in the 'Décret No. 66–450 du 20 Juin 1966 relatif aux principes généraux de protection contre les radiations ionisantes'. The equivalent Federal German law is contained in the Federal 'Atomgesetze' and the 'Strahlenschutzverordnung', 1989. In the USA the control of reactor-produced radionuclides is governed by the United States of America Atomic Energy Act 1954 and that of other radiation sources, including X-rays, microwaves and other radiation from electronic devices, by the United States of America Radiation Control for Health and Safety Act 1968. Federal regulations relating to the control of radioactive materials and radiation sources are contained in the United States of American Code of Federal Regulations. Title 10, especially Parts 30, 31 and 35; transport is covered by Title 49 of the Code.

In other countries of the world the radiation protection regulations are broadly similar. Although they may differ in content, detail and administrative arrangements, the various national laws contain essentially the same basic requirements for the health surveillance of workers, monitoring of personnel and radiation areas, maintenance of records of radioactive sources, transport, the disposal of radioactive waste, and emergency procedures to be used in the event of accidental contamination of laboratory personnel. Every person working with sources of ionizing radiation should have read the appropriate 'code of practice' and know and understand its requirements. Each establishment should draw up its own local rules or 'code of practice' which incorporate the basic official requirements and include such additional requirements as may be considered desirable in the local conditions. These rules must be brought to the attention of all who work with or come into contact with ionizing radiation and it is desirable that each of these persons should have his own copy.

Most codes of practice require that a 'radiological safety officer' shall be appointed to be responsible for the overall organization and regulation of the use of radiation and radioactive materials in each establishment. The radiological safety officer alone is responsible for radiation protection; however, although he is responsible for ensuring compliance with the legal regulations governing radiation work, an important part of his work lies in advising and instructing staff on the correct procedures for working with ionizing radiations. The radiological safety officer must always be informed of any accidental exposure to radiation, however trivial, or any spillage or personal contamination by radioactive materials.

In all work with radiation sources or with radioactive materials in any country it should never be forgotten that while the ultimate responsibility for radiation protection will almost always lie with the employing organization, the primary responsibility for protecting him- or herself and other people from radiation hazards rests with the individual worker. Consequently no-one should be permitted to begin to use radiation sources in any form until he or she has become fully acquainted with the nature of the potential hazards and the general and local rules for radiation work.

RADIOACTIVE WASTE DISPOSAL

The safe disposal of radioactive waste is a matter of considerable public anxiety at this time. While this concern lies principally with the disposal of the high-activity waste from nuclear power generation, it has important ramifications in respect to the disposal of radioactive waste from hospitals, research laboratories and other establishments, even though the amounts of radioactivity in the waste are orders of magnitude less than those from burnt-up nuclear fuels.

In all countries where there is legislation concerning work with radioactive substances there is, or should be, strict control of radioactive waste disposal, with regard to both the methods of disposal and the quantities of radioactivity which may be disposed of by each route per month or per year. The disposal methods permitted vary from country to country and reflect both local conditions and national attitudes, thus in this chapter the topic can be discussed only in broad general terms.

Radioactive waste arising from the use of radioactive materials in hospitals, laboratories or animal houses falls into one or more of the following categories:

(a) Liquid waste: this may range from simple aqueous solutions to contaminated blood or other types of sample, aqueous and non-aqueous. This type of waste includes the waste arising from liquid scintillation counting which is mainly a mixture of aqueous and non-aqueous fluids containing principally ^{14}C or ^{3}H but may include a variety of other radionuclides. Some of these waste fluids may be inflammable.

(b) Combustible solid waste: this may include contaminated tissue from human or animal sources; disposable plastic syringes and other laboratory ware; contaminated absorbent materials, paper, tissues, etc.; contaminated animal bedding; contaminated animal carcasses.

(c)   Non-combustible solid waste: this type of waste includes contaminated glassware, hypodermic needles, other types of non-combustible laboratory apparatus as well as sealed or solid radionuclide sources used in medicine or research.

For all types of waste contaminated with short-lived radionuclides, with half-lives ranging from a few hours to a few weeks, it may be practical to store the waste in a suitably shielded, locked store until the activity has decayed to an agreed negligible level and then to dispose of the material in the same way as other non-radioactive waste.

For waste containing longer-lived radionuclides other methods of disposal must be found and various options are open. For example, in some situations a controlled discharge of small quantities of aqueous liquid waste into the normal sewage system may be permitted, or inflammable liquid waste may be burnt in small quantities in oil-fired heating plants. However, in other situations all liquid waste must be specially processed, either to separate the radioactivity from the bulk solvent or water, or by solidification with concrete or other material. With combustible solid waste it is advantageous to reduce the bulk by burning; this will release relatively 'volatile' radioactive materials such as ^{14}C, ^{3}H, ^{35}S, ^{32}P, and radioiodine compounds into the atmosphere via the smoke stack and will concentrate the 'non-volatile' radionuclides in the ash. In some circumstances low-activity combustible waste may be permitted to be burnt in hospital or other domestic refuse incinerators but high-activity waste must be burnt in special incinerators with special filters and trapping systems to reduce the output of radioiodines and of radioactive fly-ash. Solid waste, including solidified liquid waste and the ash from the combustion of combustible waste, must be sealed in waterproof and relatively corrosion-proof containers and either buried in relatively shallow pits, or in suitable disused mines.

The disposal of radioactive carcasses may sometimes present problems. For small animal carcasses containing no more than moderate amounts of medium or low-toxicity nuclides, immediate disposal by incineration or by maceration and flushing into the drains may be permitted. Macerators of various sizes capable of accepting animals as large as a whole dog can be obtained. This is a very convenient way of disposing of animal carcasses. However, although the use of macerators may be authorized for the disposal of radioactive carcasses, their use for the disposal of large numbers of carcasses may be viewed with disfavour by some sewage authorities since the high biochemical oxygen demand of the macerate may cause problems at the sewage works. The disposal of the carcasses of large animals is more difficult. It may sometimes be necessary to store such carcasses for some time before their removal for destruction by other permitted procedures.

For the temporary storage of carcasses prior to disposal deep freezing at –20 °C is most convenient. Some other methods for the temporary preservation of radioactive carcasses prior to disposal are described in Appendix 7 of the Code of Practice issued by the United Kingdom Department of Employment (1968). If storage of carcasses or liquid waste is necessary, the materials should be placed in suitably shielded, leakproof containers and placed in a locked and adequately ventilated storeroom. Advice on the specific methods used for the disposal of radioactive waste in the reader's own establishment must be obtained from the radiation safety officer. It is essential that every person working with radioactive materials should know exactly how the waste arising from his or her own work is to be disposed of. Unauthorized disposal of radioactive waste via the normal drains or domestic refuse may lead to serious contamination of persons or property and in some situations may render the individual liable to prosecution.

EMERGENCY PROCEDURES

Many codes of practice require that, in their contingency planning, every establishment shall make preparations to deal with an accidental contamination of personnel. Whatever the legal requirements may be, it is a wise precaution in all laboratories or facilities which handle unsealed sources of radioactive materials to prepare plans for dealing with a spill or similar emergency and to publish these plans clearly in the local rules for the conduct of radiation work. All staff should be conversant with the procedures to be adopted should an emergency occur.

In case of a spill or radioactivity the action will depend on the activity involved and the radiotoxicity of the radionuclide. The procedure discussed below can be applied to all significant spills, which may be defined as those which involve more than about a tenth of a MBq of a medium- or low-radiotoxicity radionuclide.

Equipment should be kept readily available for use in emergency in any department where significant amounts of activity are handled. The essential items will depend on the type of work being carried out but will include protective clothing; decontamination materials; warning signs; equipment for the handling, temporary storage and disposal of contaminated articles; and portable monitoring equipment.

The following is an example of the sequence of actions which should be followed when a spill occurs.

If the accident has involved injury to staff or other persons, first aid must be administered. At the same time a person qualified or experienced in radiation protection must be called and the radiation safety officer or equivalent informed. The next concern is to stop the spread of contamination and clear people from the area of the spill. Care should be taken that people leaving the site are not contaminated, especially that they do not spread activity with their shoes. Before any further action is taken any person involved in the cleaning up operations must wear adequate protective clothing; this will involve, at the minimum, over-shoes or boots, gloves and gown. A suitable respirator may be needed.

Decontamination of persons should take priority over clearing up the spill. Protective and, if possible, other outer clothing which is contaminated with radioactive substances should be removed and left in the contaminated area. Activity in the eye should be washed out with copious amounts of saline or water. Contaminated skin must be washed thoroughly with soap and water. If this fails to remove the activity detergent may be used but any further action should only be taken with care as the skin must not become broken or porous. A shower bath may be required but only after the major areas of contamination have been cleaned. When there is any question of ingestion of radioactivity then medical advice must be sought or a whole-body count carried out.

In cleaning up spills appropriate equipment must be used. For simple spills soap, water and absorbent material may be sufficient. Commercial detergents and decontamination agents can be of great value. Contaminated articles, clothing and waste can be removed from the site of the spill in plastic or non-absorbent bags. For short-lived radionuclides, if activity still remains on a surface after decontamination, the surface should be suitably covered until the radioactivity has decayed to a sufficiently low level.

The level of spill which has to be reported to official supervisory bodies varies from country to country, but any, except perhaps the most trivial, degree of contamination must be reported to the local radiation protection officer since he or she is responsible for ensuring that adequate decontamination steps have been taken.

CONCLUSION

The use or misuse of all sources of ionizing radiation is potentially capable of causing cancer or other serious injury to the health of persons working with them. This risk is very small if both the employing organization and the individual workers cultivate an informed and responsible attitude to radiation work. The ultimate responsibility for the safe conduct of work with all forms of radiation lies with the employer but the *primary responsibility* for protecting him or herself and his or her colleagues lies with the individual worker. Thus it is essential that before commencing work with ionizing radiation every worker receives proper instruction in the general nature of radiation risks and the reasons underlying the specific safety procedures which he or she must practise.

As with all other hazardous agents, safe and trouble-free work with radioactive materials and radiation sources requires the individual worker to use care, forethought, self-discipline and, above all, common sense at all times. Familiarity with radioactive materials should never be allowed to develop into a contempt for their potential dangers and, like fire, electricity, and toxic substances in general, ionizing radiation should always be treated with respect but without fear.

LITERATURE CONSULTED

British Institute of Radiology (1979). Guidelines for the Preparation of Radiopharmaceuticals in Hospitals. Special Report No. 11, British Institute of Radiology, London

Committee of Vice-Chancellors and Principals of the Universities of the United Kingdom (1966). *Radiological Protection in Universities*. (London: Association of Commonwealth Universities)

Department of Employment (1968). *Code of Practice for the Protection of Persons Exposed to Ionising Radiations in Research and Teaching*. (London: HMSO)

Euratom Directive (1976). Council Directive of 1 June 1976 laying down the revised basic safety standards for the health protection of the general public and workers against the dangers of ionizing radiation. *Official Journal of the European Communities*, L/187, 12 July 1976 (76/579 Euratom)

Euratom (1980). Guidelines of the Council of 15 July 1980 on Revision of the Basic Safety Standards for the Health Protection of the General Public and Workers against the Dangers of Ionizing Radiation. *Official Journal of the European Communities*, L246, 17 September 1980 (80/836 Euratom)

Hughes, D. (1974). The design and installation of efficient fume-cupboards. Special Report No. 8, *Br. J. Radiol.*, **47**, 888-892

International Atomic Energy Agency (1963). *A Basic Toxicity Classification of Radionuclides*. (Technical Report Series No. 15). (Vienna: International Atomic Energy Agency)

International Commission on Radiological Protection, Publication 17 (1969). *Protection of the Patient in Radionuclide Investigations*. (Oxford: Pergamon Press)

International Commission on Radiological Protection, Publication 26 (1977). Recommendations of the ICRP. *Annals of the ICRP*, **1** (3)

International Commission on Radiological Protection Publication 34 (1982). Protection of the patient in diagnostic radiology. *Annals of the ICRP*, **9** (2/3)

Kristensen, K. (1979). Preparation and Control of Radiopharmaceuticals in Hospitals. Techn. Rept. Series No. 194. (Vienna: International Atomic Energy Agency)

Langmead, W.A. (1983). *Protection of the Patient in Nuclear Medicine. A manual of good practice*. (Oxford: Oxford University Press)

Seamer, J.H. and Wood, M. (1981). *Safety in the Animal House*, Laboratory Animals Handbook 5. (London: Laboratory Animals Ltd.)

World Health Organisation (1972). *Protection against Ionizing Radiation: a Survey of Current World Legislation*. (Geneva: WHO)

SUGGESTIONS FOR FURTHER READING

Martin, A. and Harbison, S.A. (1979). *An Introduction to Radiation Protection*. (London: Chapman & Hall)

Shapiro, J. (1972). *Radiation Protection: a Guide for Scientists*. (Cambridge, Mass.: Harvard University Press)

Sowby, F.D. (1965). Radiation and other risks. *Health Physics*, **11**, 879

Pochin, E. (1983). *Nuclear Radiation, Risks and Benefits*. (Oxford: Oxford University Press)

17 Ultraviolet Radiation Safety

B.L. Diffey

INTRODUCTION

The skin and eyes of humans are frequently exposed to ultraviolet radiation (UVR) from the sun either during everyday activity or during intentional exposure to achieve tanning. Exposure may also occur from any of a number of artificial sources which emit UVR. These include the increasingly popular commercial sunbeds and solaria used in an attempt to produce year-round tanning, the therapeutic UVR lamps used in the treatment of psoriasis and other skin diseases, welding arcs, gas discharge arc lamps, fluorescent lamps, and lasers used in industry or research. Physiological mechanisms exist to deal with the absorbed energy, but they are not totally efficient. Sufficient damage at tissue, cellular, subcellular, and molecular levels invokes an inflammatory response, repair processes, and an increase in the function of protective processes. If no further exposure occurs, these processes run a short course and then cease to act. If multiple exposures occur, the processes continue and intensify. Since neither repair nor protective process is perfect, continuing exposure can lead to long-term damage, such as skin cancer.

Table 17.1 Workers at potential risk from exposure to ultraviolet radiation

Dentists	Paint and resin curers
Hairdressers	Physiotherapists
Laboratory workers	Photographic workers
Lighting technicians	Plasma torch operators
Lithographic and printing workers	Spectroscopists
Nurses	Welders

Apart from the cosmetic and therapeutic uses of artificial sources of UVR, the exposure of people as a result of the radiation occurring will normally be as an unwanted by-product of a particular process, particularly in the context

349

of laboratory sources. Because of the harmful effects of UVR exposure in humans, it is important that occupationally exposed persons are aware of potential hazards and how to avoid them. Some of the groups of workers at potential risk from exposure to UVR are given in Table 17.1, and some devices which emit UVR are listed in Table 17.2.

Table 17.2 Some devices emitting ultraviolet radiation

Artificial weathering chambers	Mercury lamps
Bacterial lamps	Photocopying machines
Carbon, xenon and other arcs	Plasma torches
Dental polymerizing equipment	Printing ink polymerizing equipment
Fluorescence equipment	UV microscopes
Medical phototherapy equipment	Welding equipment

In addition, the general public may be affected by exposure from:
Natural UVR (sunlight)
Sunlamps and sunbeds
Welding equipment

THE ULTRAVIOLET SPECTRUM

Ultraviolet radiation is part of the electromagnetic spectrum and lies between the visible and the X-ray regions. Different wavebands in the ultraviolet spectrum show enormous variations in causing biological damage and for this reason the UV spectrum is divided into three spectral regions; UV-A, UV-B and UV-C. The notion to divide the ultraviolet spectrum into different spectral regions was first put forward at the Copenhagen meeting of the Second International Congress on Light held in August 1932[1]. It was recommended that three spectral regions be defined as follows:

UV-A	400–315 nm
UV-B	315–280 nm
UV-C	<280 nm

Various regulatory authorities including the International Commission on Illumination (CIE), the National Institute for Occupational Safety and Health (NIOSH) in the United States, and the Health and Safety Executive (HSE) and the National Radiological Protection Board (NRPB) in the United Kingdom, have by their use endorsed these regions, with the slight modification that the lower limit of the UV-C region is taken to be 100 nm by the CIE, HSE and NRPB, and 200 nm by the NIOSH. Radiation in the spectral region 100–200 nm (the vacuum UV) is readily attenuated in air with little opportunity to produce direct biological effects, and so the lower limit of the UV-C region for practical purposes is not critical.

350

The development of environmental photobiology has prompted some workers[2] to redefine the boundaries of the three spectral regions as follows:

UV-A	400–320 nm
UV-B	320–290 nm
UV-C	290–200 nm

The upper limit of the UV-B region has been extended to 320 nm, since most acute and chronic effects of sunlight exposure on biological systems are believed to occur at wavelengths less than 320 nm, whilst the division between the UV-B and UV-C regions has been set at 290 nm since the wavelength is the approximate lower limit of terrestrial radiation. Yet another publication[3] has defined the UV-B region as 280–320 nm. Although the divisions between the spectral regions are not necessarily rigid it would seem sensible to adopt international recommendations and so the convention in this chapter is as follows:

Spectral region	Also known as	Range of wavelengths (nm)
UV-A	Longwave or 'blacklight'	400–315
UV-B	Middlewave or 'erythemal'	315–280
UV-C	Shortwave or 'germicidal'	280–100

BIOLOGICAL EFFECTS OF ULTRAVIOLET RADIATION IN HUMANS

The observable biological effects in man due to exposure from external sources of ultraviolet radiation are limited to the skin and to the eyes because of the low penetrating properties of UVR in human tissues. This section will outline the recognizable short-term and long-term effects of UV exposure in the skin and the eyes.

The skin

Structure of the skin

The skin consists of a superficial layer, the epidermis, and a deeper vascular connective tissue layer termed the dermis or corium. A schematic cross-section of the superficial layers of the human skin perpendicular to the skin surface is given in Figure 17.1.

The epidermis contains no blood or lymphatic vessels and is composed of stratified squamous epithelium which varies in thickness in different parts of

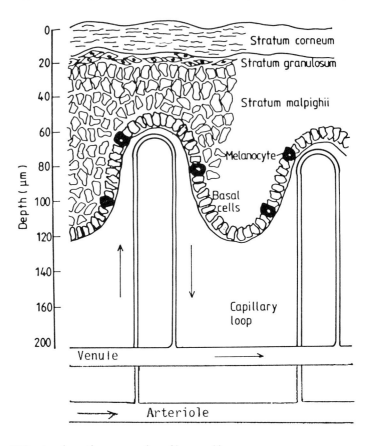

Figure 17.1 A schematic cross-section of human skin

the body. The superficial layer of the epidermis, termed the stratum corneum or horny layer, is a mechanically tough and chemically resistant layer. The epidermal cells are continually being manufactured by the keratinocytes (prickle cells) of the stratum malpighii. Keratinocytes are derived from a single germinative layer of basal cells. In normal skin it may take up to 14 days for a daughter cell of the basal layer to reach the stratum corneum and another 1–2 weeks before it is sloughed off from the skin surface. There are specialized cells called melanocytes which reside within the basal layer and produce granules called melanosomes containing the pigment melanin. Melanin is a complex macromolecular protein which strongly absorbs light and UVR and plays an important role in protecting the viable cells against damage by UVR. Below the epidermis lies the dermis, which has well-marked ridges and projections, called papillae, on its upper surface. This prevents a separation of the two layers by shearing. The dermis consists of dense connective tissue with blood vessels and lymphatics, and merges into the less

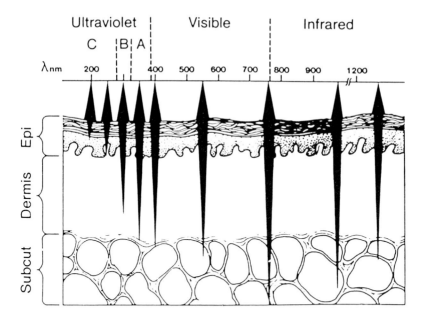

Figure 17.2 A diagrammatic summary of the penetration of optical radiation of different wavelengths into human skin. (Epi; epidermis: Subcut; subcutaneous tissue)

dense subcutaneous tissue. It is the elastic fibres present in the dermis that give the skin its characteristic elasticity.

Finally, the skin over the entire body is supplied segmentally by nerves from the spinal cord. The nerve endings, or receptors, are responsible for cutaneous sensations such as touch, pain, heat and cold.

Interaction of UVR with biomolecules in the skin

Studies on the optics of the skin present severe experimental problems. The skin is not only reflecting and absorbing, it is inhomogeneous, containing structures such as hair follicles, sweat glands and sebaceous glands, and even its dimensions are difficult to measure. UVR incident on the skin may be reflected, refracted, absorbed, scattered, transmitted or produce fluorescence. The depth of penetration of optical radiation in the skin shows a large variation with wavelength, as is illustrated diagramatically in Figure 17.2.

Only those photons that are absorbed contribute to a biological response, and the absorbing molecule is termed a chromophore. In general, only unsaturated organic compounds are good UVR chromophores at wavelengths longer than about 220 nm. These compounds usually contain alternating single and double bonds and are frequently cyclic or polycyclic.

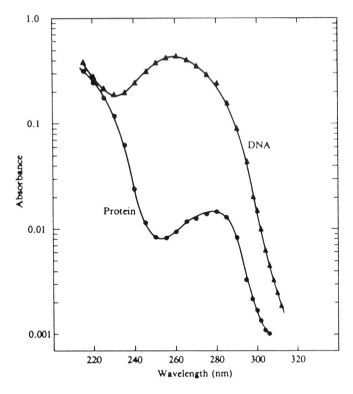

Figure 17.3 Typical absorption spectra of the important biomolecules, deoxyribonucleic acid (DNA) and protein

Important substances in the skin capable of absorbing UVR are the purine and pyrimidine bases of nucleic acids, which absorb maximally at about 260 nm; the amino acids of proteins (especially the aromatic tryptophan, tyrosine, and phenylalanine and the non-aromatic cystine and cysteine), which absorb maximally at about 280 nm (see Figure 17.3); melanin; and haemoglobin. Less important are urocanic acid, the porphyrins, riboflavin, steroids, nicotinamide adenine dinucleotide, isoprenoid quinones (such as vitamin K), betacarotene and bilirubin. Many of the major biomolecules *in vitro* absorb optimally in the UV-C region which, although outside the range of terrestrial sunlight, is often an important component of the emission spectrum of many artificial sources of UVR. Following absorption of a photon, the electrically excited absorbing molecule rapidly returns to a more stable energy state (a) by relaxation through vibrational or rotational energy levels resulting in production of heat; (b) by re-emision of a photon with lower energy in the form of fluorescence or phosphorescence; (c) by undergoing a permanent structural change; or (d) by reacting with an appropriate nearby molecule. After the initial photochemical reaction, so-called 'dark' thermal chemical reactions may cause direct tissue damage or release of mediators and result in the observable clinical response. Exact details of the photochemical and subsequent thermal chemical reactions associated with given clinical responses are not known in most cases, although there is some information concerning the products of the latter reactions.

Effects of UVR on normal skin

The normal responses of the skin to UVR can be classed under two headings: acute effects and chronic effects. An acute effect is one of rapid onset and generally of short duration, as opposed to a chronic effect which is often of gradual onset and long duration. These effects should be distinguished from acute and chronic exposure conditions which refer to the length of the UVR exposure. The acute reactions considered will be erythema (sunburn), delayed melanin pigmentation (suntan) and vitamin D production. Skin ageing and skin cancer will be discussed as those chronic reactions produced by prolonged or repeated UVR exposure.

Ultraviolet erythema (sunburn)

Exposure to UVR, particularly from wavelengths less than 315 nm, can result in erythema. The redness of the skin which is characteristic of erythema is attributable to an increased blood content by dilation of the superficial blood vessels, mainly the subpapillary venules. Sunburn caused by exposure to solar radiation normally has a latent period of a few hours. Erythema induced by artificial sources is strongly dependent on the wavelength of radiation. At 300 nm an average threshold dose or minimal erythema dose (MED) in unacclimatized white skin[4] is about 300 J m^{-2} whereas for UV-A radiation the MED is about a thousand-fold higher. Larger doses of UV-B may result in oedema, pain and blistering, although blistering seldom occurs with UV-C[5].

The vascular response due to UVR could be considered to arise from two different types of mechanism[6]. It could be from a direct action on the vessel wall itself, or indirectly from a photochemical reaction via a diffusing chemical mediator arising in the epidermis. There is recent evidence that prostaglandins, a group of long-chain fatty acids with vasoactive properties, are implicated as possible mediators or modulators of inflammation in UV-C and UV-B erythema[5]. It is observed that prostaglandin production increases following UVR exposure. However, prostaglandins are thought not to play as important a role, if any, as mediators of the UV-A-induced erythema, which may be due to a direct effect on dermal vasculature.

The evidence that UVR erythema entails diffusion of a chemical mediator from the epidermis to the dermis includes the following[7]:

1. the erythemally reactive UVR is mostly absorbed in the epidermis;
2. there is a latent period between exposure and appearance of erythema;
3. The phenomenon known as 'diffusion flush' which is that an erythema, elicited with a large dose of UVR, is after some time surrounded by a diffuse reddening, less intense than the central erythema and slowly spreading outward.

The erythema action spectrum

The ability of UVR to produce an erythema response in human skin is highly dependent upon the wavelength of the radiation and is expressed by the action spectrum. An action spectrum is a plot of the reciprocal of the dose

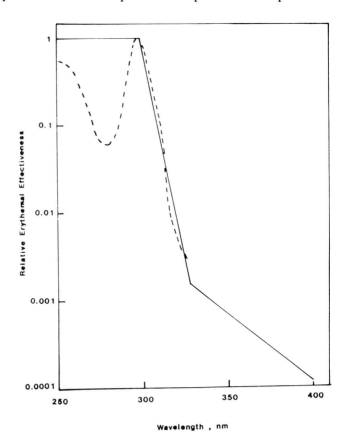

Figure 17.4 Comparison of the standard erythemal curve (CIE, 1935) and the new proposed reference erythema action spectrum[23]. Continuous line, new action spectrum; dashed line, old erythemal curve

required for a given effect against wavelength, and strictly applies only if the dose-response curves are similar at all wavelengths, which implies that the mechanism of action is the same at all wavelengths.

The effectiveness of UVR of different wavelengths in producing erythema in normal human skin has been a subject of study for about 60 years. Hausser and Vahle (1922)[8] first reported the erythema action spectrum which showed a major peak of activity at 297 nm, a minimum at about 280 nm and a second but lesser peak at around 250 nm. The general form of this curve was confirmed by other investigators in the following ten years[9-11], so much so that in 1934 Coblentz and Stair[12] proposed a 'standard erythema curve' which was subsequently published by the CIE in 1935.

Experimental data from more recent estimates of the erythema action spectrum have all differed appreciably from the CIE standard, particularly in the spectral region 250 to 300 nm[4,13-21]. All of these investigators have shown that the effectiveness of radiation at 250 nm is in fact higher than that at about 300 nm, with a less apparent, or even no, minimum at 280 nm. At wavelengths greater than 300 nm these recent results concur with earlier estimates in that the erythemal effectiveness of ultraviolet radiation drops very rapidly, falling to an efficiency at 320 nm of about 1% of that at 300 nm.

Recent quantitative work on ultraviolet erythema[22] has shown that the slopes of the erythemal response – log UV dose curves are markedly different for UV-B and UV-C radiation. This means that although smaller doses of 250 nm are required to produce a minimal erythema than from 300 nm radiation, the reverse is the case for moderate to severe erythema. As a consequence of these observations and the 'recent' erythema action spectra, a new, and simpler, reference erythema action spectrum has been proposed[23] and has now been adopted by the CIE. Figure 17.4 compares the old (1935) standard erythemal curve with the new (1987) action spectrum. The new erythema action spectrum $[\varepsilon(\lambda)]$ is considered to have the following advantages over the 1935 CIE curve:

1. It additionally covers the UV-A region;
2. It can be represented by relatively simple functions over three clearly defined and biologically different spectral regions;

$$\varepsilon(\lambda) = 1.0 \qquad 250 \leq \lambda \leq 298 \text{ nm}$$
$$\varepsilon(\lambda) = 10^{0.094(298-\lambda)} \qquad 298 < \lambda \leq 328 \text{ nm}$$
$$\varepsilon(\lambda) = 10^{0.015(139-\lambda)} \qquad 328 < \lambda \leq 400 \text{ nm}$$

Melanin pigmentation

A socially desirable consequence of exposure to ultraviolet radiation is the delayed pigmentation of the skin known as 'tanning', which becomes notice-

357

able about 2 days after exposure and gradually increases for several days. Tanning is due not only to the formation of new melanin but also to the migration of the pigment already present in the basal cells to the more superficial layers of the skin.

Production of vitamin D

The skin absorbs UV-B radiation in sunlight to convert sterol precursors in the skin, such as 7-dehydrocholesterol, to vitamin D_3[24]. Vitamin D_3 is further transformed by the liver and kidneys to biologically active metabolites such as 25-hyroxyvitamin D; these metabolites then act on the intestinal mucosa to facilitate calcium absorption, and on bone to facilitate calcium exchange.

Ageing of the skin

Chronic exposure to sunlight can result in an appearance of the skin often referred to as premature ageing or actinic damage. The clinical changes associated with skin ageing include a dry, coarse, leathery appearance, laxity with wrinkling, and various pigmentary changes[25].

Photocarcinogenesis

The idea that chronic exposure to UVR can lead to skin cancer has been evident for about 90 years following the observations of Unna (1894)[26] and Dubreuilh (1896)[27]. Since then it has gradually been accepted that sunlight, or more precisely those wavelengths less than about 320 nm (UV-B region), plays an aetiological role in the formation of skin cancer in man[28]. There appears to be little question now that the majority of squamous cell carcinomas are caused by exposure to solar UV-B, although such a clear relationship between the incidence of either basal cell carcinomas or malignant melanoma has not been demonstrated[29].

Photosensitivity

Photosensitivity is a general term describing the adverse effects of UVR on the skin. A distinction can be made between primary and secondary photosensitive conditions. Primary photosensitivity, in which the subject's response to UVR is abnormal, includes such diseases as polymorphic light eruption, chronic actinic dermatitis and solar urticaria. People suffering from these so-called 'photodermatoses' should be particularly careful to avoid unintentional exposure to artificial sources of UVR.

Table 17.3 Some common chemical photosensitizers

Hypnotics	e.g. phenobarbitone
Tranquillisers	e.g. phenothiazines, especially chlorpromazine
Diuretics	e.g. thiazides
Antibiotics	e.g. tetracyclines
Sulphonamides	e.g. sulphamethoxazole with trimethoprim
Antibacterials	e.g. nalidixic acid
Sunscreens	
Tar	
Cosmetics, due to presence of eosin or psoralens, for example	

In secondary photosensitivity the condition may be the result of some other disease such as porphyria (a disease of abnormal liver metabolism resulting in the deposition of endogeneous photosensitizing chemicals, porphyrins, in the skin), or of recognizable external factors such as drugs or chemicals which may be therapeutic, cosmetic, industrial, and so on. Chemicals which cause photosensitization may enter the body by ingestion, injection or absorption through the skin. The speed of effect and severity of the symptoms depend upon the route of entry. In general, topical substances like pitch, tar or synthetic dyes give symptoms such as erythema or oedema which can occur within minutes of exposure to the sun. Orally administered photosensitizers, such as therapeutic drugs, will not produce symptoms until an effective concentration is present in the skin and this may take several days or weeks. The principal reaction is erythema, although symptoms such as a bullous eruption may occur with some drugs, e.g. nalidixic acid. Some common chemical photosensitizers are listed in Table 17.3.

The eye

Structure of the eye

A schematic sagittal section of the human eye is illustrated in Figure 17.5. The eye is almost spherical, approximately 1 inch in diameter, but with a more acutely convex bulge at the front formed by the cornea. The neurophysiological response to photons in the visible region of the electromagnetic spectrum is relayed to the brain via the optic nerve at the back of the eye. The eyeball consists of three co-spherical layers.

1. An outer protective sclera, the opaque white of the eye surrounding the whole globe apart from where it merges into the cornea. The air-cornea interface represents the principal refracting boundary in the eye.

359

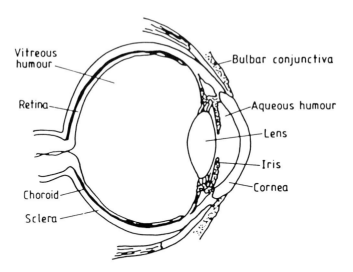

Figure 17.5 Schematic sagittal section through the human eye

2. An intermediate pigmented layer termed the choroid which is modified in front to form the iris diaphragm of variable aperture immediately in front of the lens.
3. An internal nervous layer, the retina, adapted for the reception of light stimuli.

Within the eye there are three different types of refracting media:

(a) the watery aqueous humour which fills the space between the lens and the cornea;
(b) the translucent solid lens, which can be modified in curvature so as to accommodate for near and far vision; and
(c) the thin jelly of the vitreous humour which fills the bulk of the eye.

Ultraviolet optics of the eye

Most of the measurements on the ultraviolet transmission through the eye have been performed in animals, notably the rabbit eye. This section, however, discusses UV transmission through the human eye from measurements carried out by Boettner and Wolter[30]. These investigators studied the optical properties of nine normal human eyes taken from patients varying in age

360

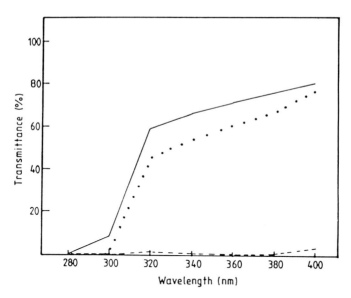

Figure 17.6   Average fraction of UVR incident on the aqueous humour (full curve), the lens (dotted curve) and the vitreous humour (broken curve) of the human eye (after Ref. 30)

from 4 weeks to 75 years during surgical operation. Immediately after enucleation of the eye it was divided into its components. The aqueous humour and vitreous humour were withdrawn with a hypodermic needle and syringe and transferred to quartz cuvettes. The cornea and lens were removed by dissection. Each component was placed in turn at the entrance aperture of an integrating sphere housed in a spectrophotometer so as to measure total transmittance, i.e. direct plus scattered radiation. Figure 17.6 illustrates the average fraction of UVR incident on the aqueous humour, the lens, and the vitreous humour. These data have been estimated from the spectral transmittance curves for each component given by Boettner and Wolter[30]. Two points are worth noting. Ultraviolet radiation with wavelength less than 310 nm is absorbed mainly in the cornea. This corresponds to the observation that acute biological effects of UV exposure to the eye are limited to the UV-B and UV-C and occur predominantly in the corneal tissue. Secondly, UV-A radiation is absorbed primarily in the lens, which supports the hypothesis that UV-A may be implicated in the production of cataracts.

Effects of ultraviolet radiation on the eye

Photokeratitis and conjunctivitis The acute effects of exposure to UV-C and UV-B radiation are primarily those of conjunctivitis and photokeratitis[2].
 Conjunctivitis is an inflammation of the membrane that lines the insides

of the eyelids and covers the cornea, and may often be accompanied by an erythema of the skin around the eyelids. There is the sensation of 'sand in the eyes' and also varying degrees of photophobia (aversion to light), lachryma- tion (tears), and blepharospasm (spasm of the eyelid muscles) may be present.

Photokeratitis is an inflammation of the cornea which can result in severe pain. Ordinary clinical photokeratitis is characterized by a period of latency that tends to vary inversely with the severity of UV exposure. The latent period may be as short as 30 min or as long as 24 h, but it is typically 6–12 h. The acute symptoms of visual incapacitation usually last from 6 to 24 h. Almost all discomfort usually disappears within 2 days and rarely does exposure result in permanent damage. Unlike the skin, the ocular system does not develop tolerance to repeated exposure to UVR. Many cases of photokeratitis have been reported following exposure to UVR produced by welding arcs and by the reflection of solar radiation from snow and sand. For this reason the condition is sometimes referred to as 'welder's flash', 'arc eye' or 'snow blindness'.

Action spectrum for corneal effects

There have been several attempts to define an ultraviolet ocular action spectrum, but in general corneal damage has been taken as the end-point for most studies of wavelengths less than 320 nm. Most published data on ocular action spectra have been obtained by using the rabbit as the experimental model, although results have also been reported for primates and for man. Criteria used to establish a threshold response have included the appearance of some or all of the following:

(a)   epithelial debris – small glistening bodies located in the pre-corneal tear layer;
(b)   epithelial haze – an irregular, crackled appearance of the anterior surface of the cornea;
(c)   epithelial granules – small, white, discrete, round spots located deep in the epithelial layer of the cornea; and
(d)   photophobia – avoidance response to light.

A comparison of the radiant exposure thresholds for rabbits, primates and man is shown in Figure 17.7[31]. Note that for all three species the minimum threshold occurs at a wavelength of 270 nm and a radiant exposure of 40 J m^{-2}.

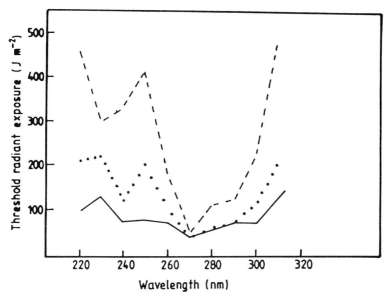

Figure 17.7 Comparison of the radiant exposure thresholds for the cornea of the human (full curve), the primate (dotted curve), and the rabbit (broken curve) (from Ref. 31 with permission)

Cataracts

A cataract is a partial or complete loss of transparency of the lens or its capsule. Most of the available data on the production of cataracts have been obtained using the rabbit. The most effective wavelengths for producing lenticular opacities appear to lie in the range 295–315 nm[32].

Chemical effects in the lens protein, tryptophan, have been shown to occur after UV-A exposure of human lenses[33]. The effects lead to the formation of chromatic photoproducts that bind to, and alter, the solubility of lens proteins, resulting in a yellowing of the lens material. While the basic biochemical mechanisms remain to be found, it is nevertheless suggested that exposure to UV-A can enhance cataractogenesis in humans.

There is scant evidence that the incidence of cataracts is increased in temperate areas[34] and is more common in outdoor, rather than indoor, workers[35]. Although circumstantial evidence does not prove a relationship between sunlight exposure and human cataracts, the evidence does suggest a causal relationship to be a likely possibility.

THE PRODUCTION OF ULTRAVIOLET RADIATION

Artificial sources of incoherent (non-laser) ultraviolet radiation may be

363

produced either by the heating of a body to an incandenscent temperature or by the excitation of a gas discharge.

Incandescence

A body heated to a high temperature radiates as a result of its constituent particles becoming excited by numerous interactions and collisions. For a perfect black body the power radiated at any wavelength from unit surface area of such a body is determined by its temperature, in accordance with Planck's law which is

$$M_e\lambda = A/\lambda^5 [\exp(B/\lambda T) - 1] \qquad (1)$$

where $M_e\lambda$ is the spectral radiant excitance at wavelength λ, T is the absolute temperature of the radiator, and A and B are constants. As the temperature is raised, not only does the maximum power radiated increase rapidly, but the peak of the emission curve λ_{max} moves to a shorter wavelength, given by Wien's displacement law as

$$\lambda_{max} = 2.898 \times 10^6/T(K)nm \qquad (2)$$

The sun, of course, is the most celebrated source of incandescent UVR, although artificial incandescent sources are not efficient emitters of UVR; the ultraviolet emission from a general-purpose tungsten filament lamp is only 0.08% of the rated power for a 40 W lamp, rising to 0.1% for a 100 W lamp and 0.17% for a 1 kW lamp. However, some tungsten halogen lamps, which operate at a colour temperature of around 3000 K, may emit sufficient quantities of UVR, particularly UV-A, to present an exposure hazard.

Gas discharges

The most usual way to produce UVR artificially is by the passage of an electric current through a gas, usually vaporized mercury. The mercury atoms become excited by collisions with the electrons flowing between the lamp electrodes. The excited electrons return to particular electronic states in the mercury atom and in doing so release some of the energy they have absorbed in the form of optical radiation – that is, ultraviolet, visible and infrared radiation. The spectrum of the radiation emitted consists of a limited number of discrete wavelengths (so-called 'spectral lines') corresponding to electron transitions characteristic of the mercury atom (see Figure 17.8), and the relative intensity of the different wavelengths in the spectrum depends upon the pressure of the mercury vapour. For low-pressure discharge tubes containing mercury vapour at about 0.01 torr, more than 90% of the radiated energy is at a wavelength of 253.7 nm.

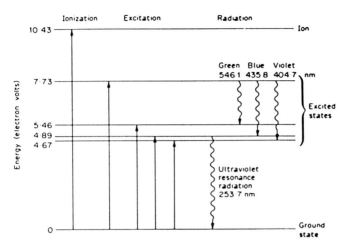

Figure 17.8 A simplified energy transition diagram for mercury (from Henderson and Marsden, 1972)

As the pressure in a discharge tube is raised to a few atmospheres, two principal changes occur:

1. the gas temperature increases due to the increasing number of collisions (mainly elastic collisions) with the energetic electrons;
2. the high temperature becomes localized at the centre of the discharge, there now being a temperature gradient towards the walls, which are much cooler.

The wall becomes much less important at high pressures, and not altogether essential: discharges can operate between two electrodes without any restraining wall, and are then referred to as arcs. At high pressures the characteristic lines present in the low-pressure discharge spectrum broaden and are accompanied by a low-amplitude continuous spectrum. By 'doping' mercury vapour lamps with traces of metal halides it is possible to enhance both the power and the width of the spectrum emitted, particularly in the UV-A and visible regions. It is also possible to produce fluorescent tubes which emit significant amounts of UVR. A fluorescent tube is a low-pressure mercury discharge lamp which has a phosphor coating applied to the inside of the envelope. Fluorescent radiation is produced by the excitation of the phosphor by the 253.7 nm radiation. The wavelength range of the fluorescence radiation will be a property of the chemical nature of the phosphor material. Phosphors are available which produce their fluorescence radiation mainly in the visible (for artificial lighting purposes), in the UV-A, or in the UV-B regions. Other man-made sources of UVR include the deuterium lamp, commonly found in spectrophotometers; and the xenon arc lamp, which is often used as a so-called 'solar simulator' because of the close agreement between its emission spectrum and the spectral power distribution of terrestrial sunlight. A full description of the various types of UV lamps and their associated hazards is given in a later section.

OCCUPATIONAL ULTRAVIOLET EXPOSURE STANDARDS

At the present time there are no internationally formally agreed limits for occupational exposure to UVR. The most comprehensive occupational exposure standard for incoherent (non-laser) UV sources which has be published is that of the American Conference of Governmental Industrial Hygienists (1976)[36]. This standard has been endorsed by the National Institute for Occupational Safety and Health (NIOSH 1972)[37] in the United States and adopted as a voluntary standard in the United Kingdom by the Health and Safety Executive (HSE)[38] and the National Radiological Protection Board (NRPB 1977)[39].

The exposure standard is considered separately for the UV-A region, and for the UV-B and UV-C regions, since most acute biological effects are initiated by wavelengths less than 315 nm.

UV-A exposure standard

For the spectral region 400–315 nm (UV-A), the total irradiance incident on unprotected eyes and skin for periods of greater than 1000 s should not exceed 10 W m^{-2}, and for exposure times of 1000 s or less than total radiant exposure on unprotected eyes and skin should not exceed 10^4 J m^{-2}.

UV-B and UV-C exposure standard

The exposure standard for the spectral region 315–200 nm (UV-B and UV-C) is based on an envelope action spectrum which combines the photokeratitis and skin erythema action spectra and which is defined as a smooth curve somewhat below the energies required for the development of observable effects[40]. The standard applies to occupational exposure during an 8 h working day and shows maximum sensitivity at a wavelength of 270 nm and an exposure dose of 30 J m^{-2} (see Figure 17.9).

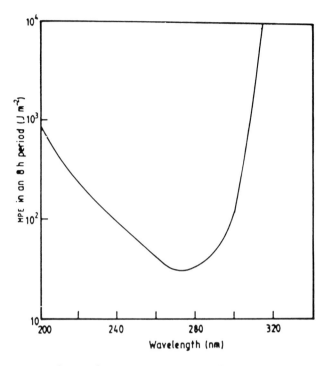

Figure 17.9 Envelope action spectrum used to define maximum permissible exposure (MPE) to ultraviolet radiation for an 8 h period (from Ref. 40)

Table 17.4 Maximum permissible exposure (MPE) for eight-hour period

Wavelength nm	MPE (Jm^{-2})	Relative spectral effectiveness, $S(\lambda)$
200	1000	0.03
210	400	0.075
220	250	0.12
230	160	0.19
240	100	0.30
250	70	0.43
254	60	0.5
260	46	0.65
270	30	1.0
280	34	0.88
290	47	0.64
300	100	0.30
305	500	0.06
310	2000	0.015
315	10000	0.003

Maximum permissible exposures (MPEs) are presented in Table 17.4, together with the spectral effectiveness of the radiation relative to a wavelength of 270 nm. The MPE for monochromatic UVR sources in the wavelength region 315–200 nm can be determined directly from Figure 17.9 or Table 17.4, but for broad-band UVR sources, an effective irradiance, E_{eff}, is calculated by summing the contributions from all the spectral components of the source, each contribution being weighted by the relative spectral effectiveness, according to:

$$E_{eff} = \Sigma E_s(\lambda)\, S(\lambda)\, \Delta(\lambda) \tag{3}$$

where E_{eff} is effective irradiance relative to a monochromatic source at 270 nm (Wm^{-2}); $E_s((\lambda))$ is the spectral irradiance at wavelength λ; $(Wm^{-2}\,nm^{-1})$; $S(\lambda)$ is the relative spectral effectiveness at wavelength λ; and $\Delta\lambda$ is the bandwidth employed in the measurement or calculation of $E_s(\lambda)(nm)$.

The maximum permissible exposure time, t_{max}, is then calculated as:

$$t_{max} = 30(J\ m^{-2})/E_{eff}(Wm^{-2})s \tag{4}$$

The method of summation described by equation (3) assumes that there are no synergistic or protective interactions between wavelengths, although it is unlikely that these assumptions are true.

For UVR sources which emit line spectra arranged in simple exposure geometries, it may be possible to assess the MPE by calculation. In most practical situations, however, recourse to measurement is probably necessary.

INSTRUMENTATION FOR ASSESSING UV EXPOSURE HAZARDS

The experimental determination of a UV exposure hazard is necessary either when the spectral power distribution of the source is unknown, or when the geometry of the source makes calculation prohibitive.

UV-B/C (actinic) radiation detectors

The most fundamental method is to measure the spectral irradiance of the source, $E_s(\lambda)$ and to combine these data with the relative spectral effectiveness, $S(\lambda)$, in order to calculate an effective irradiance, E_{eff}, as given by equation (3). However, this technique requires a spectroradiometer with high spectral resolution coupled with extremely good rejection of stray radiation, and probably demands a double monochromator.

Because of the severe experimental difficulties associated with absolute spectral radiometry, an assessment of the potential hazard from a UVR source is usually made through the use of a direct-reading instrument whose

Table 17.5 Examples of the effective irradiance in the actinic region (100–315 nm) from various sources of ultraviolet radiation (data compiled from Refs 41, 53, 58 and 64)

Source	Distance from source	Actinic ultraviolet hazard E_{eff} (Wm^{-2})	t_{max}(min)
Natural			
Solar radiation at noon midsummer, latitude 55°N	Sea-level	2×10^{-2}	30
Solar radiation at noon, midwinter, latitude 55°N	Sea-level	1.5×10^{-4}	Safe
Medical			
Kromayer lamp medium-pressure mercury vapour arc in a quartz envelope	30 cm	3	0.16
Alpine sunlamp medium-pressure mercury vapour arc in an envelope designed not to emit ozone-producing radiation	30 cm	20	0.025
Theraktin ultraviolet bath Four Westinghouse FS40 fluorescent sunlamps (1.22 m long)	30 cm	0.75	0.6
Hygiene			
Rentokil electronic fly killer	30 cm	6×10^{-4}	Safe
Insect-O-Cutor model 10-8 Mk II	30 cm	5×10^{-4}	Safe
Laboratory			
Hanovia Chromatolite, low-pressure mercury (no filter)	25 cm	4	0.125
Photo Chemical Reactor, medium-pressure mercury (100 W)	25 cm	5	0.1
Philips HPW high-pressure mercury, Wood's glass	25 cm	5×10^{-3}	100
Philips TUV 15W, low-pressure mercury	25 cm	2.6	0.2
Deuterium arc lamp (30W)	25 cm	1×10^{-2}	50
Incandescent: quartz-tungsten halide, DXW; 1 kW	50 cm	2.1×10^{-2}	24
HID fluorescent: GE, HG400DX; 400-W	50 cm	1.1×10^{-2}	46
High pressure sodium: GE Lucalox; 150-W	50 cm	8×10^{-5}	Safe
Low-pressure fluorescent			
–Cool white, GE, F40CW	50 cm	1.4×10^{-3}	360
–Blacklight, Westinghouse, F40BL	50 cm	1.2×10^{-3}	420
–Royal white, Sylvania, F403K	50 cm	1.4×10^{-3}	360
Sunlamp: Sylvania Type RSM, 275-W	50 cm	5.1	0.1
Xenon short-arc lamp: Hanovia 976C1	50 cm	6.8	0.07
Medium-pressure, clear-jacket mercury: 400-W Sylvania	50 cm	1×10^{-2}	50
Medium-pressure clear-jacket metal hallide: Sylvania 400-W Metalarc	50 cm	1.2×10^{-2}	42

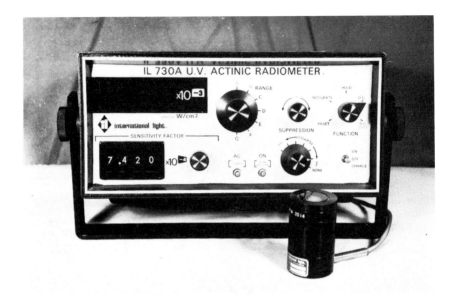

Figure 17.10 the IL730A actinic radiometer

spectral response has been designed to match the NIOSH 'hazard curve'[41].

A prototype ultraviolet hazard monitor was developed by Roach in 1973[42]. This device made use of a spectrally weighted UV filter, a silicon photodiode, and an optical chopper to reduce noise. Although the instrument was found to be quite reliable and followed the hazard action spectrum fairly accurately, it was never produced commercially since the optical filter was not available in quantity. There were several further attempts in the 1970s to develop an appropriate hazard monitor, but most failed because of the principal difficulty of combining sufficient sensitivity to UV-B and UV-C radiation with adequate rejection of longer wavelength radiation[41].

Possibly the best instrument which is commercially available at present is the IL730A actinic radiometer (see Figure 17.10), manufactured by International Light, Inc. This device incorporates a quartz wide angle diffuser, an interference filter, a blocking filter, and a 'solar blind' vacuum phototube as the detector. The published spectral response of a typical instrument is shown in Figure 17.11. The spectral response of the instrument is an adequate match to the NIOSH curve in the wavelength range 250–300 nm, but the response at longer wavelengths may give cause for concern. The solar blind vacuum phototube can exhibit variations in its long wavelength response due to changes in the photoemissivity of the cathode with time and temperature. This can give rise to severe errors when trying to estimate the actinic hazard associated with sources which have a high UV-A component but whose

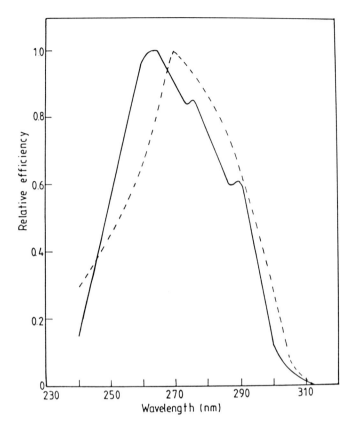

Figure 17.11   The published spectral response of the IL730A actinic radiometer (full curve) used in conjunction with a SEE240 solar blind vacuum phototube and an ACTS270 filter compared with the NIOSH relative spectral efficiency curve (broken curve)

spectral distributionin the actinic region extends only a short way below 315 nm.

Examples of the UVR hazard in the actinic region (100–315 nm) for various sources are given in Table 17.5. The levels of UVR are quoted in terms of an effective irradiance in W m^{-2} and so the maximum permissible exposure time (in seconds) is calculated by dividing this irradiance into the MPE for 270 nm radiation (30 J m^{-2}).

UV-A radiation detectors

There are several different commercially available UV-A detectors. These devices generally incorporate a solid-state photodiode, one or more optical

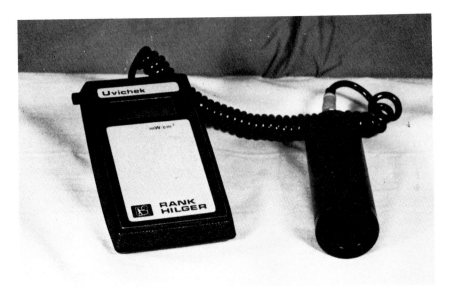

Figure 17.12 the 'Uvichek' UV-A detector

filters, some simple electronic circuitry and a display. One such UV-A detector is shown in Figure 17.12.

The properties of the optical components used typically result in a spectral response from about 300 to 400 nm, peaking at around 360 nm, and an angular response which is often a poor approximation to a cosine-weighted response[43].

The meter reading in Wm^{-2} generally refers to monochromatic irradiation at 365 nm incident normally on the sensor since calibration can be conveniently carried out using this strong mercury line. In fact, with a medium-pressure mercury vapour lamp it is possible to isolate radiation at wavelengths between 350 and 380 nm, with over 96% of the radiation coming from the group of mercury emission lines between 365 and 367 nm.

OCCUPATIONAL PROTECTION AGAINST OVEREXPOSURE TO UVR

Protection against overexposure to UVR may be achieved by a combination of administrative measures, engineering design and personal protection. It is desirable to place emphasis on administrative and engineering control measures so as to minimize the need for personal protection.

Administrative measures

Limitation of access

Only persons directly concerned with the work in hand should be permitted access to areas where there is equipment emitting UVR.

Hazard awareness

Persons working with UV equipment should be given adequate instruction as to the hazards associated with UVR. To this end 'local rules' could usefully be prepared and issued as appropriate.

Hazard warning signs and lights

Indication of the presence of a potential UVR hazard can be given by the judicious use of warning signs, and lights should be used to show when the equipment is energized.

Distance and time as safety factors

As with ionizing sources of radiation, the user should always bear in mind the protection afforded by maximising distance from the source and minimizing exposure time. As a rule of thumb, at distances in excess of twice the greatest dimension of the source the intensity falls off according to the inverse square law, whereas at shorter distances the intensity falls off approximately linearly with distance. The exposure time should be such so as not to exceed the MPE time given by equation (4).

Engineering design

Containment of the radiation

Wherever it is reasonably practicable, the UVR should be kept within a sealed housing. If exposure takes place external to the source housing, as in patient irradiation, the radiation should be contained within a screened area by using, for example, dark cotton curtains. If observation of the UV source is required, then the viewing port should be made of a material with appropriate absorbing properties. Perspex VA acrylic sheet 6 mm thick is a convenient material for this purpose since it effectively blocks UVR at wavelengths less than 380 nm[44].

Use of interlocks

Interlocks are an essential requirement on source housings containing high-intensity UV lamps in order to prevent unnecessary and excessive exposure. However, if the housing contains a high-pressure arc lamp, such an interlock will not prevent the risk of injury from flying glass due to possible explosion of the lamp envelope, should the source housing be opened before the lamp has cooled down. Particular care should also be taken when high-pressure lamps are being removed or replaced; never handle a lamp by the quartz envelope since fingerprints or other contaminants can weaken the envelope.

Minimizing reflected UVR

Many surfaces, such as polished metal, glass and high-gloss ceramic surfaces, are good reflectors of UVR. Reduction in reflected intensity can be achieved by coating the surface with a paint of low reflectance, although the ability of a material to reflect visible light is not necessarily a guide to its reflection in the UV. Table 17.6 lists the reflectance from a number of white pigments and other materials, and indicates that ordinary white wall plaster has a reflectance of 65% at 297 nm, whereas pressed zinc oxide and titanium oxide, which are equally good reflectors of visible light, reflect only 2.5% and 6% respectively at this wavelength. On the other hand, smoked magnesium oxide exhibits more than 90% reflectance throughout the UV and visible regions, and as such is sometimes used as the internal coating of integrating spheres designed for use in the ultraviolet.

Table 17.6 Reflectance of white pigments and other materials (Luckiesh, 1946)

Material	Percentage reflectance			Visible light
	254 nm	*297 nm*	*365 nm*	
Smoked magnesium oxide	93	93	94	95–97
White wall plaster	46	65	76	90
Titanium oxide	6	6	31	94
Pressed zinc oxide	2.5	2.5	4	88
Flat black Egyptian lacquer	5	5	5	5
Five samples of wallpaper	18–31	21–40	33–50	55–75

Personal protection

If adequate attention is given to administrative and engineering control measures, it may not be necessary to resort to personal protection, particularly skin protection. Nevertheless, on some occasions the nature of the work in hand demands unavoidable exposure to UVR and in these instances appropriate personal protection should be taken.

Skin protection

Protection of the skin against unnecessary exposure to UVR can be achieved by covering it with a material of suitable absorbing properties. Materials which transmit little UVR include poplin and flannelette, whereas white muslin batiste, cotton voile and nylon are relatively transparent. In general, tightly woven fabrics offer the best protection against actinic radiation, and colour and thickness are not necessarily a good guide to the suitability of protective clothing[45]. Suitable gloves and face shields can be fabricated from polyvinyl chloride.

Where it proves impossible to shield the skin by suitable clothing, protection may still be achieved by sunscreens. Sunscreens are usually classified as chemical or physical. Chemical sunscreens act by absorbing the UVR and dissipating the energy as radiation of longer wavelength, and include such agents as para-aminobenzoic acid and its esters, cinnamates and salicylates. Physical agents, such as titanium dioxide and talcum powder, act by reflecting, absorbing or scattering the radiation.

To be an effective agent for blocking incident actinic radiation the sunscreen should possess the following qualities:

1.   High attenuation for radiation with wavelengths less than 315 nm;
2.   Adherence to the skin under a variety of conditions, such as sweating, immersion of skin in water, and high and low humidity; and
3.   Cosmetic acceptability

Eye protection

Because of the sensitivity of the eye to UVR, it is good practice to wear adequate eye protection whenever there is the possibility of UV exposure (see Figure 17.13). The principal acute ocular effect is keratoconjunctivitis, which is initiated by radiation in the UV-C and UV-B regions. Chronic exposure to UV-A is thought to be a factor in producing cataracts. The counsel of perfection, therefore, is to wear glasses which are opaque to wavelengths less than 400 nm but that transmit an adequate amount of visible light so as not to be disorienting. Examples of a face shield, goggles and spectacles which meet these requirements are shown in Figure 17.14.

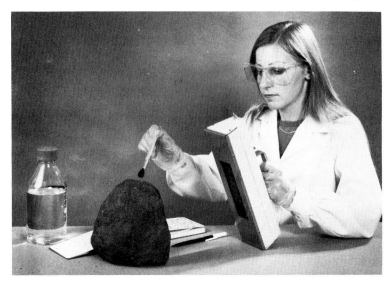

Figure 17.13 Identification of minerals on the surface of a rock. Note the eye protection with safety spectacles and hand protection with vinyl gloves (courtesy of NRPB)

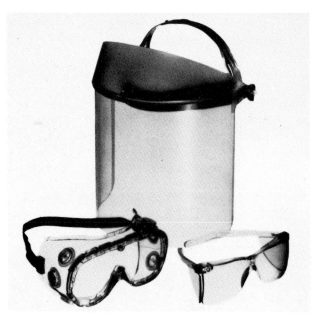

Figure 17.14 Examples of UV protective spectacles, goggles and faceshield (courtesy of UVP, Inc.)

Personal monitoring of occupational exposure to ultraviolet radiation

Personal exposure to UVR in the workplace has been monitored in a limited number of studies using the polymer film, polysulphone. The basis of the method is that when polysulphone film ($40\,\mu$m thick) is exposed to UVR at wavelengths less than 330 nm, the UV absorption of the film increases. The increase in absorbance measured at 330 nm (ΔA_{330}) increases with the UV dose, and so the film readily lends itself to application as a UV dosimeter[46]. The spectral sensitivity of the film is not an exact match to the ACGIH realtive spectral effectiveness curve (Figure 17.15) and for this reason high accuracy is achieved when the film is calibrated with the artificial light source under study. The effective irradiance is determined either by spectroradio-metry followed by weighted summation (equation 3), or by a broad band instrument of the type illustrated in Figure 17.10. Polysulphone film badges are then exposed for different known time periods and a calibration curve of ΔA_{330} against effective actinic dose constructed.

In practice, polysulphone films are held in type 110 photographic mounts and worn on the shoulder or lapel site (Figure 17.16) during working hours. Studies have been reported of monitoring occupational UVR exposure to a cinema projectionist working with a high intensity xenon arc lamp[47], workers in a paint inspection area in a car factory[48], electric arc welders[49], and nurses

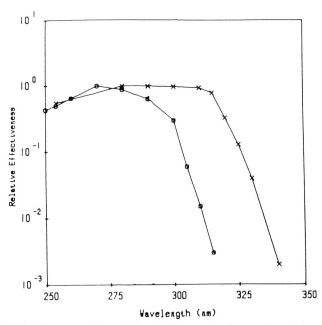

Figure 17.15 The spectral sensitivity of $40\,\mu$m polysulphone film ($\times$) and the ACGIH relative spectral effectiveness curve (o)

377

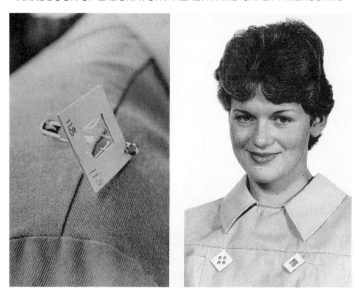

Figure 17.16 Polysulphone film badges worn on the shoulder or lapel site by occupationally-exposed workers

in a hospital dermatology department where phototherapy lamps are used[50].

Polysulphone film badges are a useful means of recording personal exposure to UVR in the workplace and are complementary to more bulky and expensive instrumentation used for surveys of environmental levels of UVR.

TYPES OF LAMPS AND THEIR ASSOCIATED ULTRAVIOLET HAZARD

The general characteristics of lamps and the pertinent data related to their ultraviolet hazard will be reviewed in this section. A diagrammatic summary of the hazards of different lamps is shown in Figure 17.17. A detailed description of the technological aspects of these lamps can be found elsewhere[51].

Incandescent lamps

Incandescent lamps emit optical radiation as the result of the heating of a filament. Modern filaments are made almost exclusively from tungsten alloys.

As the melting temperature of tungsten is 3380 °C (3653 K) the theoretical maximum possible luminous efficacy of an incandescent filament lamp corresponds to that of a perfect black-body radiator at that temperature. The

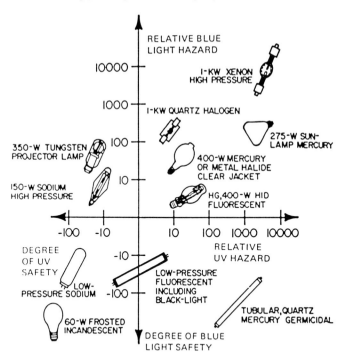

Figure 17.17 The relative ultraviolet and blue light hazards of different types of lamps (from Ref. 41)

luminous efficacies of incandescent lamps are generally much less for two main reasons: (1) with the exception of photoflood lamps, lamp filaments are generallly not heated to temperatures in excess of 3000 °C – this prolongs their useful life; (2) the spectral emissivity of tungsten varies with temperature. Incandescent lamps are made in a wide range of shapes and sizes including the simple domestic light bulb (general lighting service lamp GLS), striplights, reflective display lamps, car headlamps, panel bulbs and photoflood lamps etc. The 'glass' envelopes of low-power incandescent lamps are normally made from lead or soda glass and those of higher-power ones from silica glass or quartz. The envelopes are made either clear, or etched to produce a diffuse 'pearl' effect. However, even in the case of quartz bulbs, the levels of emission of UVR, and in particular actinic ultraviolet, from standard incandescent lamps are small enough not to constitute a potential UVR hazard.

Tungsten halogen lamps, on the other hand, usually operate at a colour temperature between 2900 and 3450 K and are much higher-power devices (up to 5 kW) than standard vacuum or gas-filled incandescent lamps. Because of their higher black-body equivalent temperature and the use of quartz as an envelope material they may emit UVR in excess of the recommended maximum permissible exposure[52].

379

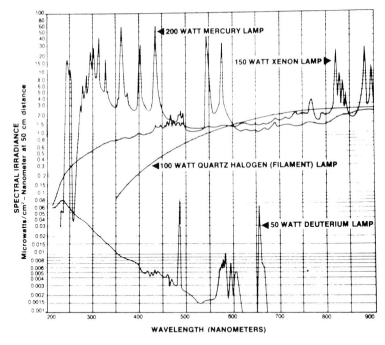

Figure 17.18 Typical spectral irradiance data for four different types of lamps (Oriel Corporation Optical Systems and Components Catalogue, with permission)

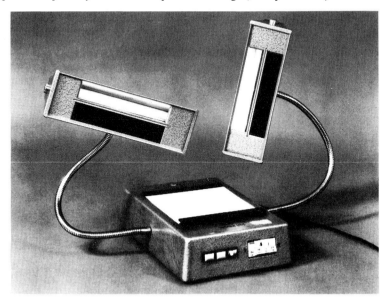

Figure 17.19 An apparatus for inspection of materials by means of fluorescence analysis. The apparatus contains both a germicidal lamp (peak emission at 253.7 nm) and a fluorescent 'black light' lamp (peak emission around 365 nm)

380

The principal applications of tungsten halogen lamps are floodlighting, projector lamps, studio and theatre lighting, car headlamps, photocopier lamps, and a wide range of optical instrument lamps. A typical spectral irradiance curve at 50 cm from a 100 W tungsten halogen lamp in a quartz envelope is shown in Figure 17.18.

Low-pressure mercury vapour discharge lamps

Germicidal lamps

The principal radiation emitted by low-pressure mercury vapour discharge lamps is at 253.7 nm. This radiation is particularly efficacious for preventing the growth of moulds and bacteria. In germicidal lamps there is no phosphor present and a fused silica (quartz) envelope is used. Therefore, such lamps are very efficient sources of 253.7 nm ultraviolet. Approximately 50% of the electrical power is converted to radiation of which up to 95% is emitted in the 253.7 nm line. Germicidal lamps are available in a range of sizes, shapes and powers. The tubular types ar the most common and they fit into standard domestic and commercial fluorescent lamp fittings (bi-pin) and operate on standard fluorescent lamp control gear. Two of the most commonly used sizes are the 15 W, 18″ and the 30 W, 36″ tubes. Small low-wattage germicidal type lamps are often used as fluorescence lamps for chromatographic analysis, and identification of minerals. A germicidal type lamp is often used in combination with a UV-A fluorescent lamp for such pruposes (see Figure 17.19). Each lamp has its own 'on/off' switch but both usually have the same type of end fittings. This allows the lamps to be interchanged and may lead to a potentially hazardous situation.

Some low-pressure mercury vapour lamps have quartz envelopes which transmit the characteristic 185 nm radiation. The interaction of this radiation with oxygen in the surrounding air results in the production of ozone, which is a powerful oxidizing agent and a toxic gas. In some lamps the production of ozone is deliberate, e.g. for air deodorization; in others it is adventitious. The detection and potential hazards of ozone are discussed later.

The monochromaticity of emission at a biologically hazardous wavelength combined with their relatively high efficiency for converting electrical power into radiation make germicidal lamps hazardous if used carelessly. They should be effectively contained within a shielded enclosure, and warning notices pertaining to the hazardous nature of the emitted radiation should be clearly displayed. Where germicidal lamps are required to be used in open situations, e.g. for room air sterilization, appropriate warning notices should also be displayed.

Fluorescent lamps

The principal application of the low-pressure discharge is the fluorescent lamp. Light is produced by conversion of the 253.7 nm mercury resonance emission radiation of a low-pressure mercury vapour discharge to longer wavelength radiations by means of a phosphor coating on the inside wall of the lamp. Fluorescent lamps are available with many different phosphors and envelopes resulting in a wide range of spectral emissions covering the visible, UV-A and UV-B regions. Since their introduction to the UK around 1940 their use for domestic, commercial, and industrial general lighting has grown enormously. This has been due to the introduction of mass-production techniques for their manufacture and testing, hence low production costs; long life and high conversion efficiency of electrical power to light, hence low running costs; flexibility of size; low surface brightness, hence reduced glare; and colour rendering properties. There are few public, commercial, or industrial premises which do not use fluorescent lamps for general lighting purposes. Fluorescent lamps have also found many specialized applications. The introduction of phosphor with enhanced UV-A emissions has led to the recent and widespread use of fluorescent lamps in sunbeds, solaria, and medical phototherapy treatment cabinets. Other phosphor-type lamps are used for a wide variety of photochemical applications including many in the printing industry. Fluorescent lamps are also available with UV-B emitting phosphors and are used as sunlamps.

General lighting fluorescent lamps

General lighting fluorescent lamps are available in a range of powers and physical dimension. A range of phosphors is available which allows a large selection of near-white and other emissions. The lamp walls are made from soda lime glass which effectively absorbs residual actinic radiation (UV-B) not already absorbed by the phosphor. The ultraviolet emissions from general lighting fluorescent lamps do not present a hazard at levels of illumination normally used in the UK.

UV-A fluorescent lamps

In recent years the use of artificial sources of UV-A radiation has increased rapidly in both the medical and the consumer fields. This has been due largely to the widespread treatment of the common skin disease psoriasis by oral psoralen photochemotherapy, and the increasing cosmetic use of sunlamps, solaria, and sunbeds[53,54]. Most commercial tanning equipment in current use exploits the divergence in the erythema and tanning action spectra[55] and

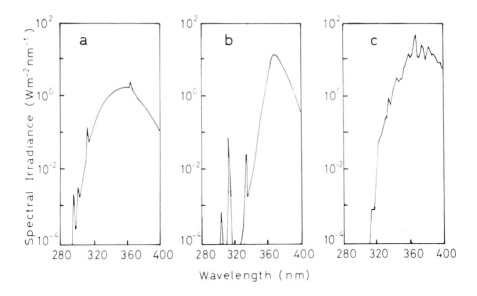

Figure 17.20 Typical spectral irradiances in the ultraviolet region from tanning appliances incorporating: (a) type 1 fluorescent lamps; (b) type 2 fluorescent lamps; (c) optically-filtered metal halide high-pressure mercury arc lamp (e.g. UVASUN 25000; Mutzhas GmbH & Co., W. Germany)

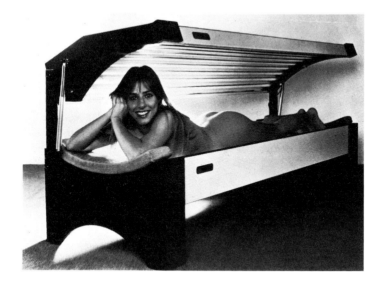

Figure 17.21 A cosmetic sunbed and sun canopy incorporating UV-A fluorescent lamps (courtesy of Nordic Saunas Ltd)

emits almost entirely UV-A radiation. The sources include the so-called type 1 UV-A fluorescent lamp (e.g. Philips TL09, Wotan L100/79), type 2 UV-A fluorescent lamp (Philips TL10R or 'RUVA tubes'), and optically-filtered, metal halide doped mercury arc lamps[56]. The spectral emissions from these three types of lamp are shown in Figure 17.20.

The UV-B content of a type 1 and type 2 UV-A fluorescent lamp as a percentage of the total UV output is about 1% and 0.05% respectively[57,58]. The UV-A irradiance at the skin surface from a typical sunbed or suncanopy containing type 1 UV-A lamps (see Figure 17.21) is around 80 W/m^2. The corresponding irradiance from a solarium incorporating type 2 UV-A lamps is typically 250 W/m^2 [58] and that from the filtered metal halide lamps may be 1000 W/m^2 or greater[56]. Solaria incorporating unfiltered mercury arc lamps are now less popular because of the relatively large quantities of actinic (UV-B and UV-C) radiation leading to the increased risk of burning and acute eye damage such a photokeratitis.

Fluorescent 'blacklight' lamps

These lamps employ a phosphor which has a peak emission in the UV-A at around 370 nm. The term 'blacklight' is almost always reserved for lamps which have a nickel/cobalt oxide glass (Wood's glass) envelope. These glasses can be nearly opaque for visible light but will transmit UV-A radiation. The lamps were developed for materials testing whereby liquid dyes penetrate surface cracks and the UV-A induces fluorescence. These are now also used in forensic, philatelic, mineralogical and similar studies and for entertainment purposes. In general, their UV-B (AGGIH weighted) and UV-A emissions are sufficiently low so that they do not present an acute hazard to either skin or eyes. The results of long-term exposure of the lens of the eye to the UV-A emission of black lights is less clear and, as with UV-A fluorescent lamps, if repeated exposure at short distances from black light sources is unavoidable then appropriate protective eyewear should be worn.

The fluorescent sunlamp

This is a low-pressure mercury discharge lamp incorporating a phosphor which is coated onto the inside of the lamp envelope. The resulting spectrum consists of a continuum from about 270 to 380 nm with a peak at 313 nm, together with the mercury characteristic lines, some of which lie in the visible region (see Figure 17.22). The fluorescent sunlamp, e.g. the Westinghouse FS20T12 and the Philips TL12 lamp, is used in physiotherapy for the treatment of certain skin diseases[53]. The high actinic content of these lamps makes them the most hazardous of all fluorescent lamps (see Table 17.5)

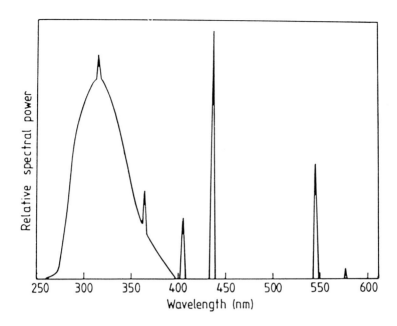

Figure 17.22 The spectral power distribution of a fluorescent sunlamp

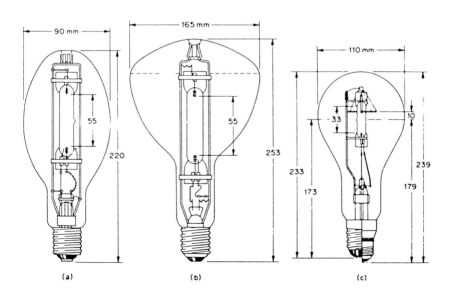

Figure 17.23 Designs of 250 W medium-pressure mercury lamps (from Henderson and Marsden, 1972): (a) MBF; (b) MBFR; (c) MBTF

Medium- and high-pressure mercury lamps

General lighting lamps

Medium-pressure (2–10 atmospheres) mercury vapour lamps (MB lamps) are widely used for industrial and commercial lighting, street lighting, display lighting and floodlighting. The spectral emission typical of a medium-pressure mercury lamp is shown in Figure 17.18. The general construction of all of these types of lamps consists of a fused silica (quartz) discharge tube containing the mercury vapour discharge. This is mounted inside an outer borosilicate (Pyrex type) glass bulb. The most common lamp of this type in use is the MBF (mercury fluorescent) lamp. The inner discharge tube emits the characteristic white light of mercury vapour together with a large amount of UVR. Phosphors coated on the inside wall of the outer borosilicate glass bulb absorb the ultraviolet and convert it to visible radiation. The phosphors chosen emit red light in the wavelength range 600–700 nm. The borosilicate glass bulb effectively absorbs any residual UVR. The quantity of potentially harmful UVR emitted by lamps of this design depends critically on the integrity of the outer bulb.

The tungsten ballasted or blended lamp (MBT) is a combination of a mercury discharge and a tungsten filament operating in series. The filament controls the discharge current and also contributes black-body emissions which are rich in red light. These supplement the predominantly blue/green light from the discharge to produce good colour rendering. They are often used for display purposes. Fluorescent versions (MBTF) are also available. MBFR lamps are similar in operation to MBF described above but have an outer bulb which is shaped and coated internally with a reflecting layer to direct most of the light downwards. The designs of the MBF, MBFR and MBFT mercury lamp are shown in Figure 17.23. Both the MB and MBT lamps are available with outer bulbs made from cobalt and nickel oxide doped glass (Wood's glass). These MBW and MBTW lamps emit predominantly UV-A 'black light' and a very small quantity of visible radiation. As they are fitted with standard domestic bayonet caps they are in widespread use for 'effect lighting' in dance halls, discotheques, clubs, bars, etc. in addition to materials testing and identification.

Under normal operating conditions the emissions from these lamps are not hazardous. However, as discussed above, if the outer bulb breaks leaving the inner discharge tube intact the lamps will emit hazardous levels of actinic UVR. Measurements at 2 m from a 400 W mercury lamp with the outer bulb removed have indicated AGGIH weighted actinic ultraviolet irradiances[59] of 0.384 mW cm^{-2}, resulting in a MPE time of only 8 seconds. These comments apply also to 'black light' type medium-pressure lamps where the hazardous nature of the emitted radiation depends critically on the continuing integrity of the outer 'Wood's glass' envelope.

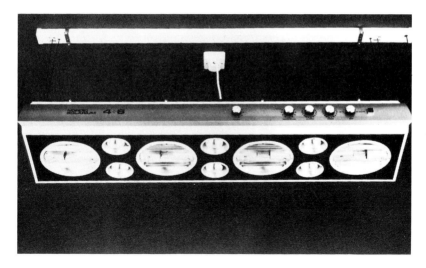

Figure 17.24 A solarium incorporating four medium-pressure 450 W mercury lamps with quartz envlelopes and six 60 W 'Warmalux' infrared lamps (courtesy of Nordic Saunas Ltd)

Special equipment lamps

A range of linear medium-pressure mercury discharge lamps is manufactured for use as original equipment for incorporation in devices such as photo-polymerizers, commercial and domestic sunlamps. Typical sunlamps use 80-300 W discharge tubes between approximately 80 and 170 mm in length and consititute lower-power examples of medium-pressure lamps (see Figure 17.24). However, all of these types of lamps emit copious quantities of UVR in the UV-B and UV-A regions and some extending into the UV-C. Medium- and high-pressure lamps used for photopolymerizing of inks, resins, etc. vary in power from hundreds of watts to many kilowatts. For very high-pressure systems, such as used in large-scale photopolymerizing equipment, the power loading on a lamp may exceed 8 kWm^{-1}. An example of a high-intensity ultra-violet source for industrial applications is shown in Figure 17.25.

Special-purpose versions of MB, MBT, and MBR lamps are available for a range of users requiring ultraviolet. MBT lamps with 'hardened glass' envelopes which transmit UVR in the range 280-400 nm are used as domestic sunlamps. These lamps (e.g. Philips MLV 300) are available fitted with either Edison screw or bayonet caps. They are potentially hazardous and should be used with the care appropriate to sunlamp systems. MB, MBT, and MBR lamps are also available with ultraviolet transmitting envelopes and are used extensively as reprographic lamps (e.g. Philips HPR 125W) in, for example, copyboard lighting and silk screen processing.

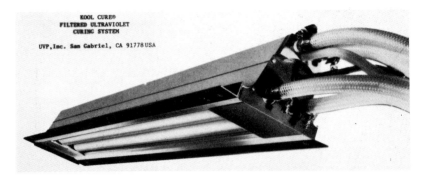

Figure 17.25 A high intensity mercury lamp with a power loading of 8 kW m^{-1} used for ultraviolet curing processes (courtesy of UVP, Inc.)

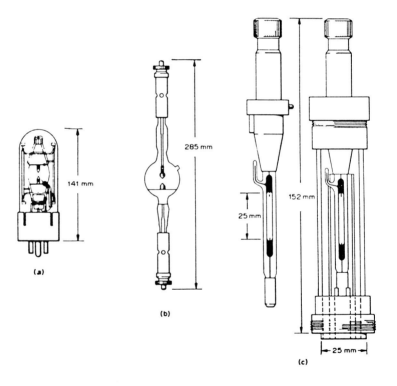

Figure 17.26 Very high-pressure mercury lamps (from Henderson and Marsden, 1972): (a) 250 W ME; (b) 1000 W ME; (c) 1000 W MD

Very high-pressure mercury lamps

In certain applications such as projection systems and photochemical reactors where a source of very high radiance/luminance, but reasonably small physical dimensions, is required, a very high-pressure mercury discharge lamp may be used. Two types are in common use: (1) the ME compact source type, and (2) the MD water-cooled tubular type as illustrated in Figure 17.26. The ME types are used typically as a projector lamps. Because of their very high operating current and pressure (20–40 atm) and high ultraviolet emission, these lamps must be contained within a protective housing. The MD water-cooled lamp, operating at pressures between 50 and 200 atm, is often used in photochemical reactors. Water cooling is achieved by using two concentric glass tubes. The cooling water initially flows between the discharge tube and the inner tube and returns between the inner and outer tubes. Both ME and MD types emit copious quantities of hazardous UVR.

Metal halide lamps

By adding a variety of metallic halides to a medium- or high-pressure mercury arc it is possible to increase the output and vary the spectral emission. Approximations can be made to the spectrum of natural daylight by using different combinations of metals. Strongly coloured light can be produced by

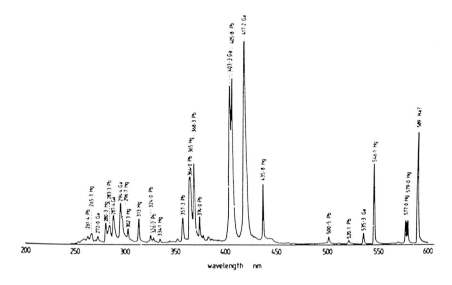

Figure 17.27 The spectral power distribution of a Philips HPM 15 metal halide lamp (from Ref. 51)

adding single metals, e.g. thallium or indium. Typical applications of medium- and high-pressure metal halide lamps include photochemical processing, graphic and photographic illumination, studio lighting, reprography, and recently UV-A solaria. The UV output of all metal halide lamps is generally high and includes UV-B and UV-C radiations (see Figure 17.27).

So varied are the designs of equipment incorporating metal halide lamps that an individual hazard assessment is required for each application. For example, the safe use of high-power metal halide lamps in a high-intensity UV-A sunlamp system will depend critically on the continuing integrity of the filter incorporated in the lamp housing. Similarly, studio lamps will be adequately shielded provided that the luminaire glass does not break. Those lamps, which are specifically chosen because they emit large quantities of ultraviolet radiation, e.g. in the photopolymerizing drying of inks, varnishes and other photochemical processes, should be effectively contained in interlocked enclosures. Care should be taken to minimize the leakage of scattered radiation through badly fitting panels or apertures.

Xenon lamps

In the xenon arc the radiation is emitted primarily as a continuum, unlike mercury lamps which essentially emit line spectra. The production of the continuum is optimum under conditions of high specific power, high current density and high internal pressure, leading to compact, bright sources. Because of high operating temperatures the lamp envelope is normally constructed from fused silica. Xenon lamps consist of an arc burning between solid tungsten electrodes in a pressure of pure xenon and may be designed to operate from AC or DC. Cold-filling pressures up to 12 atm are commonly used and as a result there exists a potential hazard from explosive failure of the lamp, although in practice lamp explosions are rare. The lamps can be of the compact form, when the bulb is nearly spherical, or the linear form which utilizes a cylindrical lamp envelope. The compact xenon arc lamp is available in power ratings from 75 W to 25 kW or more. Linear source lamps of up to 65 kW are used for floodlighting in sports stadia. Because xenon lamps contain a permanent gas filling, the full radiation output is available immediately after switching on; there is no run-up period as in arc lamps containing mercury which has to vaporize.

The spectral power distribution of a 150 W xenon arc lamp is shown in Figure 17.18. Because of the similarity of the spectrum to that of the solar spectrum, the xenon lamp has been employed as a laboratory source of sunlight, the so-called solar simulator[60]. Also because of its continuous spectrum the xenon lamp is commonly used in conjunction with a monochromator for biological action spectrum studies[53].

Deuterium lamps

The deuterium lamp in its most common form is a low-pressure, low-power (20–200 W) compact source of actinic ultraviolet radiation[51]. The arc discharge in a deuterium lamp gives a line-free continuum between 170 and 350 nm, with a peak output close to 200 nm (see Figure 17.18). The falling spectrum with increasing wavelength in the visible region gives the lamp a purplish glow when operating.

The main application of the deuterium lamp is as a source for spectro-photometers, spectrofluorimeters and spectropolarimeters. Its attractions are its point source characteristic, its line-free continuum over a wide range of UV wavelengths, and its high UV:visible ratio. Other sources of appreciable continuum, such as the compact xenon arc, have strong visible outputs which given problems with stray light when dispersing elements are used. These attractions are also the rationale for a minor, but significant, application of deuterium lamps. They are used as secondary, or transfer, standards for spectral radiance and irradiance[51]. Because of the high UV-C content of deuterium lamps they can be particularly hazardous to the eyes. However, their low power makes them relatively safe sources compared with, say, high-power, medium- and high-pressure mercury lamps with UV-transmitting envelopes.

HAZARDS FROM OZONE

Ozone is a colourless, toxic irritant gas and is formed from biatonic oxygen either by electric arc or corona discharges in air, or by a complex photochemical reaction between short-wavelength UVR and the oxygen present in the air. It is, therefore, possible to find ozone near ultraviolet lamps, especially those where radiation of wavelength shorter than about 250 nm is transmitted through the envelope of the lamp. There are many so-called 'ozone-free' lamps available nowadays in which the lamp envelope is opaque to wavelengths below about 260 nm, thus preventing shorter-wavelength UVR from forming ozone in the air.

Ozone has a characteristic pungent odour which has been described as that of new-mown hay or sparking electrical machinery. It has been claimed by workers in the USSR that ozone can be detected by smell at a concentration as low as 0.005 ppm; other workers put the limit as high as 2 ppm. Detection by smell, therefore, may not provide adequate protection against occupational exposure. Olfactory fatigue occurs but one volunteer has claimed that the ozone could still be smelt after 2 h of exposure to 1.5–2 ppm. The time-weighted average threshold limit value (TWA) for occupational exposure to ozone is currently given as 0.1 ppm by volume in air with the short-term (15 min) exposure limit tentatively set at 0.3 ppm[36]. This places ozone in the same toxicity class as carbonyl chloride (phosgene) (TWA = 0.1 ppm) and it is of higher toxicity than, for example, chlorine (TWA = 1 ppm) or carbon monoxide (TWA = 50 ppm). Exposure to ozone at a concentration of 50 ppm for 0.5 h may be fatal[61].

A simple, cheap and reliable way of estimating the concentration of ozone which may exist in the vicinity of an UVR emitting lamp is to use a Dräger tube (type ozone 0.05/a) and a Gastec pump[62]. In this method a known volume of air is drawn through a glass tube packed with indigo. Ozone decomposes indigo into isatine, which is white, and the length of whitening corresponds to the ozone concentation. The glass tube is graduated in scale values of ppm ozone when 1000 ml of air (ten strokes of the piston) are drawn through the tube. Greater sensitivity can be achieved by increasing the number of strokes. The relative standard deviation of the estimate of concentration is about 10–15%. Ozone concentration is highest immediately after an ultraviolet lamp is struck, since, as the gas pressure rises, the short-wavelength UVR which produces ozone is reabsorbed more efficiently within the lamp.

If ozone is suspected, either by measurement or smell, steps should be taken to ensure adequate ventilation in the area around a source. One way is to connect the source housing to an exit port in an outside wall by means of ducting. A fan situated appropriately in the source housing should then serve to remove ozone, whilst cooling the lamp at the same time.

TREATMENT OF OVEREXPOSURE TO UVR

Treatment of cutaneous erythema

To be most effective all treatments need to be commenced during or immediately after exposure, at which time the subject is usually not aware of the need or in reach of the treatment. Once redness and pain begin, treatment can be only symptomatic and partially effective. Most cases need only soothing creams or cooling shake lotions (e.g. calamine lotion) and mild analgesics. More severe cases can be treated with a topical preparation of non-steroidal anti-inflammatory agent such as 2.5% indomethacin in ethanol: propylene glycol: dimethylacetamide 19:19:2 by volume applied as soon as possible after irradiation and then every hour or so for 24 h[63].

Treatment of ultraviolet injury to the eyes

In terms of first aid measures for the eye, there is really very little that can be done. However, perhaps the most useful first aid measures are to secure the lids closed and this can be done with Sellotape and then lightly pad the eyes to cut down trans-lid illumination. The person then really needs to go along to an eye unit for further treatment (Marshall, 1983; personal communication).

In most eye units the treatment will consist of dilating the pupil with a mild and short-acting agent, this being done to reduce the possible problems of spasm in either the pupillary muscle or the ciliary muscle. After this, an anti-infective preparation, such as chloramphenicol, may be applied to the front surface of the eye.

ACKNOWLEDGEMENT

I am grateful to Dr A.F. McKinlay for his contribution to the section concerning types of lamps and their associated ultraviolet hazard.

LITERATURE CONSULTED

International Commission on Illumination (1935). *Comptes Rendus de la Commission Internationale de l'Eclairage, Berlin*, **9**, 624–625

Luckiesh, M. (1946). *Applications of Germicidal, Erythemal and Infrared Energy*. (New York: Van Nostrand), p. 383

Henderson, S.T. and Marsden, A.M. (eds) (1972). *Lamps and Lighting*, 2nd edn. (London: Edward Arnold)

REFERENCES

1. Coblentz, W.W. (1932). Report on the Copenhagen meeting of the Second International Congress on Light. *Science*, **76**, 412–15
2. Parrish, J.A., Anderson, R.R., Urbach, F. and Pitts, D. (1978). *UV-A: Biological Effects of Ultraviolet Radiation with Emphasis on Human Response to Longwave Ultra-violet*. (Chichester: John Wiley)
3. World Health Organisation (1979). *Environmental Health Criteria. 14: Ultraviolet radiation*. (Geneva: WHO)
4. Parrish, J.A., Jaenicke, K.F. and Anderson. R.R. (1982). Erythema and melanogenesis action spectra of normal human skin. *Photochem. Photobiol.*, **36**, 187–91
5. Warin, A.P. (1978). The ultraviolet erythemas in man. *Br. J. Dermatol.*, **98**, 473–7
6. van der Leun, J.C. (1972). On the action spectrum of ultraviolet erythema. In Gallo, V. and Santamaria, L. (eds), *Research Progress in Organic, Biological and Medicinal Chemistry*, vol. 3, pp. 711–36, (Amsterdam: North Holland)
7. Magnus, I.A. (1976). *Dermatological Photobiology*. (Oxford: Blackwell)
8. Hausser, K.W. and Vahle, W. (1922). Die Abhängigkeit des Lichterythems und der Pigmentbildung von der Schwingungszahl (Wellenlänge) der erregenden Strahlung. *Strahlentherapie*, **13**, 41–71
9. Luckiesh, M., Holladay, L.L. and Taylor, A.H. (1930). Reactions of untanned skin to ultraviolet radiation. *J. Opt. Soc. Am.*, **20**, 423–32
10. Hausser, K.W. and Vahle, W. (1927). Sonnenbrand und Sonnenbräunung. *Wiss. Veröff. Siemens Konzern*, **6**, 101–20

11. Coblentz, W.W., Stair, R. and Hogue, J.M. (1932). The spectral erythemic reaction of the human skin to ultraviolet radiation, *Proc. Nat. Acad. Sci.*, **17**, 401–5
12. Coblentz, W.W., Stair, R. (1934). Data on the spectral erythemic reaction of the untanned human skin to ultraviolet radiation. *Bur. Stand. J. Res.*, **12**, 13–14
13. Magnus, I.A. (1964). Studies with a monochromator in the common idiopathic photodermatoses. *Br. J. Dermatol.*, **76**, 245–64
14. Everett, M.A., Olson, R.L. and Sayre, R.M. (1965). Ultraviolet erythema. *Arch. Dermatol.*, **92**, 713–19
15. Olson, R.L., Sayre, R.M. and Everett, M.A. (1966). Effect of anatomic location and time on ultraviolet erythema. *Arch. Dermatol.*, **93**, 211–15
16. Sayre, R.M., Olson, R.L. and Everett, M.A. (1966). Quantitative studies on erythema. *J. Invest. Dermatol.*, **46**, 240–4
17. Freeman, R.G., Owens, D.W., Knox, J.M. and Hudson, H.T. (1966). Relative energy requirements for an erythemal response of skin to monochromatic wavelengths of ultraviolet present in the solar spectrum. *J. Invest. Dermatol.*, **47**, 586–92
18. Berger, D., Urbach, F. and Davies, R.E. (1968). The action spectrum of erythema induced by ultraviolet radiation: preliminary report. In Jadassohn, W. and Schirren, C.D. (eds), *Proc. XIII Congressus Internationalis Dermatologiae. vol. 2, pp. 1112–1117. (Berlin: Springer-Verlag)*
19. Cripps, D.J. and Ramsay, C.A. (1970). Ultraviolet action spectrum with a prism grating monochromator. *Br. J. Dermatol.*, **82**, 584–92
20. Mackenzie, L.A. and Frain-Bell, W. (1973). The construction and development of a grating monochromator and its application to the study of the reeaction of the skin to light. *Br. J. Dermatol.*, **89**, 251–64
21. Nakayama, Y., Morikawa, F., Fukuda, M., Hamano, M., Toda, K. and Pathak, M.A. (1974). Monochromatic radiation and its application - laboratory studies on the mechanism of erythema and pigmentation induced by psoralen. In Fizpatrick, T.B. (ed.), *Sunlight and Man*. (Tokyo: University of Tokyo Press), pp. 591–611
22. Farr, P.M. and Diffey, Bl (1985). The erythemal response of human skin to ultraviolet radiation. *Br. J. Dermatol.*, **113**, 65–76
23. McKinlay, A.F. and Diffey, B.L. (1987). A reference action spectrum for ultraviolet induced erythema in human skin. *CIE Journal* , **6**, 17–22
24. Holick, M.F., MacLaughlin, J.A., Parrish, J.A. and Anderson, R.R. (1982). The photochemistry and photobiology of vitamin D3. In Regan, J.D. and Parrish, J.A. (eds), *The Science of Photomedicine*, pp. 195–218. (New York: Plenum Press)
25. Giese, A.C. (1976). *Living with our Sun's Ultraviolet Rays*. (New York: Plenum Press)
26. Unna, P. (1894). *Histopathologie der hautkrankheiten* (Berlin: August Hirschwald)
27. Dubreuilh, W. (1896). Des hyperkeratoses circonscriptes. *Ann. Dermatol. Syphiligr. (Paris)*, **7** (Ser. 3), 1158–1204
28. Blum, H.F. (1959). *Carcinogenesis by Ultraviolet Light*. (Princeton: Princeton University Press)
29. Urbach, F. (1982). Photocarcinogenesis. In Regan, J.D. and Parrish, J.A. (eds), *The Science of Photomedicine*, pp. 261–292. (New York: Plenum Press)
30. Boettner, E.A. and Wolter, J.R. (1962). Transmission of the ocular media. *Invest. Ophthal.*, **1**, 776–83
31. Pitts, D.G. (1974). The human ultraviolet action spectrum. *Am. H. Optom. Physiol. Opt.*, **51**, 946–60
32. Pitts, D.G. and Cullen, A.P. (1977). Ocular ultraviolet effects from 295 to 335 nm in the rabbit eye. A preliminary report, DHEW (NIOSH) Publication No. 77–130. (Cincinatti, Ohio: National Institute of Occupational Safety and Health, Division of Biomedical and Behavioral Science)
33. Zigman, S., Griess, G., Yulo, T. and Schultz, J. (1973). Ocular protein alterations by near UV light. *Exp. Eye Res.*, **15**, 255–65

34. Duke-Elder, S. (1972). *System of Ophthalmology*, vol. 14: *Injuries*, part 2: Non-mechanical injuries. (St. Louis: C.V. Mosby)
35. Zigman, S., Yulo, T., Paxhia, T., Salceda, S. and Datiles, M. (1977). *Comparative Studies of Human Cataracts*, Abstracts of the Association for Research in Vision and Ophthalmology, Sarasota, Florida
36. ACGIH (1976). Threshold limit values for chemical substances and physical agents in the workroom environment: ultraviolet radiation. American Conference of Governmental Industrial Hygienists, Cincinnati, Ohio
37. National Institute for Occupational Safety and Health (1972). Criteria for a recommended standard occupational exposure to ultraviolet radiation. publication HSM 73-11009. (Washington, DC: US Department of Health Education and Welfare, Public Health Service)
38. HSE (1978). *Threshold Limit Values for 1978, Guidance Note EH 15*. (London: HMSO - Health and Safety Executive)
39. National Radiological Protection Board (1977). *Protection against Ultraviolet Radiation in the Workplace*. (London: HMSO)
40. Sliney, D.H. (1972). The merits of an envelope action spectrum for ultraviolet radiation exposure criteria. *Am. Ind. Hyg. Assoc. J.*, **33**, 644–53
41. Sliney, D.H. and Wolbarsht, M. (1980). *Safety with Lasers and other Optical Sources: a Comprehensive Handbook*. (New York: Plenum Press)
42. Roach, T. (1973). Final report on a method for field evaluation of UV radiation hazards, prepared by CBS Laboratories for the National Institute for Occupational Safety and Health (NIOSH), Contract No. HSM-99-72-144, NIOSH, Cincinnati
43. Stobbart, D. and Diffey, B.L. (1980). A comparison of some commercially available UVA meters used in photochemotherapy. *Clin. Phys. Physiol. Meas.*, **1**, 267–73
44. Hughes, D. (1978). *Hazards of Occupational Exposure to Ultraviolet Radiation*. Occupational Hygiene Monograph No. 1. University of Leeds Industrial Services
45. Welsh, C. and Diffey, B.L. (1981). The protection against solar actinic radiation afforded by common clothing fabrics. *Clin. Exp. Dermatol.*, **6**, 577–82
46. Diffey, B.L. (1984). Personal ultraviolet radiation dosimetry with polysulphone film badges. *Photodermatology*, **1**, 151–7
47. Challoner, A.V.J., Corbett, M.F., Davis, A., Diffey, B.L., Leach, J.F. and Magnus, I.A. (1978). Description and application of a personal ultraviolet dosimeter: a review of preliminary studies. *Nat. Cancer Inst. Monogr.*, **50**, 97–100
48. Diffey, B.L., Larko, O., Meding, B., Edeland, H.G. and Wester, U. (1986). Personal monitoring of exposure to ultraviolet radiation in the car manufacturing industry. *Ann. Occup. Hyg.*, **30**, 163–70
49. Shehade, S.A., Roberts, P.J., Diffey, B.L. and Foulds, I.S. (1987). Photodermatitis due to spot welding. *Br. J. Dermatol.*, **117**, 117–19
50. Larko, O. and Diffey, B.L. (1986). Occupational exposure to ultraviolet radiation in dermatology departments. *Br. J. Dermatol.*, **114**, 479–84
51. Phillips, R. (1983). *Sources and Applications of Ultraviolet Radiation*. (London: Academic Press)
52. Mohan, K., Knight, W., Chen, K.W., Lewin, I. and Heinisch, R. (1980). *Optical Radiation Emissions from Selected Sources*. FDA 81/36. (Maryland: Bureau of Radiological Health)
53. Diffey, B.L. (1982). *Ultraviolet Radiation in Medicine*. (Bristol: Adam Hilger Ltd)
54. Diffey, B.L. (1986). Use of UV-A sunbeds for cosmetic tanning. *Br. J. Dermatol.*, **115**, 67–76
55. Gange, R.W., Park, Y.K., Auletta, M., Kagetsu, N., Blackett, A.D. and Parrish, J.A. (1986). Action Spectra for Cutaneous Responses to Ultraviolet Radiation. In Urbach, F. and Gange, R.W. (eds). *The Biological Effects of UVA Radiation*. pp. 57–65. (New York: Praeger)

56. Mutzhas, M.F. (1986). UVA-emitting light sources. In Urbach, F. and Gange, R.W. (eds). *The Biological Effects of UVA Radiation. pp. 10–23. (New York: Praeger)*
57. Diffey, B.L. and McKinlay, A.F. (1983). The UV-B content of 'UVA fluorescent lamps' and its erythemal effectiveness in human skin. *Phys. Med. Biol.*, **28**, 351–8
58. Diffey, B.L. and Langley, F.C. (1986). Evaluation of ultraviolet radiation hazards in hospitals. Report no. 49. (London: Institute of Physical Sciences in Medicine)
59. Piltingsrud, H.V. and Fong, C.W. (1978). An evaluation of ultraviolet radiation personnel hazards from selected 400 Watt high intensity discharge lamps. *Am. Indus. Hyg. Assoc. J.*, **39**, 406–13
60. Berger, D.S. (1969). Specification and design of solar ultraviolet similators. *J. Invest. Dermatol.*, **53**, 192–8
61. EMAS (1972). *Ozone. Notes of Guidance.* (London: Chief Employment Medical Adviser, Health and Safety Executive)
62. Diffey, B.L. and Hughes, D. (1980). Estimates of ozone concentrations in the vicinity of ultraviolet emitting lamps. *Phys. Med. Biol.*, **25**, 559–61
63. Hawk, J.L.M. and Parrish, J.A. (1982). Responses of normal skin to ultraviolet radiation. In Regan, J.D. and Parrish, J.A. (eds), *The Science of Photomedicine.* pp. 219–60. (New York: Plenum Press)
64. Hughes, D. (1982). Laboratory sources of ultraviolet radiation. In Law, J. and Haggith, J.W. (eds), *Practical Aspects of Non-ionising Radiation Protection.* pp. 58–61. (London: Hospital Physicists' Association

18 Hazards of Using Microwaves and Radiofrequency Radiation

H. Moseley

Radiofrequency (RF) is a term which may be applied to electromagnetic radiation of frequency between 100 kHz and 300 GHz but generally its use is restricted to frequencies between 100 kHz and 300 MHz and the term microwave is applied to radiation of frequency from 300 MHz to 300 GHz. Frequency and wavelength are inversely related and, in free space, a frequency of 100 kHz corresponds to a wavelength of 13 km; 300 MHz is equivalent to a wavelength of 1 m and 300 GHz to 1 mm. The position which microwave and RF radiation occupies in the electromagnetic spectrum is shown in Figure 18.1.

Claims and counterclaims abound concerning the health implications of exposure to low level microwave and RF radiation. This chapter will cover biological effects, exposure levels, standards, and safety measures.

1. POSSIBLE HARMFUL CONSEQUENCES OF EXPOSURE

1.1 Important factors

The interaction between microwave or RF radiation and a body depends on electrical parameters of the exposed tissue (such as dielectric constant and conductivity), and geometrical factors (such as size, shape and orientation). Subsequent biological consequences will depend on the ways in which the species react to the absorbed radiation dose. For example, different thermo-regulatory systems will react differently to a microwave-induced heat load.

The electric field strength or intensity within the tissue depends on the strength of the external field and the degree of charge separation (or polar-

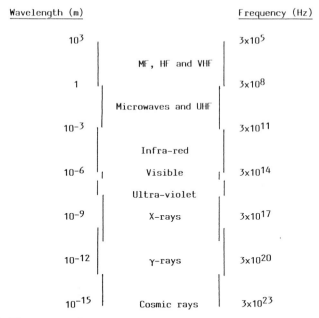

Figure 18.1   Electromagnetic spectrum

ization) within the tissue. The dielectric constant is the factor by which the electric field strength in a vacuum exceeds that in the substance. In water, a polar molecule, the dielectric constant varies between a value of 81 at D.C. to 1.8 at high frequency. Likewise, the dielectric constant of blood decreases as frequency increases, with a plateau in the frequency interval 100 MHz to 10 GHz. The dielectric constant of tissue is very much dependent on the water content. At a frequency of 900 MHz, the dielectric constant of fatty tissue with a 10% water content is 40 and that with 50% water is 12.

The power absorbed depends on tissue conductivity. Conductivity is the inverse of electrical resistance and is measured in units called siemens (S). In the case of blood, the conductivity is fairly constant up to a frequency of 1.0 GHz but at higher frequencies it increases markedly. Once again, in fatty tissue, conductivity and water content are related. At a frequency of 900 MHz, the conductivity of fatty tissue with a 6% water content is 40 Sm^{-1}, and that with 60% water is 400 Sm^{-1}.

The consequence of all this is that tissue with a high water content, such as skin and muscle, exhibits a higher absorption of microwave radiation than tissue with little water, such as fat and bone. As well as depending on electrical properties, absorption also depends on size and shape of the body and its orientation in the radiation field. It appears that an adult human operates as an efficient antenna in the frequency interval 70 MHz to 100 MHz, particularly when the long axis (head to toe) of the body is parallel to the electric field vector. A particularly useful term is the specific absorption rate (SAR),

398

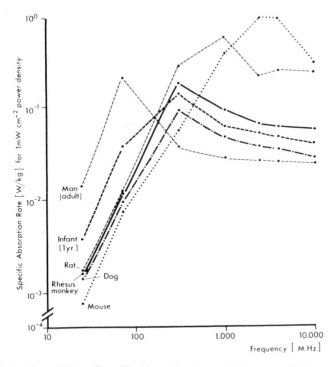

Figure 18.2 The variation of Specific Absorption Rate with frequency for humans and other animal species (from Moseley, 1988)

which is defined as the ratio of the total absorbed power to the body mass (units are watts per kilogramme). Figure 18.2 illustrates the relation between SAR and frequency in the case of an adult human under different exposure conditions. Similar data are presented for different species, with resonance occurring at higher frequencies in the case of smaller animals. In the rat, for example, maximum absorption occurs at a frequency of about 1 GHz.

1.2 Thermal and non-thermal effects

It is well recognized that microwave and RF radiation can induce a temperature rise in soft tissue as a result of increased molecular vibration and rotation. This effect is exploited in domestic microwave ovens. Exposure guidelines are largely based on limiting the heat load imposed on the body. A thermal effect might also be considered to cover the situation when the body's thermo-regulatory system is activated although there is no observable temperature rise in the tissue. An obvious example would be the increase in blood flow in the skin for the purpose of heat dissipation. In this case the altered rate of blood flow as well as changes in the associated chemical indicators would be a thermal effect even though the temperature rise might only be minimal.

A highly controversial area is the possible existence of non-thermal effects. These, if they exist, act by pathways which are not the result of an increased heatload but are due to the direct action of the radiation field on molecules or cellular components. Some investigators claim that a wide range of biological effects arise by non-thermal mechanisms at radiation levels much lower than those necessary to evoke a thermal response. Reported non-thermal responses include hallucinations, fatigability, headache, sleepiness, irritability, loss of appetite, memory difficulties, decrease in olfactory sensation and hair loss (Cleary, 1973). Whether such responses are attributable to microwave or RF radiation is highly contentious. Although some mechanisms have been proposed, none would have significant effects at the low levels of exposure at which the responses are alleged to occur. Moreover, most of the reports of non-thermal responses have not been successfully reproduced under controlled conditions. Since it is not possible to prove the absence of a hazard, argument will continue over the possible existence of a hazard from low level microwave and RF radiation.

1.3 Hyperthermia

When a body is exposed to a sufficiently high level of a microwave or RF field, its temperature may increase at a rate which exceeds its ability to dissipate heat. This condition is called hyperthermia and it can result in death. In the case of the dog, for example, whole body exposure to an RF field of frequency 200 MHz at a power density of 3000 W m^{-2} for 15 to 20 minutes will result in thermal death (WHO, 1981). The consequences of RF exposure in a species will depend on the power absorbed, the area of exposure, body cover, thermo-regulatory system, physiological condition, and the environment. In the case of partial body exposure local blood supply will influence the tissue temperature.

Calculations have been made, based on animal exposure data, to predict the thermal response of man under conditions of whole body exposure to an RF field. The predicted equilibrium core temperature is plotted against power density in Figure 18.3 for a frequency of 75 MHz, which is the frequency at which maximum absorption occurs. According to this, body temperature is maintained at a steady value up to approximately 100 Wm^{-2} but it is predicted that the human thermo-regulatory system is overloaded above 300 W m^{-2} at this frequency.

In addition to the possibility of whole body hyperthermia, the existence of localized heating must also be recognised. In the frequency interval 500 MHz to 2 GHz, hot spots may arise. For example, it has been calculated that there

400

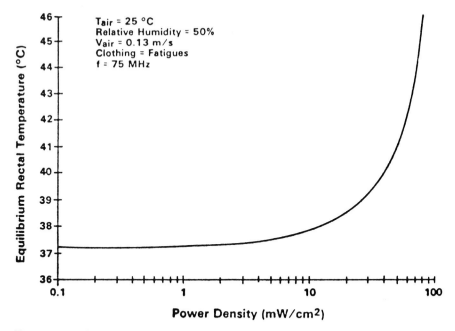

Figure 18.3 Calculated equilibrium rectal temperature in man exposed to whole body RF radiation at a frequency of 75 MHz (from Tell and Harlen 1979)

will be hot spots of 0.5 °C in a human head exposed to a power density of 100 W m^{-2} at a frequency of 2 GHz (Kritikos and Schwan, 1978).

1.4 Ocular exposure

The crystalline lens within the eye is remote from the thermo-regulatory influence of the circulation. Consequently, it is vulnerable to thermal damage. Also, since it is virtually acellular, it has only a very limited capacity for repair. Such damage may result in a lens opacity which, if it interferes with vision, is classified as a cataract.

Rabbits exposed to a microwave field at a frequency of 2.45 GHz and a power density of 1000 to 3000 W m^{-2} exhibited a latency period of between 24 and 48 hours before lens changes were detectable by slit-lamp examination (Guy *et al.*, 1975). Cataract formation occurred after exposure to a power density of 1500 W m^{-2} for 100 minutes, with higher thresholds required at shorter exposure times (Figure 18.4). Cataract induction is associated with exposure of the head or eyes alone since, in the case of the rabbit, whole body exposure at a frequency of 2.8 GHz and a power density of 1650 W m^{-2} would result in thermal death in 40 minutes. Also, there would be considerable pain

401

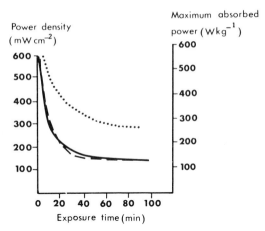

Figure 18.4 Exposure conditions for cataract induction in rabbits at a frequency of 2.45 GHz.
...... Williams *et al* (1955),   – – – Carpenter (1970),   ——— Kramer *et al* (1975)

associated with exposure to such power densities in an unanaesthetised animal as a result of the high temperature induced. There have been no reports of ocular injuries at frequencies below 500 MHz, while at frequencies above 35 GHz the threshold for keratitis (inflammation of the cornea) is lower than for cataract.

Studies have been performed which indicate that cataract induction is probably via a thermal mechanism (Baillie, 1970). However, experiments which have attempted to achieve comparable damage by microwave exposure as by simply raising the temperature of the eye have failed (Kramer *et al.,* 1975). This failure is probably due to the fact that the radiation field interacts with tissue in the eye such as to produce a temperature distribution which cannot easily be duplicated by other means. In addition, it must be recognised that biochemical and morphological changes have been observed within the lens in the absence of clinically detectable cataracts.

In conclusion, the induction of a cataract is unlikely to occur at a temperature less than 41°C. The threshold for microwave- or RF-induced cataract in man is likely to be at least 1000 to 1500 W m^{-2}.

1.5 Reproductive system

Exposure of the testes to a microwave or RF field may result in temporary sterility. The same effect can be achieved by raising the testicular temperature by a few degrees by other means. No significant pathological damage was observed and the sperm count was unaffected when experimental mice were exposed to a power density of 100 W m^{-2} (the occupational limit generally adopted in the US and Western Europe since the 1960s) for 4h 20min (Saunders and Kowalczuk, 1981). Exposure to high doses will result in testicular degeneration but no changes in rat or mouse testes were observed when the SAR was less than 4.5 W kg^{-1} (see review by Roberts *et al.*, 1986).

A significant reduction in foetal body mass was reported when pregnant adult rats were exposed to microwaves at a frequency of 2.45 GHz (O'Connor, 1980). This should not be interpreted as a low dose effect since the radiation level which produced the significant foetal abnormalities resulted in the death of 21% of the adults exposed. Reduction of foetal body mass has also been reported when pregnant adult mice were exposed to microwaves at a frequency of 2.45 GHz for 100 minutes per day throughout the gestation period (Berman *et al.*, 1978). Exposure levels in this particular study ranged up to 200 W m^{-2} (12.2 W kg^{-1}).

1.6 Neuro-endocrine system

Alteration in the hormonal status is a normal occurrence as the body tries to maintain homeostasis under conditions of a changing environment. So, it is natural that such changes will occur when animals are exposed to microwave and RF radiation.

It is likely that many observed changes arise form the body's homeostatic response to the increased thermal load. Thus, in a study on rats, the concentration of corticosterone (CS) increased with power density while that of thyroid stimulating hormone (TSH) and growth hormone (GH) decreased with power density (Lu *et al.*, 1977). In each case, hormone concentration correlated with colonic temperature as well as power density. CS is secreted by the adrenocortex, stimulation of which is generally accepted as indicating a response to thermal or other stress. More recently, exposure of the rhesus monkey to an SAR of 3.4 W kg^{-1} at 225 MHz failed to stimulate adrenocortical secretion despite causing an increase of 1.7 °C in rectal temperature (Lotz, 1985), although in earlier experiments, at a frequency of 1.29 GHz, this level of temperature rise had been shown to stimulate secretion. Clearly, at this time, there is inconsistency in results with regard to hormonal response in primates. It has been suggested that the discrepancy in the rhesus monkey experiments may be due to different baseline conditions as a result of the normal circadian rhythm (Roberts *et al.*, 1986).

A number of studies have been carried out on the influence of microwave and RF radiation on the hypothalamic-hypophysial-thyroid axis. Local thyroid exposure has been shown to cause an increase in thyroxine secretion (Magin *et al.*, 1977) whereas whole body exposure resulted in a decrease in TSH concentration, indicative of an inhibition of the hypothalamic-hypophysial-thyroid axis (Lu *et al.*, 1977). Therefore, it is believed that microwave

403

and RF exposure causes a local stimulation and axial inhibition of serum thyroxine concentration.

In conclusion, it may be said that changes in endocrine function generally require an exposure of at least 2 W kg^{-1} and correlate with changes in colonic temperature.

1.7 Central nervous system

The scientific literature of Eastern Europe contains a large number of reports on effects attributed to microwave and RF fields allegedly mediated by the central nervous system. However, exposure conditions are generally poorly controlled and, on the whole, results have not been confirmed in the West.

Electron microscopy studies of nervous tissue from hamsters have revealed changes following whole body irradiation at a power density of 100 W m^{-2} and a frequency of 2.45 GHz (Albert, 1979). Examination of the literature on frequency dependency of the SAR for a variety of species shows that the exposure conditions in the hamster experiments correspond to an SAR of 10 W kg^{-1}. Reported effects on ganglia and vagus nerves are probably due to increased temperature (Wachtel et al., 1975).

Reported effects of exposure on brain activity, as recorded on the electroencephalograph (EEG), are difficult to analyse because of the possible perturbation caused by the presence of EEG electrodes. In a carefully controlled series of experiments, mouse EEGs were normal four weeks after exposure at a frequency of 915 MHz and a power density of 50 W m^{-2} for 16 weeks (D'Andrea et al, 1980). If changes do occur at this level of exposure, they appear to be reversible. Although low level effects have been reported, it is not clear whether they are due to the direct action of the field or the result of differential heating.

1.8 Brain

The status of the blood-brain barrier after exposure to microwave or RF radiation has been the subject of a number of interesting investigations. Rats exposed for 20 minutes to a pulsed microwave field of average power density 3 W m^{-2} showed indications of altered blood-brain permeability with maximal effect occurring over a narrow range of power densities. Other studies have found that similar alterations require an SAR of at least 200 W kg^{-1} consistent with an explanation based on the effects of heat (Lin and Lin, 1982). In other experiments, permeability changes were observed at 13 W kg^{-1} but these were correlated with brain temperature (Williams et al., 1984). Possible reasons for the discrepancies may be suggested: the body temperature may be elevated due to stress; there may be resonant effects

404

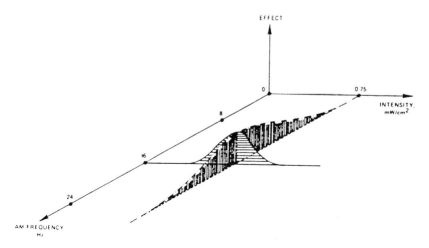

Figure 18.5 Power density and modulation frequency window for enhanced calcium ion efflux in brain tissue (from Blackman *et al* .,1979)

dependant on frequency; and local cerebral blood flow may alter. This last phenomenon has been observed in the rat as a result of irradiation with low power, pulsed microwaves (Oscar *et al.*, 1981).

Some of the most interesting findings in this area have been in connection with calcium ion efflux from the brain tissue of chicks (Blackman *et al.*, 1980). A pulsed field with amplitude modulation of 3 to 30 Hz, RF frequency of 147 MHz and power density between 5 and 20 W m^{-2} was used. It was found that optimal calcium ion efflux occurred at a modulation frequency of 16 Hz and a power density of 7.5 W m^{-2} (Figure 18.5). These findings suggest a direct interaction between the field and the tissue rather than a response to temperature elevation.

1.9 Blood

Dose-related changes in some serum components were reported when rabbits were exposed to radiation at a frequency of 2.45 GHz at power densities between 50 and 250 W m^{-2} for 2 h (Wangeman and Cleary, 1976). However, no significant alterations in blood parameters were observed when rats were exposed for 8h per day, five days per week, for 16 weeks at a frequency of 915 MHz and a power density of 50 W m^{-2}. Other studies confirm the belief that microwave and RF radiation appears to have an effect on formation of blood and this is probably due to heating.

1.10 Immunological system

A considerable number of experiments have been carried out in which immunological parameters were measured in animals following exposure to microwave or RF radiation. The significance of many of these results for humans is difficult to determine because of the marked differences in anatomy and physiology as well as physical factors relating to geometry and exposure conditions. In one study, mice were exposed to radiation at 2.45 GHz, at an SAR of 13 W kg^{-1} (Wiktor–Jedrzejczak *et al.*, 1977). This led to an increase in the relative number of splenic lymphoid cells with complement receptors compared to the control group. The ambient temperature was maintained at 25 °C with an airflow, and the rectal temperature decreased by up to 0.5 °C during the course of the experiment. These findings should be considered in the context of data from mice exposed to an SAR of 5.6 W kg^{-1} at 26 MHz (Liburdy, 1979). In the absence of forced air, core body temperature rose by 2 to 3 °C and lymphocyte, leukocyte and plasma corticoid levels were all altered. It is possible that the earlier reported increase in splenic cells with complement receptor was related to a cold stress reaction in the control animals.

In another set of experiments, an increase in lung cancer nodules in mice was reported following exposure at a frequency of 2.45 GHz and an SAR of 35 W kg^{-1} (Roszkowski *et al.*, 1980). This was most likely due to an indirect immunosuppressive effect since it was shown that the number of nodules in mice with bone marrow reconstituted from microwave-irradiated mice was greater than that in mice with bone marrow reconstituted from controls.

1.11 Cancer

A study carried out at the University of Washington at Seattle was designed to discover if prolonged exposure to low-level microwave radiation was harmful; 100 rats were exposed to radiation of frequency 2.45 GHz, power density 5 W m^{-2} (equivalent to an SAR of between 0.2 and 0.4 W kg^{-1}) for 21 h per day for 25 months. Results of 155 parameters were compared with a control group of 100 rats. Some differences between the two groups were apparent at some periods of the study but these were not of long-term significance. By contrast, there was a highly statistically significant difference in the incidence of primary malignant tumours (exposed 18; control 5). These results have been cited as evidence of a link between low level microwave radiation and cancer. However, the principal investigator has co-authored an article in which he cautions against drawing unwarranted conclusions from the study (Foster and Guy, 1986). The total number of malignant tumours in the control animals was lower than expected and the number of tumours in the exposed group did not exceed that generally observed in the particular strain. Moreover, there was no single predominant tumour type which might have pointed to a specific effect. Rather, the authors suggest that the finding of increased primary malignancy may be a statistical anomaly.

An early report which apparently showed a link between chronic exposure of mice to microwave radiation and cancer (Prausnitz and Susskind, 1962) was subsequently reassessed and the validity of the conclusions severely challenged (Roberts and Michaelson, 1983). Amongst other things, a severe infection seriously complicated the comparison between the exposed and unexposed groups.

Therefore, the case for a link between chronic low level microwave exposure and cancer has not yet been proven.

1.12 Behaviour

Effects of microwave and RF irradiation on animal behaviour have been studied by observing the animal's ability to perform learned responses. The threshold SAR is between 2 and 8 W kg^{-1} for rats exposed to continuous emission (Blackwell and Saunders, 1986). Altered behaviour using pulsed microwave emission with high peak power density may be due to auditory stimulation. This is a phenomenon whereby some individuals can sense a clicking sound when exposed to pulsed microwave radiation. The effect, due to rapid thermal expansion within the skull, is not associated with any harmful consequences.

Alterations of behaviour caused by microwave irradiation in some experiments are evidently the result of an animal's attempt to maintain a steady thermal environment. For example, it has been shown that the rate for rats, turning on an infra-red heat lamp, decreases as the microwave power density increases (Stern, 1980). Such alterations in behaviour are an effect of exposure to microwave radiation but do not necessarily imply the existence of a hazard.

1.13 Epidemiology

It is difficult to extrapolate from animal studies to man. Anatomical and physiological differences among species result in different thermo-regulatory systems. Accordingly, behavioural responses differ markedly. Physical size of the animal is important with respect to the degree of coupling with the radiation field. The SAR for the adult human peaks at a frequency of 70–80 MHz but, for smaller animals, maximum SAR is at higher frequencies (see Figure 18.2). As a result, there is merit in looking at epidemiological studies to see if any effects of microwave or RF radiation can be determined. Such studies, however, require careful analysis. In the vast majority of epidemio-

HANDBOOK OF LABORATORY HEALTH AND SAFETY MEASURES

logical studies, the level and duration of exposure are uncertain. In addition, there may be other predisposing factors present. Also, the selection of a suitable control group is of critical importance.

In the late 1970s considerable concern was expressed over allegations of irradiation of United States Embassy staff in Moscow, USSR. Exposure levels were of the order of 50 to 150 mW m^{-2}. Examination over a 23 year period showed that there were no adverse effects on mortality or morbidity. Likewise, studies carried out on US Navy personnel, who may have been exposed to radar, failed to find any detrimental effects attributable to exposure to microwave radiation (Robinette et al., 1980).

Although animal experiments have shown that microwave radiation may induce cataracts, there is no convincing epidemiological study showing increased incidence in cataract among an occupationally exposed group. It is likely that there is a threshold below which the absorbed power is too low to cause any temperature rise which may give rise to a lens opacity. One study has reported a higher proportion of retinal lesions among microwave-exposed workers (Aurell and Tengroth, 1973) but these findings have not been verified elsewhere.

2. RECORDED EXPOSURE LEVELS

2.1 Propagation

Microwave and RF radiation propagate in free space as an electromagnetic wave with the electric and magnetic field components and the direction of propagation mutually perpendicular (Figure 18.6). For such a wave there is a constant ratio between the magnitude of the electric and magnetic field strengths. Thus, the power density (W m^{-2}) can be determined by measurement of either the electric or magnetic component with an appropriate calibration factor. The power density, S (W m^{-2}), is given by the equation:

$S = E^2/377$ or
$S = H^2 \times 377$

where E (V m^{-1}) is the electric field strength
and H (A m^{-1}) is the magnetic field strength.

At distances close to the source the power density no longer follows a simple inverse square law, and this region is called the near-field. Transition from far- to near-field occurs at a distance, d given by the equation

$d < 2 l^2/\lambda$

where l is the distance between the furthest points of the source, and λ is the wavelength. Within the near-field, calculations of power density based on an inverse square approximation are invalid. At a distance closer than one

408

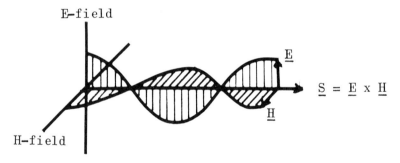

Figure 18.6 Representation of a plane-polarized electromagnetic wave in free space with the E-field and H-field mutually perpendicular

wavelength, it is necessary to measure the electric and magnetic field strengths separately because the simple relation between these components and the power density breaks down. This region is termed the reactive near field and results obtained within this zone are often very misleading.

A sensor probe in an electromagnetic field will disturb the field as will walls, floors, ceilings, metallic objects and the investigator holding the probe. Close to the source, regions of high field strength may be produced as a result of reflection between the sensor and the emitter. Metallic objects in particular will distort the field.

Due account must be taken of time-modulation of a field. Some short-wave diathermy sources used by physiotherapists have a pulsed output; also, radar antennae rotate such that the field strength at any one location varies with time. It is important, from a practical point of view, to ensure that the peak power density does not exceed the capabilities of the instrument.

2.2 Field indicators

It is possible to produce or purchase low-cost devices which may be used to indicate the presence of an RF field. Physiotherapists use neon tubes to check for leakage of RF energy from cables during short-wave diathermy therapy. The neon tube will glow provided the electric field strength is sufficiently great to cause a discharge between the electrodes through the neon gas. The threshold for discharge will depend on the geometry of the tube. Although essentially qualitative, it should function as a reliable indicator that the field strength exceeds a certain, unspecified level.

A simple diode and meter can be used to sense an electromagnetic field. Unfortunately, such a device is strongly influenced by the polarization of the field and, moreover, it will respond to a wide range of frequencies. Simple, low cost instruments which utilize diode sensors are generally unreliable. A number of such devices are available commercially and are directed towards users of microwave ovens. The use of these detectors cannot be recommended unless they can be shown to be reliable indicators of microwave radiation, and are unaffected by other factors, such as heat or 50 Hz mains radiation.

The deficiencies in some of these instruments were described in a report published by the Bureau of Radiological Health in the United States (Herman and Witters, 1979). One device indicated a "warning" which could occur at levels from 37 to 470 W m^{-2} depending on how the instrument was used. In another device, an LED was intended to light as a warning of high levels but in some instances the LED came on at levels as low as 7 W m^{-2}, while on other occasions it failed to light when the levels were much higher, 280 to 520 W m^{-2}.

2.3 Field strength monitors

Field strength monitors measure either the electric or magnetic component and present the result either as electric field strength in units of volts metre^{-1} (V m^{-1}), magnetic field strength in units of amps metre^{-1} (A m^{-1}), or power density in units of watts metre^{-2} (W m^{-2}). E-field probes contain diode dipoles and by arranging these in three mutually perpendicular planes it is possible to produce a detector with an isotropic response, i.e. the sensitivity is constant irrespective of the direction of the incident radiation. Such detectors are available, commercially, for example the isotropic probes manufactured by the Narda Microwave Corporation shown in Figure 18.7; a pre-amplifier is incorporated in the handle. In this range of instruments, the E-field probe covers the frequency range 300 MHz to 26 GHz while the lower frequencies, 10 to 300 MHz, are measured using an H-field sensor. The latter device contains three orthogonal coils to detect the magnetic component of the incident radiation. The induced current heats a thermocouple which gives a D.C. output proportional to the power in the RF field.

Detectors are available for checking microwave ovens. These come midway between the inexpensive unreliable devices and the expensive isotropic type of instruments. They incorporate a 5 cm spacer, which is the distance at which radiation leakage should be measured, according to BS 5175. They operate over a restricted range of power density, in the vicinity of 50 W m^{-2}, which is the leakage limit for microwave ovens within the United Kingdom.

All field measuring instruments should be calibrated directly or traceable to a national standards laboratory, such as the National Physical Laboratory in the United Kingdom or the National Bureau of Standards in the United States.

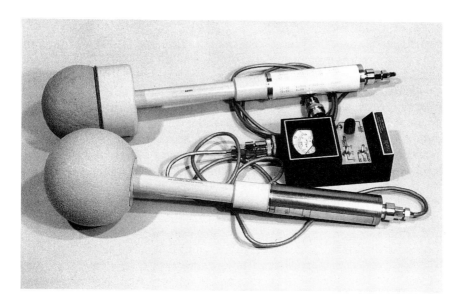

Figure 18.7 Isotropic microwave and RF radiation field probes

2.4 Radar

Radar systems generally operate in the 1–10 GHz frequency range. Several bands are designated by letters, for example, the X-band between 5.2 and 10.9 GHz. Radar installations emit beams containing high peak powers, often tens of gigawatts. In 1973, there were more than 20,000 emitters in the USA which could deliver a power density of 100 W m^{-2} at 10 m, and 565 units were capable of producing a beam with this power density at a distance of 1 km (WHO, 1981). Staff, particularly maintenance personnel, must be careful to remain without the region exposed to the beam when the radar is in operation. The main radar beam is generally emitted high above ground level and follows an elevated trajectory. In one survey, power densities at ground level were between 0.1 and 1 W m^{-2} within half a mile of the installation (Janes, 1979).

Measurements have been performed in the vicinity of low power radar sources (Janes, 1979). A power density of 135 W m^{-2} was recorded at the surface of the radome which housed an aircarft weather radar; at a distance of 1 m, it was 30 W m^{-2} or less. At the antenna turning circle radius of marine radar systems it was found to be between 0.5 and 2.5 W m^{-2}; for traffic radar devices used to measure the speed of motor vehicles, the power density at

411

the antenna surface was less than 4 W m^{-2}. It has been estimated that the occupants of cars are exposed to less than 0.01 W m^{-2} from traffic radar.

An exposure survey of civilian airport radar workers in Australia was carried out between 1983 and 1985 (Joyner and Bangay, 1986a). The primary surveillance radars investigated provide air traffic control with peak powers of nominally 2 MW and either pulse width of 2.5 μs and pulse repetition frequency (PRF) of 400 Hz or 1.5 μs and 800 Hz, respectively. In addition, secondary surveillance radar interrogate the target aircraft, and a tropospheric scatter link is used for communications. In Australia, 10 W m^{-2} is the occupational exposure limit for up to eight hours per day for frequencies between 30 MHz and 300 GHz, averaged over any 60 second period. This level was exceeded in areas around primary surveillance radar, particularly where slots were cut in the waveguide or devices were inserted through openings. No leakage radiation was detected in and around transmitter cabinets of secondary surveillance radar installations, and measured levels in and around tropospheric scatter links were well below the 10 W m^{-2} limit. For non-radiation workers, the exposure limit is 2 Wm^{-2}. This level was only slightly exceeded on the outside of the air traffic control tower at one airport. In general, both radiation and non-radiation workers would be unlikely to be exposed to levels in excess of that recommended in the Australian Standard.

In the United Kingdom, the National Air Traffic Service operates some 25 primary surveillance units with powers up to 650 kW peak and 780 W mean. Only authorised persons are permitted to enter certain areas where the power density may exceed 50 W m^{-2}. Defence radar systems operate on land, air and sea and these are surveyed regularly in order to determine exposure levels and establish safe working distances.

2.5 Industrial sources

There are several thousand industrial RF dielectric heaters in the United Kingdom. The basic principle involved in RF heating is that the material (the dielectric) is subjected to an RF field which causes oscillation of the molecules and resultant frictional heating. Although the risks of electric shock and burns have been known for some time, more recently, attention has been directed towards hazards associated with exposure to stray radiation.

Industrial RF heaters are used in plastic welding, woodworking, fibre drying, food processing, paper and box and other manufacturing processes. In a survey of RF plastic sealers performed in the United States, 60% of the units checked emitted electric field strengths greater than 200 V m^{-1} and 29% exceeded a magnetic field strength of 0.5 A m^{-1} (Cox *et al*, 1982); 10% of the operators were exposed to fields in excess of 1000 V m^{-1}. In surveys reported from other countries, equivalent power densities greater than 100 W m^{-2} have been measured at sites normally occupied by operators. In a

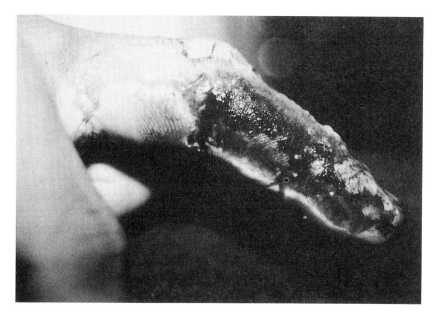

Figure 18.8   Acute injury to the hand caused by accidental exposure to the field of a 10 MHz industrial heater (from Nicholson *et al.*, 1987. Photgraph courtesy of Dr J.C. Grotting)

Swedish study of four plastic welding machines operating at 27 MHz, the electric field strength was found to be greater than 900 V m^{-1} (equivalent to 2100 W m^{-2}) and the magnetic field strength was at least 2.8 A m^{-1} (2900 W m^{-2}) incident on the operator (Mild, 1980). A further hazard arises from the cables feeding the emitter since these can also function as radiators.

More recently, a survey of 101 RF heaters operating in the frequency range 11 to 50 MHz has been carried out in Australia (Joyner and Bangay, 1986b). Results were analysed with reference to the Australian Exposure Standard: for frequencies between 30 MHz and 300 GHz, the limit is 10 W m^{-2}, with higher power densities permitted at lower frequencies. They found that 61% of the heaters surveyed exposed the operators to levels in excess of the recommended limits. In general, the closer the operator position to the weld head, the higher was the exposure. Also, shielding of the weld head greatly reduced the operator exposure.

A case report has been published concerning an acute injury to the hand suffered by a man working on a 10 MHz RF heater (Nicholson *et al.*, 1987). This type of injury contrasts with the potential hazards from chronic exposure and occurred when the heater was accidentally activated while the man was placing laminated board in the machine. The patient was wearing rubber gloves, which were partially destroyed (Figure 18.8). Immediate numbness and tingling were followed after 20 minutes by excruciating pain which was relieved with analgesics. The patient sustained second- and third-degree burns. Excision and coverage using a cross-finger flap resulted in full return of the function.

A useful document on safety in the use of RF dielectric heating equipment has been published by the Health and Safety Executive in the United Kingdom (HSE, 1986). They recommend a properly designed and installed shielding enclosure to reduce emission of RF radiation; if this is not done correctly, the screen may act as an antenna. The detailed construction of the screen will depend on the configuration of the heater. For installations where it is not possible to reduce RF emission to recommended levels, systems of work should be introduced so that personnel exposure is within acceptable limits. In this case a Controlled Area should be designated within which exposure to the field should be limited and distance between operator and machine increased to bring exposure within acceptable limits. It is permissible when assessing exposure to take into account the reduction in occupational exposure by timer-averaging when the power is off while the operator is repositioning the piece of work. A programme of routine monitoring should be established and adequate instruction and training given. In addition, a "responsible person" should advise on measures necessary to ensure safe use of RF equipment.

2.6 Radio & TV communications

Several European radio-stations transmit amplitude modulation (AM) broadcasts at effective radiated powers of 2 MW, with stations in the UK operating at up to 500 kW. Frequency modulation (FM) radio broadcasts in the UK are transmitted at effective radiated powers of up to 120 kW and ultra-high frequency (UHF) television transmission at up to 1 MW. Antennae are generally of the order of 500 m above ground-level and persons at ground-level are outside the main beam, although they may be exposed to side lobes. Satellite communications systems are now in regular use and these operate at the gigawatt (10^9 watts) and terawatt (10^{12} watts) level. Intensities are such that one system has been cited where the power density is 100 W m^2 at a distance of 100 km (WHO, 1981). At the opposite extreme, citizens' band radio utilizes a band of frequencies between 27 and 28 MHz at a legal maximum of 4 W in the UK.

Measurements made on a broadcasting tower in Sweden showed that there was an electric field strength of 400 V m^{-1} and a magnetic field strength of 2.3 A m^{-1} at places where maintenance workers might require to go (Mild, 1980). The Canadian Health Directorate have published their findings from surveys on a tele-communications tower from which several stations broadcast at effective radiated powers of up to 2.1 MW (Canada, 1982). The highest level found in the general access areas was an E-field of 32 V m^{-1}

(equivalent to 3 $W m^{-2}$). Power densities in excess of 200 $W m^{-2}$ were recorded in areas normally locked with leakage levels up to 1000 $W m^{-2}$ close to some components. The survey led to the correction of some of the leakage sources and the deliniation of limited occupancy areas.

Lower power sources may be hazardous if the operator's head is close to the transmitted beam. A survey of radio-equipped vehicles has shown that there is a wide range of field strengths, up to 1350 $V m^{-1}$, recorded at a distance of 0.5 m (Janes, 1979). In addition, levels in excess of 200 $V m^{-1}$ were measured at a distance of several centimetres from hand-held walkie-talkies.

Measurements of electric field strength have been made in the UK around two UHF transmitters. One had an effective radiated power of 100 kW and the highest electrical field strength at ground level, measured 0.8 km from the base of the mast, was equivalent to a power density of $4 \times 10^{-4} W m^{-2}$ (Allen and Harlen, 1983). The other was a 1000 kW transmitter 2 m above ground level, the power density with all channels operating was $2.6 \times 10^{-2} W m^{-2}$ at distances of 80 m and 300 m. Measurements at VHF, HF and MF transmitters confirmed the potential hazard to antenna riggers, with field strengths of the order of several hundred $V m^{-1}$

2.7 Hospital sources

Physiotherapists use microwave diathermy, usually at a frequency of 2.45 GHz, less commonly 915 MHz, or short-wave RF diathermy at 27 MHz, to produce heat at depth in soft tissue. In microwave therapy, the RF field is radiated from an antenna towards the treatment site, some 0.15m away. In the case of short-wave therapy, the part of the body to be treated forms part of a tuned circuit and the patient is coupled either capacitatively via two condenser plates or inductively by coiled cable or specially designed electrode. In all cases it is important that RF-carrying cables do not come into contact with metal objects and that connectors are tightly joined since they are liable to emit stray radiation. Power levels are governed by the patient's perception of heat and typically microwave power levels of the order of 50–100 W are utilized whereas in the case of short-wave RF, power is in the region of 200–300 W. Patients with cardiac pacemakers or metal implants should not be treated.

The question arises as to whether physiotherapists are likely to be exposed to fields which exceed the permissible levels. A number of investigations have been carried out among which that of Stuchly et al. (1982) into short-wave RF diathermy at 27 MHz is particularly extensive. Both electric and magnetic field strengths decreased rapidly with distance. A phantom was used in place of a patient. Electric field strength was greater than 200 $V m^{-1}$ near the applicator. Also, the cables were a significant source of radiation, with levels of 300 $V m^{-1}$ being measured at up to 0.4m, and 0.8 $A m^{-1}$ at 0.25 m for electric and magnetic field strengths, respectively. The conclusion was reached that the physiotherapist standing at the console for a few minutes per treatment would be unlikely to exceed the permitted level. In Canada, where the investigation was carried out, the limit for one hour is 50 V m^{-1} and 0.5 A m^{-1}.

A study of stray microwave radiation was carried out in a U.K. hospital (Moseley and Davison, 1981). Based on these measurements, it was concluded that the exposure of physiotherapists would not exceed 100 W m^{-2} which was at that time widely adopted as a maximum for 8-hour exposure, provided reasonable care was taken. Furthermore, it is likely that physiotherapist exposure will not exceed the current lower limits because of the limited occupancy in the vicinity of the radiation field. However, in some cases additional precautions may be advisable. For example, results from a survey carried out by the author in a hospital in Glasgow are given in Tables 18.1 and 18.2.

Table 18.1 Field power density (W m^{-2}) measured at several locations during treatment of knee using transverse capacitative electrodes

A: Continuous mode, position 4
B: Pulsed mode, 62 Hz, 600W – mean power 14.9 W
C: Pulsed mode (max), 200 Hz, 1000 W – mean power 80 W

Part 1: Position of Probe	Power Density (W m^{-2})		
	A	B	C
Console (cable end)	400	40	200
Console (opposite end)	20	10	15
Console (operator eye level)	20	10	15
Treatment site (vicinity of cables)	> 1000	100	> 1000
Treatment site (away from cables)	250	25	100
Patient eye level	15	2	5
Cable	> 1000	> 1000	> 1000

Part 2: Power Density	Distance from cable (m)		
	A	B	C
100 W m^{-2}	0.5	0.2	0.5
50 W m^{-2}	0.75	0.3	0.8
10 W m^{-2}	1.5	0.5	1.5

Table 18.2 Field power density (W m^{-2}) measured at several locations during treatment of knee using the circuplode applicator

A: Continuous mode, position 6
B: Pulsed mode, 62 Hz, 800W – average power 19.8W
C: Pulsed mode (max), 200 Hz, 800W – average power 64W

Part 1: Position of Probe

	Power Density (W m^{-2})		
	A	B	C
Console (cable end)	30	3	5
Console (opposite end)	3	2	2
Console (Circuplode connector)	> 1000	90	400
Console (operator eye level)	3	3	2
Patient eye level	3	2	2
Cable	80	5	25

Part 2: Power Density

	Distance from cable (m)		
	A	B	C
100 W m^{-2}	0.1	0.05	0.05
50 W m^{-2}	0.2	0.06	0.06
10 W m^{-2}	0.5	0.10	0.15

These relate to equipment operating at a frequency of 27 MHz which can be used with different types of treatment applicators and in different operating modes. If the limits recommended by the National Radiological Protection Board of the U.K. (NRPB 1989) are adopted, the occupational limit at 27 MHz is 10 W m^{-2} averaged over 0.1 h. When the capacitative electrodes are in use, this may be exceeded in the example cited, at distances within 1.5 m of the cables, at the console, at operator eye level when the operator is standing at the console and at patient eye level. When the inductive electrode is in use, levels in excess of 10 W m^{-2} may be found at distances within 0.5m of the cable and at the console, but not at patient eye level nor at operator eye level when the operator is standing at the console. A source of leakage was identified at the cable connector at the console.

Radiofrequency or microwave radiation is often used to produce hyperthermia as an adjunct to radiotherapy in the treatment of cancer. Power levels may be 1 kW or more and studies of stray radiation have shown that, generally, exposure will be less than 50 W m^{-2} provided the operator maintains a distance of at least 1m from the electrodes. If the area in which the hyperthermia treatment is given is not carefully screened, it may cause interference with other equipment. In one reported case, the interference led to false dosimetry readings on a nearby linear accelerator.

The electron beam in a linear accelerator is subjected to an electromagnetic field produced by a magnetron. While looking for arcing between high-voltage cables, service personnel often operate the accelerator with the metal covers removed from around the magnetron. Under such circumstances, we have measured power densities greater than 600 W m^{-2} at a frequency of 3 GHz within 1m of the magnetron at hospital installations. With the metal covers in place, leakage levels were reduced to below 0.2 W m^{-2} and so the potential hazard from stray radiation only existed when the metal covers were removed.

Surgical diathermy units are used to cut and coagulate tissue. E-field intensity measured at a distance of 0.16m from the active lead has been reported to be between 210 and 1000 V m^{-1} (Ruggera, 1977); magnetic field strength was found to range between 0.06 and 0.71 A m^{-1}. A report has recently been published of field strength measurements made at the position normally occupied by the head of the operator during electrosurgery (Paz *et al.*, 1987). Electric field strength for bipolar units had a peak value of 300 V m^{-1} and magnetic field strength was as high as 1.9 A m^{-1}. These levels exceed the limits recommended by the American National Standards Institute and so this may be an area that requires further investigation.

2.8 Microwave ovens

Microwave ovens operate at a frequency of 2.45 GHz. In order to avoid interference with telecommunications transmissions, there are limits on permitted leakage levels at higher harmonic frequencies. From the point of view of radiation safety, it is the limit at the fundamental frequency which is important. In the British Standard (BS 5175), the maximum allowed is 50 W m^{-2} at 5 cm.

BS 5175 is an emission standard and should be distinguished from an exposure standard. An emission limit refers to an item of equipment and is such that personnel exposure will be within the recommended exposure limit during normal operation of the equipment. The results of a total of 662 radiation leakage surveys performed annually on microwave ovens located in hospitals in the West of Scotland are summarised in Table 18.3.

Levels in excess of 50 W m^{-2} at 5 cm were recorded from ovens operating with the door closed on seven occasions from six different ovens (maximum: 200 W m^{-2}); levels recorded while opening the door exceeded 50 W m^{-2} on ten occasions from seven different ovens (maximum: 600 W m^{-2}). A hazard analysis showed that on no occasion would staff exposure have exceeded the permitted maximum (taken to be 50 W m^{-2}).

Table 18.3 Microwave radiation leakage measurements at 50 mm (from Moseley and Davison, 1989)

A. Oven operating with door closed

Power density (W m^{-2})	1980	1981	1982	1983	1984	1985	1986	1987
<2.0	22	32	42	44	53	48	33	57
2.0–20	24	24	21	29	44	49	53	52
21–50	3	6	6	3	2	7	0	2
51–100	0	3	0	0	0	2	1	0
>100	0	0	1	0	0	0	0	0
Total	49	65	69	76	99	106	87	111

B. Oven operating with door held slightly open

Power density (W m^{-2})	1980	1981	1982	1983	1984	1985	1986	1987
<2.0	29	37	44	48	74	55	41	73
2.0–20	17	17	20	21	19	44	44	37
21–50	2	8	3	7	4	6	1	1
51–100	0	1	1	0	1	0	1	0
>100	1	2	1	0	1	1	0	0
Total	49	65	69	76	99	106	87	111

Hazards of a different kind have been reported in connection with the use of microwave ovens. For example, the food may catch fire. The operator has to take account of the amount of food put in for cooking; a small amount will heat up much more rapidly than a large amount. Also, users need to be aware that some food will be much hotter in the centre than on the outside. Reported cases include the youth who burned his mouth from a microwave-heated jam-filled doughnut (Perlman, 1980), and the boy who sustained injury to the eye and peri-ocular region on opening a bag of microwave-popped popcorn (Routhier *et al*, 1986)

2.9 Video display terminals

Fears have been expressed that operators using video display terminals (VDTs) are at risk from exposure to ionising and non-ionising radiation. Concern has been fuelled by reports of increased incidence of miscarriages among VDT operators in some places of work. No link with VDT usage has been established. The Council on Scientific Affairs of the American Medical Association has reported on health effects of VDTs (AMA, 1987). They concluded that no association has been found between radiation emissions and reported spontaneous abortions, birth defects, cataracts or other injuries. They observed that complaints of health effects were more likely to be ergonomically or stress related.

Several studies have been conducted to measure radiation levels from the terminals (see, for example, Murray *et al.*, 1981). These have reported X-ray levels at or near background, and no measurable levels of ultra-violet or RF radiation. Some radiation has been measured at frequencies below 100 KHz from some fly-back transformers. This was of no biological significance and the electrical component could easily be shielded. The conclusion from examination of the published data is that there is no electromagnetic radiation hazard to the operator working at or near a VDT. It follows that there is no requirement for any sort of protective wear, either special glasses or clothing. There may be discomfort caused by posture, or eye fatigue, and this can be reduced by good diffuse ambient lighting, anti-reflection screens, an ergonomically designed work-station, and a working practice which permits the operator sufficient opportunity to relax their concentration on the screen.

To prevent low frequency radiation being emitted from the VDT and interfering with the functioning of other equipment, it may be necessary to fit shielding. This is often available as a retrofit from the manufacturer; alternatively, it can be constructed from a copper screen with a wire to ground. Screen shields are available commercially.

3. STANDARDS

A number of national and international microwave and RF radiation exposure standards have been formulated. The large differences which existed (up to a factor of 1000) between standards adopted in the USA and Western Europe, compared to those of Eastern Europe are being reduced.

Different limits may reasonably be applied depending on whether exposure is occupational or otherwise. For the former, personnel can be instructed on risks, hazards and safety precautions and can have access to an expert adviser; the general population, however, are not expected to take precautions against microwave and RF exposure in their normal everyday life. Differences will exist between the period of exposure for staff, usually a maximum of eight hours per day, and the public, which may be 24 hours per day. Account must also be taken of people in "at risk" categories, such as wearers of cardiac pacemakers.

Since the early 1960s, and until recently, the exposure limit generally adopted in the West was 100 W m^{-2}. The thinking behind this was that an additional heat load equivalent to a doubling of the basic metabolic rate could easily be tolerated since this occurred naturally while performing light work. This was equivalent to a load of 100 W or 100 W m^{-2} on half of the body

420

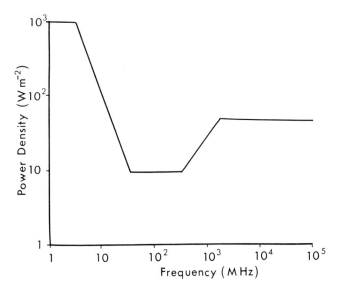

Figure 18.9 Exposure limits recommended in the ANSI (1982) standard

surface - the normal exposure condition. Studies in animals showed that it was unlikely for a cataract to be induced below 1000 W m^{-2} and so there was a safety factor of 10 or more incorporated in the 100 W m^{-2} limit.

This value contrasted markedly with the 100 mW m^{-2} limit which was adopted in the USSR in 1959. The rationale behind the Soviet standard was that the permitted exposure level should be reduced below that at which harmful effects have been alleged to occur. Exposure limits were based on empirical animal experiments or investigations of the health status of persons exposed to microwave and RF radiation. Similar standards have been adopted in other Eastern European countries. The USSR standard has recently been revised such that exposure to a power density of 10 W m^{-2} is now permitted for a period of 20 minutes or less.

Standards now being promulgated by many bodies utilize the concept of the specific absorption rate (SAR). The SAR takes account of frequency-dependance of absorption. The current recommendations of the American National Standards Institute (ANSI, 1982) sets a limit on the SAR of 0.4 W kg^{-1} averaged over the whole body. Examination of published experiments show marked inconsistencies in reported effects at an SAR below 6 W kg^{-1}, with few properly conducted studies, indicating an effect below 0.4 W kg^{-1} (Cahill, 1983). It is also the case that a heat load equivalent to an SAR of 0.4 W kg^{-1} averaged over the whole body would activate the thermo-regulatory system in an adult.

The ANSI (1982) exposure standard is shown in Figure 18.9. In the frequency interval 300 kHz to 3 MHz, the power density limit is 100 W m^{-2}.

Between 3 MHz and 30 MHz, the maximum power density P_{max} (W m^{-2}) is given by the equation:

$$P_{max} = 9000/f^2$$

where f is the frequency (MHz).

From 30 MHz to 300 MHz the limit is 10 W m^{-2}. Between 300 MHz and 1.5 GHz the maximum power density, P_{max} (W m^{-2}) can be calculated from the formula $P_{max} = f/300$ where f is the frequency (MHz) as before. Above 1.5 GHz up to 300 GHz, the power density limit is 50 W m^{-2}.

The limits are averaged over any 0.1h period. Provided the mean SAR does not exceed 0.4 W kg^{-1}, the SAR in any part of the body may be higher, up to 8 W kg^{-1}. Many hand-held walkie-talkies are automatically exempted since the standard excludes devices which radiate 7W or less at a frequency, below 1 GHz.

Other similar standards are based on a limit of 0.4 W kg^{-1} on the SAR. In the United Kingdom, the 100 W m^{-2} limit which was adopted by the Home Office in 1960, has been replaced by an SAR limit of 0.4 W kg^{-1} (NRPB, 1989). The gross difference between standards adopted in the West and in Eastern European countries are diminishing. Accordingly, Czerski (1985) concluded his review of exposure limits in Czechoslavakia, Poland and the USSR by commenting that complete agreement on exposure limits on an international basis did not seem to be very far away.

Recommendations applicable during magnetic resonance imaging have been published in the United Kingdom (NRPB, 1983). The static magnetic field should not exceed 2.5 T for patients, 0.02 T for staff whole body exposure and 0.2T for staff exposure of arms or hands. For periods of less than 15 minutes, staff exposure limits may be increased by a factor of 10. There are also limits on the rate of change of the magnetic field. If the period of change is greater than 10 ms, the limit is 20 Ts^{-1} RMS; if it is less than 10 ms, the rate of change (dB/dt) is given by the equation:

$$(dB/dt)^2 t < 4$$

where t is the time (sec). The RF field is restricted to a maximum SAR of 0.4 W kg^{-1}, whole body, and 4 W kg^{-1} to any mass of tissue not exceeding 1 g.

4. PRECAUTIONS

Responsibility for the health and well-being of staff lies with the employer. Where there is a possibility that staff may be exposed to hazardous levels of microwave or RF radiation, a survey should be performed by a competent person. During the investigation, equipment should be operated under a variety of conditions. The radiation levels measured should be assessed in relation to the permitted exposure levels, using the appropriate national standard, if one exists. In the absence of a national guideline, it would be reasonable to adopt the ANSI (1982) standard or, in the UK, the NRPB (1989) proposal. Advice should then be issued so that staff levels are kept within the recommended exposure limits.

Four categories of protection have been recognised and these are listed in order of desirability:

(1) *Engineering design.* Look first at the source of radiation leakage to see if it can be eliminated. This may be achieved by proper shielding or fitting an interlock to a removable screen. This has the added benefit of eliminating a potential source of electromagnetic interference.

(2) *Siting of equipment.* Many microwave and RF sources are what is called "deliberate emitters" where containment of the field is not possible. Examples are radio transmitters and microwave or short-wave diathermy applicators. Where possible, such items should be positioned such as to minimise unintentional exposure.

(3) *Administrative control.* If there is an area in which persons may be exposed to radiation levels in excess of the maximum permissible levels, the area should be controlled and rules drawn up specifying restrictions on occupancy. Adequate information should be available. Staff should be instructed not to override interlocks unless under approved procedures.

(4) *Personal protection.* The donning of protective clothing should be the final line of defence. In general, this should not be necessary if the engineering design, equipment siting and administrative control are adequate. A situation where it may be useful is in hospital physiotherapy departments. Here, wire mesh goggles may be used to attentuate the radiation field, significantly reducing the chance of stray radiation causing ocular damage. They are particularly desirable for use by patients if the field is close to their eyes.

REFERENCES

1. Albert, EN (1979). Evidence of neuropathology in chronically irradiated hamsters by 2450 MHz microwaves at 10 mW/cm^2. In *USNC/URSI National Radio Science Meeting Bioelectromagnetics Symposium, Seattle, Washington*, p355. US National Committee of the International Union of Radio Science, National Academy of Sciences.
2. Allen, SG and Harlen, F (1983). Sources of exposure to radiofrequency and microwave radiations in the UK. National Radiological Protection Board, Chilton, Didcot, Oxon, UK, NRPB-R144
3. AMA (1987). Health effects of video display terminals. *J.A.M.A.*, **257**, 1508
4. ANSI (1982). Safety levels with respect to human exposure to radio-frequency electromagnetic fields, 300 kHz to 100 GHz. C95.1. New York: American National Standards Institute
5. Aurell, E and Tengroth, B (1973). Lenticular and retinal changes secondary to microwave exposures. *Acta Ophthalmol.*, **51**, 764
6. Baillie, HD (1970). Thermal and non-thermal cataractogenesis by microwaves. In *Biol-*

ogical Effects and Health Implications of Microwave Radiation, ed. Cleary, SF. HEW Publication BRH/DBE 70–2, p59: US Department of Health, Education and Welfare

7. Berman, E, Kinn, JB and Carter, HB (1978). Observation of mouse fetuses after irradiation with 2.45 GHz microwaves. *Health Phys.*, **35**, 791

8. Blackman, CF, Elder, JA, Weil, CM, Benane, SG, Eichingen, DG and House, DE (1979). Induction of calcium efflux from brain tissue by radio-frequency radiation: Effects of modulation frequency and field strength. *Radio Sci.*, **14**, 93

9. Blackman, CF, Benana, SG, Elder, JA, House, DE, Lampe, JA and Faulk, JM (1980). Induction of calcium ion efflux from brain tissue by radiofrequency radiation. *Bioelectromagnetics J.*, **1**, 35

10. Blackwell, RP and Saunders, RD (1986). The effects of low-level radio-frequency and microwave radiation on brain tissue and animal behaviour. *Int. J. Radiat. Biol.*, **50**, 761

11. B.S. 5175 (1976). Specification for safety of commercial electrical appliances using microwave energy for heating foodstuffs. London: British Standards Institution

12. Cahill, DF (1983). A suggested limit for population exposure to radiofrequency radiation. *Health Physics*, **45**, 109

12. Canada (1982). A survey of radiofrequency and microwave radiation at and near the CN tower. Environmental Health Directorate, Health and Welfare Canada Publication 83-EHD-78

13. Carpenter, RL (1970). Experimental microwave cataract: a review. In *Biological Effects and Health Implications of Microwave Radiation*. Ed. Cleary, SF. HEW Publication BRH/DBE 70–2, 76: US Department of Health, Education and Welfare

14. Cleary, SF (1973). Uncertainties in the evaluation of the biological effects of microwave and radiofrequency radiation. *Health Phys.*, **25**, 387

15. Cox, C, Murray, WE and Foley, ED (1982). Occupational exposures to radiofrequency radiation (18–31 MHz) from RF dielectric heat sealers. *Am. Ind. Hyg. Assoc. J.*, **43**, 149

16. Czerski, P (1985). Radiofrequency radiation exposure limits in Eastern Europe. *J. Microwave Power*, **20**, 233

17. D'Andrea, JA, Gandhi, OP, Lords, JL, Durney, CH, Astte, L, Steneaas, LJ and Schoenberg, AA (1980). Physiological and behavioural effects of prolonged exposure to 915 MHz microwaves. *J. Microwave Power*, **15**, 123

18. Foster, KR and Guy, AW (1986). The microwave problem. *Sci. Amer.*, **255**, 28

19. Guy, AW, Lin, JD, Kramer, PO and Emery, AF (1975). Effects of 2450 MHz radiation on the rabbit eye. *IEEE Trans. Microwave Theory Tech.*, **MTT-23**, 492

20. Herman, WA and Witters, DM (1979). Inexpensive microwave survey instruments: an evaluation. Rockville, US Department of Health, Education and Welfare. HEW Publication (FDA) 80–8102

21. HSE (1986). Safety in the use of radiofrequency dielectric heating equipment. Guidance Note PM51. Her Majesty's Stationery Office: London

22. Janes, DE (1979). Radiation surveys – measurement of leakage emissions and potential exposure fields. *Bull. N.Y. Acad. Med.*, **55**, 1021

23. Joyner, KH and Bangay, MJ (1986a). Exposure survey of civilian airport radar workers in Australia. *J. Microwave Power*, **21**, 209

24. Joyner, KH and Bangay, MJ (1986b). Exposure survey of operators of radiofrequency dielectric heaters in Australia. *Health Phys.*, **50**, 333

25. Kramer, PO, Harris, C, Guy, AW and Emery, A (1975). Mechanisms of microwave cataractogenesis in rabbits. In *Proc. URSI/USNC Ann. Meeting*. Boulder, CO, p40. Washington DC: International Union of Radio Science, National Academy of Sciences

26. Kritikos, HN and Schwan, HP (1978). Potential temperature rise induced by electromagnetic field in brain tissues. *IEEE Trans. Biomed. Eng.*, **BME-26**, 29

27. Liburdy, RP (1979). Radiofrequency radiation alters the immune system: modulation of T- and B-lymphocyte levels and cell-mediated immunocompetence by hyperthermic radiations. *Radiat. Res.*, **77**, 34

424

28 Lin, JC and Lin, MF (1982). Microwave hyperthermia-induced blood-brain barrier alterations. *Radiat. Res.*, **89**, 77
29. Lotz, WG (1985). Hyperthermia in radiofrequency exposed rhesus monkeys: A comparison of frequency and orientation effects. *Radiat. Res.*, **102**, 59
30. Lu, ST, Lebda, N, Michaelson, SM, Pettit, S and Rivera, D (1977). Thermal and endocrinological effects of protracted irradiation of rats by 2450 MHz microwaves. *Rad. Sci.*, **12**, supp., 147
31. Magin, RL, Lu, S-T, Michaelson, SM (1977). Stimulation of dog thyroid by local application of high intensity microwaves. *Amer. J. Physiol.*, **233**, E363
32. Mild, KH (1980). Occupational exposure to radiofrequency electromagnetic fields. IEEE 68, 12
33. Moseley, H and Davison, M (1981). Exposure of physiotherapists to microwave radiation during microwave diathermy treatment. Clin. Phys. Physiol. Meas., 2, 217
34. Moseley, H (1988). Non-ionising radiation. Adam Hilger: Bristol
35. Moseley, H and Davison, M (1989). The results of radiation leakage surveys performed annually on microwave ovens. *J. Radiol. Protection* (in press)
36. Murray, WE, Moss, CE, Parr, WH and Cox, C (1981). A radiation and industrial hygiene survey of video display terminal operations. *Hum. Factors*, **23**, 413
37. Nicholson, CP, Grotting, JC and Dimick, AR (1987). Acute microwave injury to the hand. *J. Hand. Surg.*, **12A**, 446
38. NRPB (1983). Revised guidance on acceptable limits of exposure during nuclear magnetic resonance clinical imaging. *Br. J. Radiol.*, **56**, 974
39. NRPB (1989). Guidance on standards: Guidance as to restrictions on exposures to time varying electromagnetic fields and the 1988 recommendations of the International Non-Ionizing Radiation Committee. London: HMSO
40. O'Connor, ME (1980). Mammalian teratogenesis and radiofrequency fields. *Proc. IEEE* **68**, 56
41. Oscar, KJ and Hawkins, TD (1977). Microwave alteration of the blood-brain barrier systems of rats. *Brain Res.*, **126**, 281
42. Oscar, KJ, Gruenau, SP, Folker, MT and Rapoport, SI (1981). Local cerebral blood flow after microwave exposure. *Brain Res.*, **204**, 220
43. Paz, JD, Milliken, R, Ingram, WT, Frank, A and Atkin, A (1987). Potential ocular damage from microwave exposure during electrosurgery: dosimetric survey. *J. Occup. Med.*, **29**, 580
44. Perlman, A (1980). Hazards of a microwave oven. *New Eng. J. Med.*, **302**, 970
45. Prausnitz, A and Susskind, C (1962). Effects of chronic microwave irradiation on mice. *IRE Trans. Biomed. Electron.*, **9**, 104
46. Roberts, NJ and Michaelson, SM (1983). Microwaves and neoplasia in mice: analysis of a reported risk. *Health Physics*, **46**, 430
47. Roberts, NJ, Michaelson, SM and Lu, S-T (1986). The biological effects of radiofrequency radiation: a critical review and recommendations. *Int. J. Radiat. Biol.*, **50**, 379
48. Robinette, CD, Silverman, C, Jablon, S (1980). Effects upon health of occupational exposure to microwave radiation (radar) 1950–1974. *Am. J. Epedemiol.*, **112**, 39
49. Roszkowski, W, Wrembel, JK, Roszkowski, K, Janiak, M and Szmigielski, S (1980). The search for an influence of whole-body microwave hyperthermia on anti-tumor immunity. *J. Cancer Res. Clin. Oncol.*, **96**, 311
50. Routhier, P, Mathin, AH and Ishman, RE (1986). Eye injury from microwave popcorn. *New Eng. J. Med.*, **315**, 1359
51. Rugerra, PS (1977). Near-field measurements of RF fields. In *Symposium on Biological Effects and Measurements of Radio Frequency/Microwaves.*, ed. Hazzard, DG. HEW Publication (FDA) 77–8026, p104
52. Saunders, RD and Kowalczuk (1981). Effects of 2.45 GHz microwave radiation and heat on mouse spermatogenic epithelium. *Int. J. Radiat. Biol.*, **40**, 623

425

53. Siu, V and Kisson, N (1987). Hazards of microwave ovens. *Pediatr. Emerg. Care*, 3, 99
54. Stern, S (1980). Behavioural effects of microwaves. *Neurobehav. Toxicol.*, 2, 49
55. Stuchly, MA, Repacholi, MH, Lecuyer, DW and Mann, RD (1982). Exposure to the operator and patient during short wave diathermy treatments. *Health Phys.*, 42, 341
56. Tell, RA and Harlen, F (1979). A review of selected biological effects and dosimetric data useful for development of radiofrequency safety standards for human exposure. *J. Microwave Power.*, 14, 405
57. Wachtel, H, Seaman, R and Joines, W (1975). Effects of low intensity microwaves on isolated neurons. *Ann. N.Y. Acad. Sci.*, 247, 46
58. Wangeman, RF and Cleary, SF (1976). The *in vivo* effects of 2.45 GHz microwave radiation of rabbit serum components and sleeping times. *Radiat. Environ. Biophysics.*, 13, 89
59. WHO (1981). Environmental Health Criteria 16. Radiofrequency and Microwaves. Geneva: World Health Organisation
60. Wiktor-Jedrzejczak, W, Ahmed, A, Sell, KW, Czerski, P and Leach, WM (1977). Microwaves induce an increase in the frequency of complement receptor-bearing lymphoid spleen cells in mice. *J. Immunol.*, 118, 1499
61. Williams, DB, Monaham, JP, Nicholson, WJ and Aldrich, JJ (1955). Biologic effects of studies on microwave radiation time and power thresholds for production of lens opacities by 12.3 cm microwave. *AMA Arch. Ophthalmol.*, 54, 863
62. Williams, RJ, McKee, A and Finch, ED (1975). Ultrastructural changes in the rabbit lens induced by microwave radiation. In: *Biological Effects of Non-ionizing Radiation*, ed. Taylor, P. *Ann. N.Y. Acad. Sci.*, 247, 166
63. Williams, WM, Hoss, W, Formaniak, M and Michaelson, SM (1984). Effect of 2450 MHz microwave energy on the blood-brain barrier to hydrophilic molecules. A. Effect on permeability to sodium fluorescein. *Brain Res.*, 319, 165

19 Applications of Ultrasound and their Potential Hazards

A.R. Williams

INTRODUCTION

The diverse and ever-expanding application of ultrasound in medicine, dentistry, the laboratory, industry, commercial premises and even the home means that the majority of the population is exposed to ultrasound at some time in their life (frequently without realizing that they are being exposed). It is often argued that the majority of these ultrasound exposures are not associated with any known risk. However, in many instances this complacency may be based upon the fact that we have not yet examined the most sensitive end-points, or that we have been unable to detect a relatively small change in a population having a large inherent variability, or even that suitable investigative trials have simply not been performed. It is therefore desirable that people should be aware of when they are being exposed to ultrasound and if the potential hazards which could result from that particular exposure are potentially hazardous, then relatively simple precautionary measures can usually be taken to minimize or eliminate these adverse effects. In the case of the industrial and laboratory applications of ultrasound (where some of the most serious potential hazards are to be found) it should be the responsibility of the employer, as well as the employee, to ensure that adequate safety measures are carried out. However, other exposure systems, such as the use of low-frequency airborne ultrasound as rodent repellers or burglar alarms in shops, art galleries and other buildings open to the general public, are more insidious. Here, the adverse effects may be psychological, more difficult to demonstrate, and also affect only a small proportion of the population. In this case public pressure may have to be brought to bear on both the manufacturers and users of these devices to ensure that the general public is not unnecessarily exposed to what could be an unpleasant or even a distressing level of ultrasound exposure.

DIVERSE APPLICATIONS OF ULTRASOUND

Figure 19.1 outlines some of the common applications of ultrasound in medicine and industry, many of which will be discussed in more detail later. It is apparent from this brief but diverse catalogue that ultrasound can produce a number of effects that one would not normally associate with sound waves. Since each of these separate effects may give rise to a different type of biological hazard, it would be appropriate to begin this review with a brief description of the physical properties of ultrasonic waves and to indicate how the ultrasonic energy can produce these unusual effects.

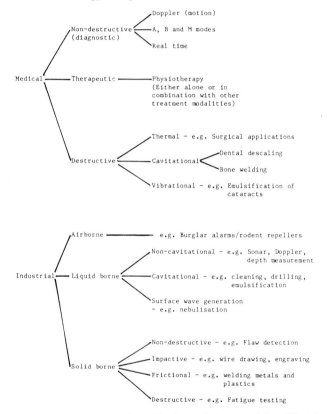

Figure 19.1 Some common uses and applications of ultrasound (modified from Williams, 1983)[1]

PHYSICAL PROPERTIES OF ULTRASOUND

Ultrasound is defined as sound waves having frequencies above the upper limit of detection by the human ear. This is commonly taken to include all sound waves having frequencies greater than 16 to 18 kHz (i.e. 16 000 to18 000 cycles per second). However, most children and many adults can detect sounds having frequencies of the order of 20 kHz at sound pressure levels of about 50 dB, and many adults complain of a sensation of pressure or 'fullness of the ears' at these same frequencies when the intensity or 'loudness' of the sound is increased.

There is no abrupt change in the physical properties of sound waves as you move from the audible to the inaudible frequencies. The velocity of sound in any given medium is independent of the frequency of that sound and so the wavelength of sound must decrease as its frequency is increased, as shown by the relationship:

$$V = f\lambda \tag{1}$$

where V is the velocity of sound, f is its frequency and λ its wavelength. The velocity of sound in air is about 340 m/s and so 20 kHz sound has a wavelength of about 1.7 cm. The velocity of sound in water is about 1500 m/s and so this same 20 kHz sound in water now has a wavelength of 7.5 cm.

POINT SOURCES AND BEAMS

Any acoustic generator whose dimensions are smaller than the wavelength of the sound it produces must emit spherical waves (i.e. waves whose leading edge is the surface of a sphere). The surface area of the spherical wave increases as it propagates away from its sources so that the power density (or intensity) of that wave must decrease as the same amount of energy is distributed over a larger area. However, a large generator which emits an acoustic wave having a wavelength much smaller than itself (e.g. a 1 inch diameter flat therapeutic transducer operating at 1 MHz in water, where the wavelength is only 1.5 mm) would emit a cylindrical beam of ultrasound. The distribution of the acoustic energy within this beam is very complex[1] but all of the energy stays within this beam unless it is lost by absorption or scattering. If a beam of ultrasound encounters a concave reflector, or if the generator itself is concave, or if the sound passes through a lens, then the ultrasound energy will be brought to a small focus where its energy density or intensity can be extremely high (of the order of thousands of W/cm^2).

PROPAGATION OF ULTRASOUND

Sound energy cannot propagate through a vacuum, and it propagates through other media by imparting energy to the particles or molecules of that medium causing them to be set into oscillation. These oscillating molecules collide with adjacent molecules passing on the energy of the wave and causing those molecules to be driven to oscillate in turn. The maximum peak-to-peak displacement of any vibrating particle is decreased as its frequency of vibration is increased (for the same input of energy). Thus, at frequencies greater than about 10^5 Hz the vibratory excursion of any molecule of a gas can be less than the average distance between the molecules of that gas. The oscillating gas molecules therefore cannot collide with other gas molecules to pass on the energy, and so the wave cannot propagate. Thus, air becomes progressively less efficient at conducting ultrasound as the frequency is raised above 20 kHz until at frequencies of several hundred kHz it may be regarded as essentially non-conducting.

ACOUSTIC MISMATCH

When a sound wave travelling in one medium encounters an interface with a different medium then the energy of that sound wave is usually partitioned such that some of it is reflected and some of it will enter the other medium. The ratio between the two is determined by the ratio of the acoustic impedances of the two media bounding that interface[2]. The acoustic impedance (Z) of a medium is defined as the product of the density of that medium times the speed at which sound travels within it; some representative values for common materials are presented in Table 19.1. The partitioning of the intensity of the transmitted wave (I_t) relative to that of the incident wave (I_i) for a sound beam encountering a large flat interface at normal incidence is given by:

$$\frac{I_t}{I_i} = \frac{4 \cdot Z_2 \cdot Z_1}{(Z_2 + Z_1)^2} \tag{2}$$

Where Z_2 and Z_1 are the acoustic impedances of the far and incident media respectively. Thus, there is 100% transmission of the sound energy if Z_2 equals Z_1, but there is progressively more reflection (and hence less transmission) as Z_2 becomes greater or less than Z_1. It is this property of generating echoes at mismatches in acoustic impedance which enables ultrasound to be used diagnostically in medicine and for flaw detection in industry or for detecting shoals of fish or submarines with Asdic or Sonar. If the reflecting surface is irregular (particularly if its dimensions are comparable with the wavelength of the sound) then the reflected acoustic wave is scattered in all directions.

ABSORPTION

The amount of energy in a uniform beam of ultrasound progressively decreases with increasing distance from its source. This loss of energy is called attenuation and is composed of the sum of scattering component described above and true absorption whereby some of the acoustic energy is converted into heat. The physical mechanisms responsible for absorption are complex

Table 19.1 Physical properties of some common materials (from Williams, 1983[1])

Material	Density (kg/m^3)	Sound velocity (m/s)	Acoustic impedance (kg/m^{2}s)	
Air (dry at STP)	1.293	331.5	429	Gases
Carbon dioxide	1.977	259	512	
Water (distilled)	0.998 x 10^3	1497	1.494 x 10^6	
Water (salt)	1.025 x 10^3	1530	1.568 x 10^6	
Ethanol	0.79 x 10^3	1210	0.956 x 10^6	
Castor oil	0.969 x 10^3	1207	1.170 x 10^6	Liquids
Chloroform	1.49 x 10^3	987	1.471 x 10^6	
Carbon tetrachloride	1.595 x 10^3	926	1.534 x 10^6	
Glycerol	1.26 x 10^3	1900	2.394 x 10^6	
Mercury	13.6 x 10^3	1450	20.0 x 10^6	
Polyethylene	0.90 x 10^3	1950	1.755 x 10^6	
Neoprene rubber	1.33 x 10^3	1600	2.128 x 10^6	
Polystyrene	1.10 x 10^3	2670	2.937 x 10^6	
Epoxy resin	1.2 x 10^3	2800	3.36 x 10^6	
Polymethylmethacrylate	1.19 x 10^3	2680	3.20 x 10^6	
Glass (crown)	2.24 x 10^3	5100	11.424 x 10^6	Solids
Glass (pyrex)	2.32 x 10^3	5640	13.085 x 10^6	
Glass (flint)	3.88 x 10^3	3980	15.442 x 10^6	
Aluminium	2.71 x 10^3	6420	17.398 x 10^6	
Brass	8.60 x 10^3	4700	40.42 x 10^6	
Stainless steel (347)	7.9 x 10^3	5790	45.74 x 10^6	

and not fully understood[1] but each tissue has its own characteristic absorption coefficient so that different tissues are heated by different amounts during a physiotherapeutic treatment. The absorption coefficient of a tissue increases with increasing frequency so that the same intensity of a higher-frequency ultrasonic beam will heat superficial tissues more than a lower-frequency beam of the same dimensions. At very high acoustic intensities the ability of water to transmit ultrasound becomes markedly non-linear, which results in the conversion of some of the ultrasonic energy to higher-frequency compo-nents[3] which are then absorbed at a faster rate than the original wave.

SURFACE WAVES AND ATOMIZATION

An ultrasonic wave propagating through a liquid will cause surface waves to be formed on any gas interface in its path. The wavelength of this surface wave (λ_s), is given by the equation derived by Lang[4] which is:

431

$$\lambda_s = \left(\frac{8\,\pi\,\sigma}{\rho f^2}\right)^{1/2} \tag{3}$$

where σ is the interfacial surface tension, ρ the density of the liquid and f the frequency of the acoustic wave. The displacement amplitude of this surface wave increases as the intensity of the driving frequency is increased. Figure 19.2 depicts three stages during one half-cycle of this surface wave. In Figure 19.2i one half-wavelength of the surface wave is moving out into the gas. In Figure 19.2ii the direction of motion is reversed, but the tip of the liquid column tends to continue and is only restrained by surface tension forces. At a high enough displacement amplitude, these forces are overcome and a droplet of the liquid breaks free and enters the gas as is shown in Figure 19.2iii. A similar process may occur during the next half-cycle of the surface wave which may result in a bubble of gas being formed within the liquid. It has been determined experimentally that the diameters of liquid droplets produced by this mechanism are roughly 0.34 times the wavelength of the surface wave providing that only small quantities of liquid are being atomized.

ACOUSTIC CAVITATION

Acoustic cavitation is a general term describing a wide range of oscillatory behaviour in gas- and/or vapour-filled bubbles in response to the large pressure changes caused by the sound wave as it passes through the fluid[5]. At one extreme, gas bubbles merely undergo a cyclical volume change (called 'breathing oscillation') at the same frequency as the low-intensity ultrasonic

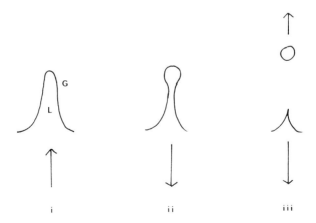

Figure 19.2 A schematic representation of the mechanism of formation of droplets of liquid (L) in a gas (G) as a result of high-amplitude surface wave activity (from Williams, 1983)[1]

source - this is commonly called 'stable cavitation'. At the other extreme, a high-intensity sound field causes minute gas bodies called 'micronuclei' to grow and then they implode violently as the acoustic pressure amplitude rises again. This latter activity is commonly called 'transient' cavitation and is associated with highly destructive shock waves and large hydrodynamic shear stresses in its immediate vicinity. It is predominantly transient cavitation which is responsible for the erosion of ships' propellers and the use of ultrasound in cleaning baths and in drilling holes in glass and diamonds. In addition to generating those highly destructive mechanical forces, a collapsing transient 'cavity' or void converts some of the incident ultrasonic energy into lower-frequency acoustic components which are re-radiated as audible 'white noise'.

At the instant of its collapse, the contents of a transient cavity may attain a temperature of several thousand degrees centigrade[6]. At these high temperatures molecules of gas and vapour will be thermally dissociated (pyrolized), yielding highly reactive free radicals. Most of these will recombine with each other within the gas phase (sometimes emitting visible light – a phenomenon called sonoluminescence), but some free radicals will persist after the cavity has collapsed and initiate various chemical reactions in the liquid phase. It is these secondary chemical reactions which form the basis for the chemical dosimetric techniques for quantifying the amount of cavitational activity which has occurred within a given medium.

STANDING WAVES

A beam of continuous-wave ultrasound in a liquid which encounters a plane interface having a large mismatch in acoustic impedance will be reflected. At normal incidence, the beam will retrace its original path and the incident and reflected beams will interfere with each other to give a standing wave field. As well as increasing the rise in temperature within the medium (since the beam now passes through each portion of the medium twice) the standing wave field also greatly amplifies the effects of radiation pressure forces[1]. These forces can cause blood cells within small blood vessels *in vivo* to be concentrated into stationary bands spaced one half-wavelength apart[7] and can greatly increase the probability of generating cavitational activity by optimizing the conditions for the growth of micronuclei[1].

DOSIMETRY OF ULTRASOUND

As with any other physical agent, the magnitude of any effects produced by ultrasound grow with increasing energy density or intensity. In fact, certain interaction mechanisms (for example, atomization or transient cavitation)

433

appear to have a 'threshold' intensity which has to be exceeded before their occurrence can be demonstrated. If we are to be able to predict the possibility of a potentially hazardous interaction, it is imperative that adequate dosimetry be performed of the relevant acoustic power densities and associated parameters at the site of their interaction with the most susceptible biological tissue.

Unfortunately, there are many inherent problems to be overcome before an 'adequate' dosimetric protocol can be decided upon. For example, the energy density of low-frequency airborne ultrasound required to damage the ear would have a negligible effect on, say, the thigh muscle if that same wave was propagating through water. This difference in biological sensitivity also illustrates the fact that ultrasound can be coupled into the human body through the air, through a liquid or by direct contact with a vibrating solid. Each different propagation medium has its own preferred range of detection systems which usually measure different parameters of the acoustic wave and consequently express the energy density of the ultrasound in different units as described in more detail below.

DOSIMETRY OF AIRBORNE ULTRASOUND

Ultrasonic microphones measure changes in air pressure caused by the passage of an acoustic wave. Recent advances in microphone technology have resulted in electrostatic types[8] with linear frequency ranges up to a few hundred kHz, and piezoelectric ceramic types with quarter-wavelength matching to air and resonant frequencies[9] up to 400 kHz. The ratio of the measured pressure (p) to that of some arbitrary reference pressure (p_r) gives the sound pressure level (SPL) according to the equation:

$$SPL \ (dB) = 20 \log_{10} \left(\frac{p}{p_r} \right) \qquad (4)$$

Where the reference pressure (p_r) is usually taken as 20μPascals or 20μNewtons/m^2. (i.e. the minimum detectable audible frequency sound level; which is equivalent to an acoustic intensity of 10^{-12} W/m^2). The actual determination of decibel levels at various positions in an airborne ultrasound field can be made with several commercially available systems[10,11]. These normally include a capacitor microphone sensing element having a flat frequency response within the range of interest, and signal processing circuitry. Usually, this circuitry includes a set of one-third octave filters, so that the additive SPL within any particular one-third octave frequency range is indicated on the meter. A spectrum of SPL as a function of frequency (to one-third octave resolution) can be obtained by 'stepping through' the filter set. When making

434

SPL measurements, humidity and temperature conditions should be taken into account[12].

DOSIMETRY OF LIQUID-BORNE ULTRASOUND

Many approaches have been employed for the measurement of ultrasonic power, intensity and other field quantities such as pressure, particle displacement and particle velocity of ultrasound traversing a water bath[2,12-14]. By tradition, the ultrasound exposure is expressed in terms of an intensity parameter (which is obtained by averaging some measure of the acoustic power emitted by the transducer over a given area) and the duration of the ultrasonic exposure. These intensity parameters are specified in most standards, e.g. AIUM–NEMA (1981)[15], Japanese standards for diagnostic equipment (JIS, 1981)[16], and the Canadian (1981)[17] and American (FDA, 1978)[18] standards for the performance of ultrasound therapy equipment.

The complexities in the definitions of the various intensity parameters arise from the fact that a beam of megahertz ultrasound is markedly non-uniform[1], and from the fact that the ultrasound can be delivered either as a continuous wave or chopped up into discrete pulses which may be non-uniform in the time domain as well as spatially. In the simplest case, a point detector (e.g. a piezoelectric transducer having dimensions of the order of a millimetre) can be used to obtain the cross-sectional distribution of energy in a continuous-wave beam at the region of interest, i.e. the beam profile. If the total amount of ultrasonic energy within the beam is measured by means of some averaging system (e.g. a radiation force technique) then this value can be divided by the area of the beam (derived from the beam profile) to obtain the spatially averaged intensity. The spatial peak intensity at the centre of this beam is typically 3 to 6 times larger than the spatial average intensity. If this same beam is now chopped into pulses, then the spatial average time average intensity (I_{SATA}) includes the off time of the transducer whereas the spatial average temporal peak intensity (I_{SATP}) remains the same as that of the original continuous wave beam provided that each pulse had a rapid rise and fall time. A similar pair of temporal average and temporal peak intensities may be defined for the spatial peak intensity giving I_{SPTA} and I_{SPTP} respectively. By way of an example, the I_{SPTP} of a manual compound scanner diagnostic unit can be up to about 200 watts/cm^2 whereas the I_{SPTA} of the same device may be only 10 to 100 milliwatts/cm^2.

DOSIMETRY OF SOLID-BORNE ULTRASOUND

It is not practicable to measure the pressure changes within a homogeneous solid as an acoustic wave propagates through it. One alternative is to clamp

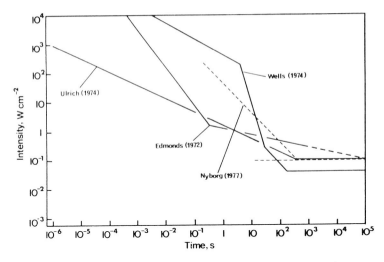

Figure 19.3 A compilation of the most commonly quoted 'threshold' or 'boundary' curves for liquid-borne exposure to megahertz ultrasound (from Williams, 1983)[1]

or cement an accelerometer to the vibrating surface (if it is large) and to measure the acceleration of the radiating surface. Another is to directly measure the displacement amplitude of the vibrating surface (i.e. half its maximum peak-to-peak excursion). The displacement amplitude may be measured optically, or by means of a strain gauge or by the changes in the inductance or impedance induced within a solenoid.

Because of the very large mismatch in acoustic impedance between steel and water or steel and air (c.f. Table 19.1), most of the ultrasonic energy within a waveguide or probe will be reflected back into the metal so that the amount being radiated is small even though the displacement amplitude of the interface may be large. In the case of a metal probe vibrating at high displacement amplitudes in water, transient cavitational activity occurs close to the interface, which further lowers the perceived impedance of the liquid. This results in even more of the incident wave within the metal being reflected, a phenomenon commonly called 'cavitation unloading'.

RECOMMENDED EXPOSURE LIMITS FOR LIQUID-BORNE MEGAHERTZ ULTRASOUND

Several authors have compiled the positive bioeffect results known at that time and displayed the data on a single graph where one axis is a measure of the acoustic intensity to which that biological system had been exposed while the other is a measure of the duration of the exposure (see Figure 19.3). A series of lines were then drawn below that portion of the intensity/time

436

domain where positive results had been reported. It is presumed that the acoustic exposure conditions below these lines represent a 'safe' region where biological tissue can be exposed without producing a biological effect or potential hazard. It is further presumed that the position of the boundary zone will be progressively lowered to smaller intensity/time combination as more sensitive biological end-points are investigated. It should be noted that the positive bioeffect data points used to define the position of each curve in Figure 19.3 represent the intensity/time combinations which happened to be used by those authors for their experiments, and generally do not represent the minimum or 'threshold' exposure conditions below which that observed bioeffect did not occur. In addition, most of the data points have not been confirmed in an independent laboratory.

However, the most serious criticism of these curves is that the data used to compile them usually employed continuous-wave ultrasound. Thus, a pulsed ultrasonic field having a long interpulse interval (e.g. pulse-echo diagnostic equipment) would have a time-averaged intensity which would be well below any of the curves in Figure 19.3 while the intensity within each pulse could perhaps be high enough to produce a biological effect. This may be reflected in a number of recent bioeffect reports which describe changes in living systems following exposure to pulsed diagnostic ultrasound fields[1]. Most of these articles were not available when the curves presented in Figure 19.3 were compiled. While it is not possible to single out any one of these recent articles using pulsed ultrasound as proof that diagnostic intensities of ultrasound may be hazardous, when viewed as a whole they suggest that the so-called 'threshold' curves derived from continuous-wave ultrasound exposures may not be applicable to pulsed ultrasound.

The bioeffects committee of the American Institute of Ultrasound in Medicine issued a statement in 1976 (and reaffirmed it in 1978 and 1982), which was essentially a verbal description of the curve of Nyborg[5] presented in Figure 19.3. The statement is:

Statement on mammalian in vivo ultrasonic biological effects (1976, 1978, 1982)

In the low megahertz frequency range there have been (as of this date) no demonstrated significant biological effects in mammalian tissues exposed to intensities* below 100 mW/cm^2. Furthermore, for ultrasonic exposure times less than 500 seconds and greater than 1 second, such effects have not been demonstrated even at higher intensities when the product of intensity and exposure time† is less than 50 Joules/cm^2

* Spatial peak, temporal average intensity as measured in a free field in water (using a miniature hydrophone whose sensitive area is smaller than the distance over which the local value of the ultrasonic field intensity shows a significant variation).
† Total exposure time: this includes off time as well as on time for a repeated-pulse regime.

Despite the clear instructions of its authors, this statement is frequently used out of context as 'proof' that diagnostic intensities of ultrasound are 'safe', even though it suffers from the same limitations as the 'threshold' curves in Figure 19.3.

The major disadvantage of statements such as the one above, or the 'threshold' curves of Figure 19.3, is that they tend to be adopted by the regulatory agencies of various national governments and incorporated into legislation as the 'scientific basis' for a maximum upper limit of emission from diagnostic devices. This is disturbing because there would be a tendency for instrument manufacturers to increase their power output (so as to obtain better-quality images) and to converge towards the permitted maximum. This could be particularly hazardous in the case of pulsed-mode devices because their 'threshold' intensity for the production of adverse effects could be much less than that of continuous-mode devices, especially if the mechanism of interaction is different and the crucial physical parameter is peak pressure amplitude and not time-average intensity.

RECOMMENDED EXPOSURE LIMITS FOR AIRBORNE ULTRASOUND

The acoustic power densities for airborne ultrasound are usually so much lower than that commonly encountered with liquid-borne ultrasound, and the impedance mismatch between air and skin is so large (more than 99% reflection), that it is unlikely that enough airborne acoustic energy will enter the human body (other than through the ear) to produce any adverse biological effects. This is not true for small fur-bearing mammals where the fur can act as an impedance matching layer and absorb enough ultrasound to raise the whole body temperature to a lethal level[10].

The ear-drum and middle ear apparatus forms an efficient impedance transformer between air and the fluid-filled cochlea, and while its transmission properties generally decrease with increasing ultrasonic frequency, it still delivers appreciable (though not accurately quantified) amounts of ultrasonic energy to the cochlea. The human cochlea does not have specific receptors for ultrasonic frequencies and so it is presumed that the ultrasound either 'enhances the sensitivities' of the sensory cells to other lower-frequency audible sounds or that some of the energy of the ultrasound is converted into subharmonics and other lower-frequency components (as a result of non-linearities in the behaviour of the eardrum and the propagation medium) which the cochlea can then detect[19-21]. However, several researchers in this field have come to the conclusion that the dominant factor responsible for the range of auditory and subjective effects following exposure to high levels of airborne ultrasound is not the ultrasound itself but the associated high levels of high-frequency audible sound[10,22,23].

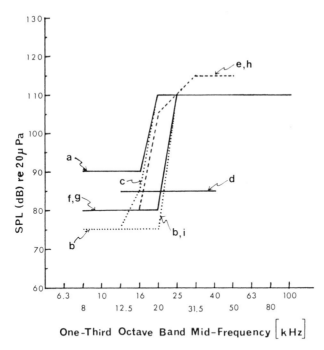

Figure 19.4 A graphical compilation of the maximum occupational exposure limits recommended for airborne ultrasound by:
a (Japan, 1971)[52]; **b** (Acton, 1975)[53]; **c** (USSR, 1975)[54]; **d** (USAF, 1976)[56]; **e** (Sweden, 1978)[56]; **f** (Canada, 1980)[57]; **g** (IRPA, 1981)[24]; **h** (ACGIH, 1981)[58]; and **i** (IRPA, 1984)[25]

Figure 19.4 presents a graphical compilation of the maximum SPL exposure limits in dB (relative to 20 μPascals) as a function of frequency, which have been adopted or proposed by various regulatory bodies and national governments. The experimental evidence upon which these curves are based is reviewed in Refs. 10, 24 and 25. These values refer to the maximum permitted levels for a person who is exposed to that particular frequency during the course of their employment for a total of 4 hours or more each day. Shorter periods of exposure, or exposure to an intermittent ultrasonic source, permit higher SPL values, usually rising by 3 dB if the daily exposure is between 2 and 4 hours, by 6 dB if between 1 and 2 hours, or by 9 dB if the daily exposure is less than 1 hour[25]. Since different countries may use different maximum exposure limits and also have different scaling factors for short-time or intermittent exposures, any interested party is advised to contact their own regulatory agency for the regulations which apply in their own country.

Table 19.2 presents the SPL limits for continuous exposure of the general population to airborne ultrasonic energy as recommended by the International Radiation Protection Association[24,25]. It should be noted that an

439

increase in the SPL of 3 dB is equivalent to doubling the acoustic pressure at that site.

PRECAUTIONS TO BE TAKEN IN THE MEDICAL APPLICATIONS OF ULTRASOUND

Diagnostic devices

A representative range of the ultrasonic intensities emitted by some common diagnostic devices is presented in Table 19.3. It can be seen that the space-averaged – time-averaged intensities range from extremely low values (especially for those devices which emit short pulses of ultrasound) up to about 400 mW/cm^2 for some peripheral vascular doppler units. Recent measurements (not included in Table 19.3) on doppler devices which are used to measure various indices of fetal blood flow show that many emit ultrasonic intensities greater than the value quoted in the AIUM statement presented above[13]. Thus, while there is no direct evidence that humans exposed to diagnostic ultrasound devices have suffered any adverse effects[1] the time-averaged intensities emitted by some of these units fall within the range where biological effects have been observed under laboratory conditions.

Table 19.2 Recommended limits of continuous airborne ultrasound exposure to the general public

Mid-frequency of one-third octave band (kHz)	SPL within one-third octave band (dB re: 20 μPa)		
	IRPA, 1981[24]		IRPA, 1984[25]
	Day	Night	
8	41	31	—
10	42	32	—
12.5	44	34	—
16	46	36	—
20	49	39	70
25	110	110	100
31.5	110	110	100
40	110	110	100
50	110	110	100
63	—	—	100
80	—	—	100
100	—	—	100

Table 19.3 Range of acoustic output parameters from medical-diagnostic equipment (compiled from the data of Carson et al.[34], Hill[59] and Rooney[60])

Equipment type	Frequency range (MHz)	Total power output (mW	Spatial average time average (SATA) (mW/cm^2)	Spatial peak temporal peak (SPTP) (mW/cm^2)	Typical duty factor
Pulse/echo	1–20	0.3–20	0.2–10	5×10^2–2×10^5	0.001
Fetal heart (doppler)	2–4	1–40	0.2–20	1–60	1
Peripheral vascular (doppler)	5–10	1–40	40–400	1–2×10^3	0.01–1

In an endeavour to minimize the possibility of risk, humans should be exposed to diagnostic ultrasound only where there is a valid medical reason for its use. Thus, individuals should not be encouraged to use themselves as convenient 'test objects' when servicing or repairing equipment or for the commercial demonstration of new devices or ultrasonic techniques. It is recommended that the organizers of major clinical meetings forbid the use of human models (and pregnant women in particular) and encourage the use of inanimate phantoms (which can be a more rigorous and objective evaluation of the performance of any instrument) and the use of prerecorded audiovisual displays.

Each diagnostic instrument should clearly display its output characteristics[15] in a standardized format so that the operators may elect to choose the device which emits the least acoustic power. Ideally, each instrument should be equipped with an adjustable power output control knob so that the clinician can use the minimum acoustic exposure necessary to obtain the relevant diagnostic information. If it is found that a certain diagnostic procedure requires a relatively high acoustic exposure, then all the preliminary site detection and alignment procedures should be performed at a lower exposure level and the higher value used only for the data gathering portion of the investigation.

In the interest of patient safety, the duration of ultrasonic investigation and the 'dwell time' of the transducer (i.e. the residence time of the ultrasonic beam on any given organ or region of interest) should be kept as low as is practicably possible. All of these recommendations are directed towards the goal of obtaining the least patient exposure compatible with retaining the optimum diagnostic information.

Therapeutic devices

These devices pose particular problems for the various regulatory agencies because they emit acoustic intensities up to about 3–4 W/cm^2, i.e. well within the exposure range where numerous undesirable biological effects have been reported. According to Lehmann and de Lateur[26] the fibrous connective tissues have to be heated to temperatures within the range 42-45 °C (i.e. to a temperature where a prolonged exposure would result in thermal damage) before there is evidence of a beneficial therapeutic effect. If these devices are restricted to the same maximum-intensity output as diagnostic devices then they are unlikely to be of any therapeutic value. There must therefore be an element of risk associated with any effective therapeutic ultrasound exposure. This can only be offset if the real or presumed benefits of the treatment are significantly greater than any potential risk. Unfortunately, physiotherapists have generally been reluctant to carry out well-controlled trials to evaluate the effectiveness of their treatment. As a consequence, it is not possible to quantify the beneficial effects of therapeutic ultrasound despite the fact that many experienced therapists frequently quote spectacular results which have convinced them that their ultrasonic treatments are extremely effective. On the other hand there is as yet no evidence of adverse sequelae resulting from therapeutic exposures. This stalemate situation, where one is trying to balance or equate two unquantified parameters, is unsatisfactory in that any study which clearly indicates that there is a significant hazard associated with therapeutic treatments will probably lead to the banning of therapeutic ultrasound. It is therefore recommended that physiotherapists devise well-controlled clinical trials to evaluate the effectiveness of their ultrasonic treatment while they still have the opportunity to do so[1]. Another advantage of conducting trials is that ineffective treatment can be identified and either modified so as to be effective or replaced with an alternative treatment regime.

In practice, patients generally receive space- and time-averaged intensities significantly less than 3 W/cm^2. Providing that the patient has normal sensation and is fully conscious, the ultrasonic intensity is gradually raised until the patient experiences a sensation of mild warmth. If a tingling sensation of pain is experienced in the area of treatment then the power level must be reduced. This approach is preferable to the one adopted by many physiotherapists whereby the same extremely low 'dose' is recommended for all patients having a given 'condition'. This has the twin disadvantages that the patient may be exposed to any hazards associated with the use of ultrasound whilst at the same time receiving an ultrasonic 'dose' which may be too low to be effective.

Patients who are anaesthetized or who have an impaired ability to detect or express the sensation of pain ought not to be exposed to therapeutic ultrasound. Liberal amounts of coupling medium should be used to ensure efficient acoustic transmission and the transducer ought to be kept in motion throughout the duration of the treatment. The use of a stationary transducer ought to be strongly discouraged as it may result in the formation of standing waves and the development of cavitational activity as well as possibly over-heating the tissues. Another disadvantage of using a stationary transducer mounted in a clamp or rack is that the therapist may be distracted or even leave the treatment room so that the patient who is experiencing discomfort (caused by too high an intensity) has no-one to complain to and bears the pain until the therapist returns, with consequent thermal damage.

The major contraindications for the use of therapeutic intensities of ultrasound are: (1) the fetus should not be exposed under any circumstances and so ultrasound should never be used to alleviate back pain of muscular origin during pregnancy; (2) the beating heart should not be irradiated; (3) if possible, the irradiation of blood pools and major blood vessels should be avoided in patients with a history of thrombophlebitis or thromboembolic disorders; (4) the irradiation of tissues which have an ineffectual blood supply with high intensities of ultrasound should be avoided; and (5) the subjection of the epiphyses of children's bones to excessive intensities should be avoided as this may restrict their rate of growth. Damage to bone is of particular concern in physiotherapy because not only does bone have a high absorption coefficient so that it is heated more than the surrounding soft tissues, but also the acoustic impedance mismatch at the bony interface results in some mode conversion to shear waves which deposits a lot of energy as heat within the periosteum[1]. It is presumably this periosteal heating which gives the sensation of pain if a hand is inadvertently placed in a moderately intense beam of ultrasound.

Therapists ought to ensure that they do not expose themselves unnecessarily to ultrasound, by refraining from immersing their hands at any point in the water bath during a treatment period. Similarly, therapists ought not to use any portion of their anatomy as a portable 'meter' to check that their transducer is emitting acoustic energy. They should also report any device which is behaving abnormally (i.e. it elicits a feeling of warmth at an unusually low output intensity or else is unable to produce a feeling of warmth even at its maximum output). A therapist complained that one European device was unpleasant to operate in that her fingers tingled and became stiff after treating two or more patients consecutively. On examination it was found that due to a faulty design of the transducer mounting, the acoustic intensity at a portion of the therapist's fingertips was greater than that received by the patient[27].

Dental devices

Despite the large number of patients each year whose teeth are descaled using an ultrasonic device, there has been relatively little research on the effects of the treatment on the tooth, and most of this has been concerned with the efficiency of the cleaning process. Ultrasonic descalers are potentially hazardous in that they operate at low ultrasonic frequencies (*ca*. 15–40 kHz) where the threshold for the generation of cavitational activity is much lower than that at megahertz frequencies. In fact, these devices utilize the cavitational activity produced within their cooling spray to assist in the removal of calcified plaque and other surface debris[28]. It has been shown that dental descaling devices are efficient initiators of thrombus formation within mammalian blood *in vitro*[29], but it is not known if this ultrasonic energy may be conducted through the tooth and possibly initiate thrombus formation within the blood vessels of the pulp cavity. This is currently under investigation. It is nevertheless reassuring to know that despite the inherently destructive nature of this ultrasonic technique, there have been no reports of adverse sequelae[30,31] provided that the temperature rise within the pulp cavity is minimized by cooling[32].

The other potential hazards associated with the use of ultrasonic dental descaling devices include: (1) thermal damage resulting from a suboptimal flow of cooling water; (2) 'gouging' of the surface of the enamel if the vibrating tip is not kept in motion; (3) conduction of the ultrasonic energy through the tooth and into the surrounding bone where it may initiate deleterious changes; and (4) damage to the structures of the inner ear. The sensory elements of the cochlea and vestibule are normally protected from high displacement amplitude airborne sounds having frequencies of the order of tens of kilohertz by the relatively high absorption coefficient of air and by the inefficient mechanical conduction system of the eardrum and the ossicles of the middle ear. However, ultrasonic descaling circumvents this inbuilt protective mechanism and couples the ultrasonic energy directly to the bones of the skull via the tooth. Despite the high attenuation coefficient of bone (which is much less at kilohertz frequencies than it is at megahertz frequencies) and the diverging nature of the acoustic beam (i.e. the probe tip acts as a point source of ultrasound), the displacement amplitudes of the acoustic waves transmitted to the inner ear by bone conduction may be high enough to damage the sensory structures (especially while descaling the upper molars and premolars). This potential hazard has not been adequately investigated, but it has been reported[33] that some patients complained of tinnitus and exhibited temporary threshold hearing shifts (a commonly accepted index of early damage to hearing) after their maxillary teeth had been descaled using an ultrasonic device.

Another potential hazard associated with ultrasonic descaling which has received scant attention is the damage to the soft tissues at the gingival margins. Ultrasonic cavitation within the cooling water in the vicinity of the gingivae could produce petechial lesions[34] and also drive small particles of dislodged calculus (and bacteria) into the gingival tissues. Also, accidental contact with the probe tip results in areas of necrosis which may become infected. It is not known if the gingival damage associated with careless descaling results in an increased incidence of gingival infection.

There has been some concern that the electrical or magnetic fields produced by dental descaling devices may interfere with the discharge rate of cardiac pacemakers[35]. In an early report[36], where one dog fitted with a pacemaker was exposed to an ultrasonic scaler no change in its output was detected. Luker[37] immersed a cardiac pacemaker in a saline water bath and found that its output was not affected by magnetostrictive or piezoelectric descaling devices. However, it has been shown[38] that magnetostrictive devices could change the discharge rate of cardiac pacemakers if they were within 6 cm of each other; piezoelectric devices having no effect. This apparent change in discharge rate may be the result of a demand type of pacemaker switching over to a fixed-mode output in response to the electrical interference induced by the descaler[39].

Finally, there is a hazard associated with the aerosol or fine mist of droplets of the cooling water generated by surface wave activity during the descaling process. Oral bacteria may be incorporated within these airborne droplets and their inhalation may result in an increased incidence of respiratory infections for both operator and patient[40,41]. This risk may be minimized by the use of an adequate suction apparatus close to the tip of the ultrasonic probe and/or the use of a face mask having a small pore size[42].

Surgical devices

Several patents have been filed in many countries for a sharp cutting blade[43] to be driven to vibrate in its longitudinal mode at 20 to 30 kHz. The advantages claimed for these 'ultrasonic scalpels' are that the small-scale 'sawing' action cuts the tissues cleanly without tearing them and that the blade cauterizes the tissues so that the normal microvascular blood loss is reduced or absent. No detailed histological comparisons of the healing rates of wounds made by the ultrasonic and conventional scalpels have been reported and it must be presumed that these devices do not offer a substantial improvement in surgical procedure since they have not been adopted into common use.

Analogous devices employing an ultrasonically vibrating saw blade have been advocated for use in the cutting of bone. Grasshoff[44] has compared the rates of healing of bones cut with these ultrasonic saws with bones cut using conventional saws, and concluded that on average bone repair occurred more slowly after ultrasonic osteotomy even though the results were highly variable. This delayed repair may be a reflection of increased thermal damage to the bone resulting from frictional contact during the cutting process.

Low-frequency ultrasound (*ca*. 20-30 kHz) may also be used as part of the procedure used in what is commonly called bone welding. This technique is used to fuse the pieces of a broken bone together under conditions where it is not possible to mechanically hold them together by means of a splint or a plaster cast. The bone is surgically exposed in the vicinity of the fracture and a fluid paste composed of a mixture of bone powder and a monomer which polymerizes by a free radical mechanism is forced into the fissure of the fracture and around a splint of bone or an inert solid material. The region is then subjected to low-frequency ultrasonic vibration from a hand-held probe whose tip is vibrating longitudinally[45] with displacement amplitudes as high as 45 μm. The free radicals generated by transient acoustic cavitation and the high local temperatures produced by frictional contact with the vibrating tip cause the monomer to polymerize. Preliminary clinical trials using this technique are claimed to be successful[46,47], but the long-term effects of the permanent polymeric mass on the strength of the bone and the local and systemic effects of any non-polymerized monomer have not been fully investigated. In view of the many potential sources of biological damage associated with this technique, it should not be used until further investigative studies have been performed, and only then if there is no other practicable means of holding the broken edges of the bone in opposition[1].

Wells[2] describes many other surgical applications of low-frequency ultrasound, including its use in the fragmentation and disruption of kidney stones and gall-bladder calculi. However, the only technique which has achieved any measure of popularity has been the phacoemulsification procedure devised by Kelman[48] for the *in situ* liquefaction and aspiration of cataractous lenses. In common with many other ophthalmological procedures, great care must be exercised so as not to damage the sensitive epithelium lining the anterior chamber and to prevent contact between the cornea and any vibrating portion of the probe.

PRECAUTIONS TO BE TAKEN IN THE LABORATORY USES OF ULTRASOUND

The major applications of ultrasound in the laboratory are in cleaning baths (originally designed for washing and degreasing glassware and intricate metal components) or in tissue disruptors for homogenizing tissues and rupturing the tough capsules of yeasts and bacterial cells. Both of these devices are now also used for a variety of other applications. For example, some laboratories use the cavitational activity occurring within a cleaning bath filled with an aqueous biocidal agent as an adjunct to greatly improve the efficiency of cold sterilization of thermolabile materials. Other applications of cleaning baths include: (1) the disaggregation of granular or particulate material prior to its use, (2) the disaggregation of clumps of viral particles prior to their enumeration, and (3) to accelerate the penetration of the liquid within the bath into

446

an inert porous solid. The tissue disruptors are also used for a variety of functions in addition to the ones for which they were originally designed; these include: (1) the emulsification of immiscible liquids, (2) the degradation of long-chain polymeric materials to shorter fragments, (3) the formation of lipid miscelles, and (4) to cold-weld plastics together.

Other laboratory sources of airborne ultrasound can arise from the use of some electronic equipment, from high-speed drills and motors, or from whistles (or even leaks) when high-pressure gas systems are being employed. Some laboratories use ultrasonic nebulizers to atomize liquids, as for example when one wishes to have small droplets containing a drug for inhalation therapy in a hospital or for delivering a substance by a respiratory route to an animal in a toxicology laboratory. Laboratories may also be fitted with ultrasonic intruder alarms or rodent repellers, but these ought not to be emitting ultrasound during the period when the laboratory is being occupied. The most common high-intensity sources of ultrasound in the laboratory environment are therefore the cleaning bath and the ultrasonic disruptor.

Ultrasonic cleaning baths

These are usually metal baths having a low-frequency (15-40 kHz) transducer attached to the underside of the bath by means of an epoxy resin. The bath is filled with an aqueous medium which usually contains a detergent or a caustic material to aid cleaning, and the mixture is driven to cavitate. The potential hazards of these devices fall into two distinct categories; one is the damage to the sensory structures of the inner ear resulting from airborne acoustic waves, and the other is the debridement of skin by the cavitation-induced streaming.

The airborne ultrasound emitted at the fundamental frequency of the device is not likely to pose a significant threat to hearing because of the relatively high attenuation coefficient of the air to the ultrasound and the inefficient mechanical transmission characteristics of the middle ear. However, the transient cavitation re-radiates a substantial amount of energy as white noise and also an intense 'peak' at the first subharmonic of the driving frequency. This intense subharmonic signal is usually within or close to the audible range and consequently poses a significant threat to hearing unless the bath is located within a sound-proofed cabinet, or some form of ear protection is worn.

Operators of ultrasonic cleaning baths ought not to immerse their bare hands in the bath while it is cavitating. The acoustic energy is efficiently coupled from water into soft tissues and so cavitational activity may be generated within the tissues of the hand even though this was not detected in the hazardous experiments reported by Fishman[49]. Cavitational activity within the bath may produce petechial lesions on bare skin[34] and will also

447

remove the outermost layers of the epidermis exposing the more permeable cells which enables molecules of detergent or caustic material to penetrate the skin and initiate an allergic dermatitis. It is therefore recommended that rubber gloves must be worn if the hands have to be immersed in the bath while it is cavitating. The layer of air trapped between the glove and the fingers acts as an efficient barrier to acoustic transmission as well as the glove itself preventing debridement of the outer epithelial layers.

Another potential hazard of ultrasonic cleaning baths which is usually neglected is the formation of an aerosol at the liquid/air interface by surface wave activity. Baths which are correctly filled and have adequate cavitational activity to scatter and absorb the acoustic energy should not form aerosols. However, baths containing too little liquid, or solid bodies which can either reflect or act as an acoustic lens and focus the ultrasound at the surface can result in the formation of an aerosol. These small airborne droplets will contain the detergent or caustic material used as a cleaning agent (and may also contain bacteria living in the bath and using these substances as a food source) and so can cause a variety of unpleasant sequelae if inhaled. It is therefore recommended that these cleaning baths are well ventilated and/or are supplied with a close-fitting lid.

The ideal site for a small-scale ultrasonic cleaning bath is within a sound-proofed cabinet or box which is vented with negative pressure ventilation (preferably into a fume cupboard) when the access door is opened.

Cell disruptors

These are usually robust low ultrasonic frequency (15–30 kHz) magnetostric-tive or piezoelectric transducers coupled to titanium or stainless steel velocity transformers or probes[2]. The free tip of the probe may be pointed or chisel-shaped (as for some plastic welding applications) or left flat if it is to be immersed in a solution or slurry. Aqueous media are driven to cavitate vigorously near the face of the probe and therefore radiate intense subhar-monic and white noise extending into the audible region. Many of these devices are supplied with a soundproofed cabinet which should be closed when the instrument is being operated. It is strongly recommended that the users of hand-held devices wear some form of effective hearing protection if they are going to use these devices for more than a few seconds or on a routine basis.

The vibrating probe should not be brought into direct contact with the skin. A sliding contact can give a severe friction burn in less than a second (depending upon the displacement amplitude), while direct contact normal to the face of the probe can generate cavitational activity within the skin leading to severe subcutaneous tissue damage[50]. It has been shown[51] that the application of a hand-held 25 kHz device to the outside of an intact vena cava

448

in a rabbit resulted in the formation of an intravascular blood clot even when the instrument was detuned, i.e. driven at a minimal power setting.

Other hazards associated with the use of these cell disrupters are similar to those described above for the ultrasonic cleaning baths. Cavitational activity can remove the outer layers of the skin and facilitate chemical agents in the cavitating liquid to penetrate the skin. The uptake of chemical agents may be directly assisted by the acoustic wave - a phenomenon called 'phono-phoresis'[1]. Care should therefore be exercised to ensure that the hand is not immersed in, or is even holding, the vessel in which the oscillating probe is being used.

The possibility of aerosol formation is even greater with these probe devices than it is with the cleaning baths. Suitable protective measures must therefore be taken whenever hazardous chemical or infective organisms are being irradiated.

General conclusion

This article indicates some of the major potential hazards arising from the laboratory uses of ultrasound. Apart from the potential damage to hearing, the main sources of hazard arise from negligent experimental technique (i.e. touching probes or inserting one's hand into a cleaning bath) or inhaling an aerosol which contains a potentially irritating or noxious material. These devices therefore ought not to be used by untrained personnel.

PRECAUTIONS TO BE TAKEN IN THE INDUSTRIAL APPLICATIONS OF ULTRASOUND

The enormous diversity of the industrial uses of ultrasound means that it is not practicable to discuss the safety precautions which ought to be applied to each individual application. Instead, those devices having common sources of potential hazard will be grouped together and some elementary precautions will be indicated.

Many industries use ultrasonic cleaning baths for washing and degreasing intricate or delicate components. The potential hazards and safety precautions to be applied with these devices are the same as those described above for their laboratory applications.

Similarly, many industrial processes use a device similar to a tissue homogenizer to generate intense cavitational activity for the large-scale disruption of bacterial or fungal cells (prior to the extraction of antibiotics, etc.), or for drilling holes in hard metals, glass or diamond (aided by the use of an abrasive slurry), or for homogenizing fruit extracts so that they can be super-concentrated. The major potential hazards are again the high levels of audible 'white noise' and the first subharmonic of the driving frequency radiated by the cavitating bubbles or cavities, as well as the possibility of aerosol formation.

Both longitudinal and torsional modes of vibration are used to weld plastics and some metals by causing friction at the point of contact of the two workpieces. Once the temperature is high enough to melt the materials at the interface, the molten surfaces fuse together and so eliminate the interface. The ultrasonic wave would then propagate through the new weld without depositing any more energy so that the weld rapidly cools down. The potential hazards arising from the use of these welding devices are that ultrasound may enter the operator's hand if either of the workpieces is being held, or that audible subharmonics may be generated during the transduction process, especially in the case of magnetostrictive transducers. Also, the airborne ultrasound levels in the vicinity of the transducer may exceed the levels indicated in Figure 19.4, particularly for the metal-to-metal welding devices used in the automotive industry. The obvious protective measures are to eliminate the possibility of direct contact with the workpieces or the vibrating probe (or to issue gloves if this is not practicable) and to recommend that ear protection effective at ultrasonic frequencies be worn. Similar potential hazards arise in the use of high amplitude longitudinal vibrations in a standing-wave mode for the fatigue testing of metal components. Here direct contact with the operator's hand is likely to result in a severe friction burn.

Less common applications of high-amplitude, low-frequency ultrasound are to drive a wire-drawing die to vibrate in a radial mode so as to reduce the tension which has to be developed to pull the wire through the die, and to drive the cutting tool on a lathe in its longitudinal mode to aid the machining of very hard materials. There is the possibility of the direct coupling of some ultrasound into the operator's body through the machine housing in both cases, but this is not usually likely to be a significant health hazard. However, a more serious potential threat is posed by the possible atomization of the cutting oils and cooling emulsions by the ultrasound. These materials are of petrochemical origin and usually contain small quantities of potentially carcinogenic materials which should not be inhaled. These devices ought therefore to be fitted with some form of extraction/ventilation system if there is any evidence of atomization of the cutting or cooling lubricants.

Ultrasonic engraving tools should be designed so that the amplitude of vibration of the handpiece is close to zero. This should be checked if the operator complains of excessive fatigue or exhibits symptoms of Raynaud's disease (i.e. vibration white finger syndrome). An additional absorbent rubber overgrip should eliminate any problems. Of more concern is the possibility of direct coupling of the ultrasound into the operator if the workpiece is hand-held (this may be overcome by the use of a glove), and the potential audiological hazard of the airborne ultrasound. It would be expected that the levels or airborne ultrasound generated during the engraving process would be quite high because of the additional radiation from the impactive or 'chipping' action of the tool tip on the metal workpiece.

High-frequency ultrasound in the megahertz range is also used in industry in a manner analogous to its use in diagnostic medicine. It is commonly used for a variety of applications including the detection of flaws and cracks in metal castings and the measurement of the rate of decrease of wall thickness in a metal tube transporting a corrosive liquid. It is unlikely that the low acoustic powers used in these devices will pose any significant hazard to the operator or his neighbours even if they come into contact with the metal workpiece being examined.

PRECAUTIONS TO BE TAKEN IN THE COMMERCIAL APPLICATIONS OF ULTRASOUND

By far the most widespread domestic application of ultrasound is the use of quartz chips and metal tuning forks as the resonators in clocks and watches. However the low amplitude of oscillation and the large impedance mismatch between these resonators and air means that the levels of airborne or solid borne ultrasound emitted by these devices is so low that it is unlikely that they pose any health hazard. Ultrasonic rangefinders in cameras also emit very little ultrasonic energy.

Similarly, the domestic uses of ultrasonic channel selectors to remotely control TV sets or other electronic equipment only pose a low potential hazard in view of their low power output and intermittent use. However, they may still prove to be a source of annoyance to some people who can hear a little in that frequency range, or to household pets, e.g. dogs, who may respond by barking.

Significantly higher sound pressure levels of airborne ultrasound are radiated by intrusion or burglar alarms[11]. These devices work by transmitting a spherical wave and 'tuning' the detector to ignore the echoes from the room's contents. Any new source of echoes disturbs this balance and triggers the alarm. Preliminary surveys of the power outputs emitted by these devices by the then Bureau of Radiological Health in Rockville, Maryland, USA, showed that several units which were mounted in public places such as department stores exceeded the airborne ultrasound exposure limits presented in Figure 19.4[11]. This would not be viewed as a potential public health hazard were it not for the fact that many of these same devices were found to be emitting ultrasound 24 hours per day, i.e. even when the alarm circuit had been cancelled. This is an example of extremely bad engineering practice whereby a large number of people are needlessly exposed to a potentially unpleasant if not distressing environment. It is the responsibility of the management of all public places which utilize these intruder alarms to ensure that they do not emit these high levels of airborne ultrasound during the period that their premises are open to the general public.

Some commercially available devices emit even more airborne acoustic energy, i.e. significantly above the limits recommended or proposed in Figure 19.4. These devices are sold as rodent repellers to be mounted in premises where food is stored. They ought only to be activated as the premises are about to be vacated because many people report severe discomfort in their vicinity (whereas others seem to be unaware that the device has been switched on). Analogous devices emitting equivalent high intensities of acoustic energy are sold as dog repellers; these are portable units which are activated by pressing a spring-loaded switch if you are being harassed by a dog. The short duration of each ultrasonic exposure means that it is unlikely that there will be any long-term damage to the hearing of humans. Some estimate of the power output from these devices may be gauged from the fact that during a test a colleague sitting in a different room 40 feet from the source complained of severe discomfort when the device was activated[11].

The military use of liquid-borne ultrasound for communication between submarines or for the detection of underwater obstacles (i.e. Sonar and Asdic) are well known. What is sometimes not appreciated is that in order to increase the range of detection or communication, you have to increase the ultrasonic power output up to the point where the water is about to cavitate. Since water is much more efficient than air at conducting ultrasound into the body, it would be inadvisable for a swimmer wearing only a bathing costume to enter one of these beams. Fortunately, these devices are usually operated in deep water under conditions were casual swimmers are unlikely to be present. If for some reason a swimmer has to be in the water when these devices are being operated or tested then it is advisable that their body be completely enclosed in a waterproof suit so that there is a layer of air trapped between the suit and the skin to minimize coupling.

Of more concern to the general public is the fact that 'smaller scale' underwater ultrasonic detection systems are being sold commercially to fishermen for the detection of shoals of fish. These units can be fitted to any boat and there is nothing to prevent an owner using or testing his device while at anchor or while passing a bathing beach. I am unaware of any measurements of the acoustic power densities in the emission from these devices, or their directionality, but it is certainly an area where a regulatory body ought to take an interest, even if only to formulate a 'code of practice' whereby these units are only operated in deep water.

REFERENCES

1. Williams, A.R. (1983). *Ultrasound: Biological Effects and Potential Hazards*. (London: Academic Press)

2. Wells, P.N.T. (1977). *Biomedical Ultrasonics*. (London: Academic Press)
3. Muir, T.G. and Carstensen, E.L. (1980). Prediction of nonlinear acoustic effects at biomedical frequencies and intensities. *Ultrasound Med. Biol.*, **6**, 345-357
4. Lang, R.J. (1962). Ultrasonic atomization of liquids. *J. Acoust. Soc. Am.*, **34**, 6-8
5. Nyborg, W.L. (1977). Physical mechanisms for biological effects of ultrasound. United States Department of Health, Education and Welfare publication. (FDA) 78-8062, pp. 1-59
6. Noltingk, B.E. and Neppiras, E.A. (1950). Cavitation produced by ultrasonics. *Proc. Phys. Soc. (Lond.)*, **B63**, 674-685
7. Dyson, M., Woodward, B. and Pond, J.B. (1971). Flow of red blood cells stopped by ultrasound. *Nature (Lond.)*, **232**, 572-573
8. Frederiksen, E. (1977). Condenser microphones used as sound sources. *Brüel und Kjaer Tech. Rev.*, **3**, 3-32
9. Kleinschmidt, P. and Magori, V. (1981). Ultrasonic remote sensors for noncontact object detection. *Siemans Forsch. Entwickl. Ber.*, **10**, 110-118
10. Michael, P.L., Kerlin, R.L., Bienvenue, G.R. and Prout, J.H. (1974). An evaluation of industrial acoustic radiation above 10 kHz. Final report on United States Department of Health, Education and Welfare contract number HSM-99-72-125. pp. 1-200
11. Herman, B.A. and Powell, D. (1981). Airborne ultrasound: measurement and possible adverse effects. United States Department of Health and Human Services publication. (FDA) 81-8163, Washington D.C., pp. 1-11
12. WHO (1982). Ultrasound. World Health Organisation Environmental Health Criteria document No. 22, Geneva, pp. 1-199
13. NCRP (1983). Biological effects of ultrasound: mechanisms and clinical implications. National Council on Radiation Protection and Measurement report number 74, Bethesda, Maryland, U.S.A., pp. 1-266
14. O'Brien, W.D. Jr. (1978). Ultrasonic dosimetry. In Fry, F.J. (ed.), *'Methods and Phenomena-Ultrasound: Its applications in Medicine and Biology'*, Part II. (Amsterdam: Elsevier Scientific)
15. AIUM-NEMA (1981). American Institute of Ultrasound in Medicine-National Electrical Manufacturers Association publication ULI-1981. Washington DC
16. JIS (1981). Methods of measuring the performance of ultrasonic pulse-echo diagnostic equipment. Japanese Industrial Standards, Tokyo, Japan
17. Canada (1981). Ultrasonic therapy devices regulation. Department of National Health and Welfare. *Canada Gaz.*, Part II, **115**, 1121-1126
18. FDA (1978). Performance standard for ultrasonic therapy products. United States Food and Drug Administration Federal Regulations, 43 (34), pp. 7166-7172
19. Gierke, H.E. von (1950). Subharmonics generated in human and animal ears by intense sound. *J. Acoust. Soc. Am.*, **22**, 675(a)
20. Eldridge, D.H. Jr. (1950). Some responses of the ear to high frequency sound. *Fed. Proc.*, **9**, 37(a)
21. Parrack, H.O. (1966). Effect of air-borne ultrasound on humans. *Internat. Audiol.*, **5**, 294-308
22. Acton, W.I. and Carson, M.B. (1967). Auditory and subjective effects of airborne noise from industrial ultrasonic sources. *Br. J. Ind. Med.*, **24**, 297-304
23. Grigor'eva, V.M. (1966). Ultrasound and the question of occupational hazards. *Maschinstreochiya*, **8**, 32. Abstract in *Ultrasonics*, **4**, 214 (1966)
24. IRPA (1981). Guidelines on limits of human exposure to airborne acoustic energy having one-third octave bands with mid frequencies from 8 to 50 kHz. International Radiation Protection Association/International Non-Ionizing Radiation Committee publication (IRPA/INIRC), Nov. 1981
25. IRPA (1984). Interim guidelines on limits of human exposure to airborne ultrasound. *Health Physics*, **46**, 969-974

26. Lehmann, J.F. and de Lateur, B.J. (1982). Therapeutic heat. In *Therapeutic Heat and Cold*, 3rd edn. (Baltimore: Williams and Wilkins)

27. Oosterbaan, W.A. (1981). A potentially harmful aspect of ultrasonic therapy transducers. In Kurjak, A. and Kratochwill, A. (eds.), *Recent Advances in Ultrasonic Diagnosis - 3*. pp. 27-8. (Amsterdam: Excerpta Medica)

28. Walmsley, A.D., Laird, W.R.E. and Williams, A.R. (1984). A model system to demonstrate the role of cavitational activity in ultrasonic scaling. *J. Dent. Res.*, **63**, 1163-1165

29. Williams, A.R. and Chater, B.V. (1980). Mammalian platelet damage *in vitro* by an ultrasonic therapeutic device. *Arch. Oral. Biol.*, **25**, 175-179

30. Goldman, H.M. (1961). Histologic assay of healing following ultrasonic curettage versus hand-instrument curettage. *Oral Surg.*, **14**, 925-928

31. Zach, L., Morrison, A. and Cohen, G. (1959). Ultrasonic cavity preparation: histopathologic survey of effects on mature and developing dental tissues. *J. Am. Dent. Assoc.*, **59**, 45-55

32. Frost, H. (1977). Heating under dental scaling conditions. In Hazzard, D.W.G. and Litz, M.L. (eds.), *Symposium on Biological Effects and Characterization of Ultrasound Sources*. Department of Health, Education and Welfare publication. (FDA) 78-8048, pp. 64-76

33. Möller, P., Grevstad, A.O. and Kristoffersen, T. (1976). Ultrasonic scaling of maxillary teeth causing tinitus and temporary hearing shifts. *J. Clin. Periodont.*, **3**, 123-127

34. Carson, T.E. and Fishman, S.S. (1976). Biological effects of ultrasound: skin and cutaneous blood vessels. *Proc. West. Pharmacol. Soc.*, **19**, 36-39

35. Griffiths, P.V. (1978). The management of the pacemaker wearer during dental hygiene treatment. *Dent. Hyg.*, **52**, 573-576

36. Simon, A.B., Lindhe, B., Bonnette, G.H. and Schlentz, R.J. (1975). The individual with a pacemaker in the dental environment. *J. Am. Dent. Assoc.*, **91**, 1224-1229

37. Luker, J. (1982). The pacemaker patient in the dental surgery. *J. Dent.*, **10**, 326-332

38. Adams, D. Fulford, N., Beechy, J., MacCarthy, J. and Stephens, M. (1982). The cardiac pacemaker and ultrasonic scalers. *Br. Dent. J.*, **152**, 171-173

39. Mokrzycki, J. (1982). The cardiac pacemaker and ultrasonic scalers. *Br. Dent. J.*, **153**, 250 (letter)

40. Larato, D.C., Ruskin, P.F. and Martin, A. (1967). Effect of an ultrasonic scaler on bacterial counts in air. *J. Periodontol*, **38**, 550-554

41. Holbrook, W.P., Muir, K.F., MacPhee, I.T. and Ross, P.W. (1978). Bacterial investigation of the aerosol from ultrasonic scalers. *Br. Dent. J.*, **144**, 245-247

42. Muir, K.F., Ross, P.W., MacPhee, I.T., Holbrook, W.P. and Kowolick, M.J. (1978). Reduction of microbial contamination from ultrasonic scalers. *Br. Dent. J.*, **145**, 76-78

43. Balamuth, L. (1972). Ultrasonic cauterisation. US Patent No. 3,636,943. Jan. 25.

44. Grasshof, H. von (1982). Der einfluss der Ultraschallsäge auf Knochenwachstum und-reparation. *Z. Exper. Chirurg*, **15**, 358-366

45. Neumann, A. Müller, Th. and Wehner, W. (1980). Physical and technical problems of bone welding. Paper E.20 at the Ultrasound Interaction in Biology and Medicine Symposium, Reinhardsbrunn, G.D.R.

46. Brug, E., Braunsteiner, E. and von Gemmern, C. (1976). Ultrasonic welding of bones. Preliminary results. *Chirurg*, **47**, 555-558

47. Volkov, M.V. and Shepeleva, I.S. (1974). The use of ultrasonic instrumentation for the transection and uniting of bone tissue in orthopaedic surgery. *Reconstr. Surg. Traumatol.*, **14**, 147-152

48. Kelman, C.D. (1967). Phaco-emulsification and aspiration. *Am. J. Ophthal.*, **64**, 23-25

49. Fishman, S.S. (1968). Biological effects of ultrasound; *in vivo* and *in vitro* haemolysis. *Proc. West. Pharmacol. Soc.*, **11**, 149-150

50. Fishman, S.S. and Willis, J.N. (1977). Development of a stress test by exposing the arm

to cavitating ultrasound: an application for thermography. *Proc. West. Pharmacol. Soc.*, **20**, 221-226

51. Chater, B.V. and Williams, A.R. (1982). Absence of platelet damage *in vivo* following the exposure of non-turbulent blood to therapeutic ultrasound. *Ultrasound Med. Biol.*, **8**, 85-87

52. Japan (1971). Airborne ultrasound standard. Guidelines on the use of ultrasonic welder. Circular 326 of the Japanese Ministry of Labour, Labour Standard Bureau, Tokyo, Japan

53. Acton, W.I. (1975). Exposure criteria for industrial ultrasound. *Ann. Occup. Hyg.*, **18**, 267-268

54. USSR (1975). USSR Health Standards for Occupational Exposure - Ultrasound. USSR State Committee for Standards GOST 12.1.001-75, Moscow, p. 9

55. USAF (1976). Hazardous noise exposure. United States Air Force regulation AFR 161-35, pp. 7-26

56. Sweden (1978). Infrasound and ultrasound in occupational life. *Liber. Foerlag.*, **162**, 89. Publication No. 110: 1-1978, Vaellingby, Sweden

57. Canada (1980). Guidelines for the safe use of ultrasound. Part I - Medical and paramedical applications. Safety code 23. Department of National Health and Welfare publication. Canada, 80-EHD-59

58. ACGIH (1981). Threshold limit values for physical agents. American Conference of Governmental Industrial Hygienists, Cincinnati, Ohio, USA

59. Hill, C.R. (1977). Ultrasound. In *Manual on Health Aspects of Exposure to Non-Ionising Radiation*. WHO Regional Office in England, ICP-CEP 803

60. Rooney, J.A. (1973). Determination of acoustic power in the microwatt and milliwatt range. *Ultrasound Med. Biol.*, **1**, 13-16

61. Edmonds, P.D. (1972). Interaction of ultrasound with biological structures - a survey of data. In Reid, J.M. and Sikov, M.R. (eds.), *Interaction of Ultrasound and Biological Tissue*. Department of Health Education and Welfare Publication/ (FDA) 73-8008, pp. 299-317

62. Ulrich, W.D. (1974). Ultrasound dosage for nontherapeutic use on human beings - extrapolations from a literature survey. *IEEE Trans. Biomed. Eng.*, **BME-21**, 48-51

63. Wells, P.N.T. (1974). The possibility of harmful biological effects of ultrasonic diagnosis. In Reneman, R.S. (ed.), *Cardiovascular Applications of Ultrasound*. (Amsterdam: North Holland), pp. 1-17

20 Safety Aspects of Laboratory and Clinical Nuclear Magnetic Resonance and Magnetic Fields

Margaret A. Foster

INTRODUCTION

Nuclear magnetic resonance (NMR) is a technique for interrogating certain nuclei to obtain information about the concentration of these nuclei in the sample and about their local molecular or crystal lattice environment. The property of the NMR-sensitive nucleus which is exploited is its spin. This spin causes the nucleus to act like a magnetic dipole and in the presence of an external magnetic field it aligns with the applied field direction in one of two orientations which have an energy difference between them (effectively north pole to south pole – low energy, or north to north – high energy). In the presence of an applied magnetic field, therefore, fairly standard absorption spectroscopy experiments can be performed, but using the magnetic aspect of the electromagnetic (EM) radiation rather than its electric component. The energy (or frequency) of the EM radiation needed to bring about a spin orientation change is directly related to the total magnetic field strength experienced by the nucleus. This field is a product of the external field applied by the investigator and any local fields produced by other nuclei or electrons in the immediate molecular environment. If the applied field is stable, therefore, examination of the various components of the EM absorption spectrum yields information about the other magnetic components in the vicinity of the interrogated nucleus and in doing so provides a considerable amount of chemical and biophysical information about the sample as a whole.

NMR has played a major role in chemistry and biochemistry for over 30 years but during the past decade the possibility has been explored for the application of NMR techniques to the study of living organisms. After a limited number of early reports, the major expansion of NMR methods into biology began in the early 1970s when various workers realized that a more detailed understanding of the form of water within tissue could lead to a better understanding of the life processes. Most of the early studies were concerned with the NMR properties of the hydrogen protons of either water or mobile lipid molecules, and particularly of the ways in which the NMR spin lattice and spin-spin relaxation times of these protons varied between different tissues. Many properties of the tissue can affect the relaxation times, including water content, the amount and proportion of the macromolecular components and the presence of paramagnetic substances such as copper or iron atoms. Although it is not possible to identify a tissue positively by its NMR proton relaxation times, tissues which are anatomically close are often very different in their NMR properties, e.g. grey and white brain tissue. It was also found that many pathological conditions can affect the normal NMR relaxation properties of tissues. For example, tumours normally have considerably longer NMR relaxation times than the equivalent normal tissue and oedamatous or inflamed tissues show similar increases. Unfortunately most of these changes are non-specific and are not reliable as direct medical diagnostic aids if only small pieces of excised tissue are examined. To make NMR a useful medical tool it was necessary to find a method for examining the relaxation characteristics *in situ* within the living body.

The development of NMR imaging methods arose from the realization that spatial information about the concentration and relaxation properties of the NMR-detectable protons could be obtained if the test object (e.g. a living human body) was placed in a carefully controlled inhomogeneous magnetic field – usually a simple field gradient. In such a case different proton populations are subjected to different applied magnetic field strengths and detailed analysis of the EM signal from the object (usually by means of Fourier transform methods) could yield information about the exact position of the protons within the body.

NMR imaging paved the way for the expansion of NMR from a laboratory technique into the general clinical situation. The hydrogen proton, however, is not the only nucleus available for NMR study. Many nuclei have spin and quite a number of these are biologically relevant. Certain carbon and nitrogen isotopes have been used in biological studies and sodium-23 can also be observed and even imaged, although its NMR sensitivity is low. In general, biological studies with these other nuclei have been of the 'spectrum' type rather than of their relaxation properties, and one of the most useful nuclei for spectral biological NMR work is phosphorus-31. This nucleus has a fairly high NMR sensitivity and a relatively simple NMR spectrum in most tissues. A good tissue ^{31}P NMR spectrum can be obtained despite the many constraints placed on the NMR experiment due to the use of biological material for a sample (i.e. low concentration, wet sample, need to maintain life processes, etc.). Phosphorus is intimately concerned in energy metabolism and the ^{31}P NMR spectrum yields information about the metabolic activity of the cells. It has been possible to observe ^{31}P NMR spectra from living tissues *in situ* in the human body. The technique, called topical magnetic resonance or TMR, involves the use of strong, specially shaped magnetic fields and surface coils. It has proved valuable in the examination of medical conditions such as forms of muscular weakness arising from energy metabolism defects, and also in studying neonatal ischaemia.

From this introduction it will be realized that NMR equipment can be used for various purposes. It is common in chemical and biochemical laboratories and increasingly common in certain types of biology laboratory. It has spread into clinical laboratories and even into the general hospital where it is likely to be found in departments of nuclear medicine or radiology. Within the hospital it will often be used by experimentalists as well as for routine patient work. Although the special safety precautions which are necessary for medical equipment and patient handling are outside the cover of this chapter, medical NMR equipment and NMR imaging systems are still so experimental and in such demand for research studies that it is essential to consider the general safety precautions needed in their use.

Although this chapter will be approached from the point of view of NMR, all points made about magnets used in NMR studies are applicable to the general use of magnets and magnetic fields in any laboratory.

THE TECHNIQUES

To understand fully the sources of hazards which may arise in the NMR laboratory it is necessary to look in a little detail at the techniques of NMR spectroscopy and NMR imaging. The relationship between the nuclear spin and an external magnetic field has already been mentioned. The energy difference between the spin states is dependent upon the applied field strength; the stronger the field, the greater the difference. The local field effects, which lead to the multiplicity of lines in the absorption spectrum, are superimposed on this applied field and are in relation to it. Spectral splitting in NMR is normally described in terms of parts per million, i.e. the distance between two lines in the spectrum is so many parts per million of the total field or frequency. It follows, therefore, that the stronger the applied magnetic field, the greater will be the separation between the lines in terms of Tesla or Hertz. The greater the separation, the more readily can the lines be measured and so there is considerable advantage, for conventional NMR studies, in using the strongest possible external magnetic field.

The NMR experiment can be performed using fairly low fields obtained from conventional electromagnets. Indeed, NMR studies have been made using only the earth's magnetic field. For really high resolution, however, it is most common to use the very high fields produced by cryomagnets which utilize the superconducting properties of certain metal alloys when exposed to very low temperatures in liquid helium. *In vivo* spectroscopy and some developments of NMR imaging also use high fields produced by superconducting magnets and safety must be a major consideration for these instruments where the bore of the magnet may be sufficiently large to accommodate the entire human body.

In addition to the main magnetic field, and any hazards which may arise from it, we must also consider the EM radiation needed to induce spin orientation changes. In conventional NMR spectroscopy this is unlikely to produce hazard since it is confined to the NMR probe and not accessible to the experimenter. In NMR imaging or *in vivo* spectroscopy on humans, however, the EM radiation must penetrate the subject being imaged and will often be accessible to the experimenter positioning the sample or patient. Potential hazards from this radiation, which is usually in the radiofrequency range, must be considered for *in vivo* studies.

In NMR imaging a third magnetic field type is encountered. It has already been mentioned that positional information is obtained by the use of field gradients. These gradients are produced by extra windings inside the main field and to obtain the spatial information it is necessary to switch the gradients (usually three orthogonal gradients working separately) on and off. The actual field strength, even at the high point of the gradient, is small compared with the main field strength but hazards may arise from the switching process, which generates eddy currents in conductive material such as the human body.

In addition to consideration of possible hazards arising from the three types of magnetic field, it is necessary to consider other aspects of laboratory NMR. For example, a wide range of special chemicals are used in NMR spectroscopy. These include solvents used in sample preparation, a variety of compounds used as NMR standards and substances such as deuterium oxide which is frequently used to exclude the hydrogen of water from the sample, especially when performing proton NMR experiments.

In NMR studies the potential hazards fall into four categories:

(a) use of potentially harmful chemicals;
(b) use of potentially harmful biological materials;
(c) hazards arising indirectly from the presence of magnets in the working environment;
(d) direct biological effects of the various types of magnetic field.

In the following sections we shall consider categories (a) and (b) briefly but our main attention will be given to categories (c) and (d).

CHEMICAL HAZARDS

Proton NMR studies can be severely upset by the presence of water in the sample. The hydrogens of water produce a very large NMR signal which distorts or obliterates the signal from other –OH groups which may be of greater interest. For this reason samples for NMR spectroscopic examination are frequently prepared in non-aqueous solution (or are dried if all extraneous protons are to be eliminated). The organic solvents are those in common use in chemical studies and present the hazards common to most solvents, e.g. inflammability, easy evaporation and biological effects such as short-term effects on the skin of some workers and the general and widespread possibility of damage to certain organs, especially the liver (e.g. carbon tetrachloride) and carcinogenicity. More detailed discussion of hazards associated with such solvents is not relevant to this chapter but in general, where use of solvents cannot be avoided completely, they should be handled with appropriate care, preferably in a fume cupboard or other device to prevent their open loss into the atmosphere.

Deuterium compounds are widely used in NMR and these also must be treated with respect. Deuterium oxide (D_2O) is often used instead of water to exclude hydrogen. In small quantities D_2O is not very harmful but it is potentially capable of upsetting certain systems because of the greater size of the deuterium atom. As with organic solvents it is suggested that D_2O is handled in an isolated area and, because of its exchangeable nature with water, all samples or sources of D_2O should be very clearly labelled and stored in such a way that they cannot be mistaken for ordinary water.

All the general precautions of a chemical laboratory should be enforced in the NMR laboratory, e.g. no eating, drinking or smoking, the use of dispensers rather than oral pipetting, full labelling of all samples, bottles, etc., extreme tidiness in the work area, etc.

BIOLOGICAL HAZARDS

The application of NMR techniques to biological and medical problems can lead to a potential source of hazard to laboratory workers. Certain biological materials can transmit bacterial or viral infection to humans. If a research worker is studying a pathogen directly, the harmful nature of that pathogen will presumably be known, and the laboratory will be properly equipped to deal with material of that type. A more subtle danger, however, can arise from the handling of biological tissues, especially if these are of human origin. Any research workers who has not previously handled human material would be strongly advised to seek expert advice from a pathologist before embarking on such studies.

Many dangers are not obvious and very ordinary material can be hazardous whilst extremely abnormal or even necrotic tumours or other tissues will often hold little danger. An important example of hidden danger is the handling of human blood samples. The blood is the carrier of many diseases but the chief hazard to laboratory workers is perhaps from hepatitis. This can be present in the blood without either the patient (or 'healthy' volunteer) or the physician being aware of it. Hepatitis is an extremely unpleasant and dangerous disease and even after recovery the affected individual will be a carrier of the disease for many years and so may be limited in his or her movement within a hospital (e.g. there will be automatic exclusion from a renal dialysis unit).

Blood is not the only carrier of disease and even if no hazard has been reported, the laboratory worker should always treat human tissue with care. Human blood should not be poured into the general drainage system, nor should human tissue be put into unrestricted waste disposal systems (e.g. laboratory waste bins). Disposal of this waste should be done by incineration or double bagging it and storage frozen until it can be taken to a local hospital for disposal in their specialist facilities. Benches should be covered with absorbent material and all procedures carried out in trays. All paper tissues or towels which have been in contact with the human material should be incinerated and all glassware and surgical instruments either autoclaved or thoroughly cleaned with an alcohol-based disinfectant solution. Anyone handling human material is strongly advised to wear gloves and a buttoned laboratory coat is essential. A disposable plastic apron is an asset when handling human material.

INDIRECT MAGNET HAZARDS

Into this section are grouped all problems arising from the presence of magnets or magnetic fields in the working environment except the direct action of magnetic fields on body tissues. It may seem inappropriate to class effects such as attraction of small tools as indirect effects but we are examining hazards to someone in the laboratory and if injuries arise from the flight of a pair of scissors across the room the direct harm is from the scissors and the role of the magnet in attracting the object is an indirect source of harm to the injured party. This explanation has served to illustrate one of the most important potential sources of hazard from laboratory magnets, namely their ability to attract ferromagnetic materials. This is, however, not the only problem and this section will deal with hazards in the following categories:

(a) attraction of external objects;
(b) interference with electrical or electronic systems;
(c) effects on metallic implants;
(d) quenching of superconducting magnets.

Attraction of external objects

The ability of a magnet to attract an external ferromagnetic object, i.e. the extent and strength of its fringe fields, is related both to the design of the magnet and its field strength.

Permanent magnets are rarely used in conventional NMR spectroscopy or imaging. The main problem, for NMR studies, is the huge size and weight of magnet needed to produce a field of usable strength. One commercial permanent magnet NMR imager, marketed by the Fonar Corporation, is reputed to weigh 100 tonnes although the same field strength can be produced by lighter designs. If it was not for their weight, permanent magnets would have some attractions such as their good field stability. They can be designed to have very low fringe fields and hence produce less hazard to workers or equipment in the vicinity. This is generally achieved by using a yoke-type design similar to that of standard electromagnets. Certain permanent magnet designs, e.g. the Watson-type magnet, do have substantial fringe fields so even permanent magnets should be carefully checked in this respect.

Most standard laboratory magnets are of the yoke-type design. In this type the electric coils are wound round pole pieces, generally thick iron rods. The adjacent ends of the pole pieces (the pole faces) have a high magnetic field between them but simply left like this there would be a strong peripheral field from the outer ends of the pole pieces. In practice, however, these outer ends are linked by a strong ferromagnetic yoke which serves the dual purpose of a mechanical support and providing a magnetic link round the outside of the poles. This greatly reduces fringe fields, as can be seen by taking a Gauss meter reading in the vicinity of any standard electromagnet used in NMR or electron spin resonance.

The resistive magnets used in NMR imaging are of a very different design with no external links and they produce significant fringe fields. In general the fringe field of an imaging resistive magnet is less than that of a superconducting magnet used to produce the same field over the same internal volume. This is because of the different coil design – the resistive magnet is smaller and generally of an overall spherical or near-spherical configuration whilst the superconducting magnet is bulkier and cylindrical.

Superconducting or cryomagnets are the general work-horses of modern NMR spectroscopy and are also used in a number of commercial NMR imaging systems and all TMR systems. These magnets work almost like permanent magnets once the field is established but they always produce strong fringe fields. The fringe field is spheroidal in shape with its long axis down the bore of the magnet. Spectroscopy magnets generally have a vertical bore and extension of fringe fields to floors above and below the magnet laboratory must be considered when high field cryomagnets are installed. For superconducting NMR imaging magnets the long axis of the ellipse will be horizontal but the fringe field is generally so great that other floors may also

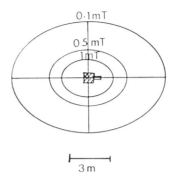

3 m

Figure 20.1   Contour map of fringe field strength from a 0.5 T superconducting magnet designed for NMR imaging

be affected. The fringe field strength is directly related to the internal field strength of the magnet and typical field/distance contour plots are shown in Figure 20.1.

Fringe fields can be a major problem in the siting of high field-strength magnets. The Federal Drug Administration (FDA), which is the body governing many aspects of laboratory and clinical safety in the United States, has suggested that the fringe field outside the 'controlled area' of an installation such as an NMR imager, should be no more than 5 Gauss (0.0005 Tesla). From Figure 20.1 it may be extrapolated that for an imaging cryomagnet of field strength 1.5 Tesla this means that the controlled area must extend out to about 40 feet on each side along the long axis and 30 feet along the short axis. So a controlled area of minimum floor area 80 feet by 60 feet would be required and it must be borne in mind that there will be a 5 Gauss field for 30 feet above and 30 feet below the magnet.

The 5 Gauss ruling is with regard to access by the general public. The strength of field required to attract metallic objects will not be met until one approaches closer to the magnet. The magnetic attraction on a small ferromagnetic object such as a screwdriver, scalpel or pair of scissors depends not only on the field strength but on the steepness of the magnetic gradient. A long thin object will more easily become a projectile than something like a ball bearing because the difference in field from one end to the other will be much greater if the object is long. A much steeper field gradient would be needed to make the ball bearing fly. Steep field gradients are met close to large cryomagnets and it is strongly recommended that some form of barrier be put round any magnet which produced sufficient fringe field to 'snatch' objects. Such a precaution would have prevented accidents such as those which involved in one case a floor polisher and in another an oxygen cylinder trolley being pulled into large bore superconducting magnets. Prohibition of entry through the barrier of all except trained personnel, and large notices stating field strength and possible hazards, should reduce problems of this

464

type. In some NMR imaging laboratories metal detector arches have been installed, of a similar type to those seen at many airports. Unfortunately these are rarely sensitive enough to react to the small items such as hypodermic needles which are frequently overlooked even by aware personnel, but which can cause considerable injury if they become projectiles. As an alternative to, or in conjunction with, warnings and restricted access it is sometimes possible to screen off the fringe fields to some extent. A 1/2–inch thick iron sheet 10 feet from the magnet will reduce fringe fields substantially from a 0.35 Tesla cryomagnet, but it would need to be thicker and at a greater distance for a high field system. Effective close screening is difficult for high field magnets.

The above remarks have been based on observations on NMR imaging systems because it is from these systems, which have to be installed in busy and crowded hospital environments, that most information is available. All these problems, however, are met when standard NMR spectrometers are installed in the laboratory and the same precautions should apply. It should also be borne in mind that when cryomagnets are used, they are always at full field and do not just come on when the instrument is in operation, as an electromagnet does. The precautions are needed, therefore, on a 24-hour, 7-day week basis and service staff such as cleaners and night porters must either be excluded from the vicinity of the magnets or informed about the hazards.

Fringe fields at an equal distance from most spectrometer cryomagnets are much smaller than for the imaging superconducting magnets. As a rough rule of thumb it can be said that the fringe field at a given distance is proportional to the volume of the magnet multiplied by the main field. Laboratory cryomagnets, producing their main field over a much smaller internal volume, are considerably smaller than imaging magnets and hence produce smaller fringe fields since the volume of the magnet is the dominating influence, as can be seen if we take generalized figures:

1. for an imaging cryomagnet of length 7.5 feet, radius 6 feet and producing an internal field of 2 Tesla. The fringe field at a specified distance, d, will be proportional to:

$$3.14 \times 6^2 \times 7.5 \times 2 = 1696$$

2. for a laboratory cryomagnet of length 3 feet, radius 2 feet and producing the same field strength as (1). The fringe field at d will be proportional to:

$$3.14 \times 2^2 \times 3 \times 2 = 75$$

So if the fringe field at d is 100 Gauss in case (1) it will be 4.4 Gauss for (2).

Interference with electrical or electronic systems

Two groups of hazard can be put under this heading; namely hazard to equipment and hazard to the person. In the first group are problems with magnetic media, cathode ray tubes, etc. and in the second group we have direct human hazards due to interference with electronic implants such as heart pacemakers.

The circuitry of most electronic equipment is relatively insensitive to the presence of magnetic fields and so power supplies, amplifiers, etc. can be used in fairly close proximity to powerful magnets. Displays based on liquid crystals or light-emitting diodes are also insensitive and function close to or even inside the high field magnets. The same is true of many modern electronic watches. Some parts of the laboratory equipment, however, are magnetically sensitive and this includes all the 'magnetic media' of the computer age. Although computer circuitry will operate adjacent to a large cryomagnet, there may be problems with data storage on magnetic discs or tape. The sensitivity of hard or floppy discs and magnetic tape depends on the nature of the coating. Some coatings can withstand higher fields, e.g. the 'chrome' coating found on some cassette tapes is only affected when the field exceeds 0.04 to 0.05 Tesla. In general the coating of floppy discs and standard magnetic tape is of the ferric type and this has a lower tolerance - errors will occur in tapes or discs subjected to about 0.02 to 0.025 Tesla. It should also be noted that the magnetic strips on credit cards are of the ferric material so these should never be subjected to fields of 0.02 Tesla or above. Because of the possibility of local effects and problems arising from transport of magnetic media within the field, many manufacturers of magnet systems recommend that magnetic media are not exposed to fields any higher than 20 to 30 Gauss (0.002 Tesla).

One of the most magnetically sensitive items of laboratory equipment is the cathode ray tube. If unprotected a standard monochromic display can be disturbed by a field of only 5 Gauss (0.0005 Tesla) whilst as little as 1 Gauss is required to cause misalignment of the electron beams and hence colour distortion to a colour display (as can be seen by placing a colour TV set too close to a loudspeaker in the home). Many modern cathode ray monitors have a special casing to reduce the effects of magnetic fields and it is necessary to ensure that such protection is fitted before purchasing monitors for use in a magnet laboratory. Hospital equipment based on accurate positioning of electron beams and items such as gamma camera imaging systems can also be affected by low magnetic fields.

Some makes of cardiac pacemakers are highly sensitive to magnetic fields. For example, it has been reported that the operating state of the CPI Command P5 Model 0530 can be changed by placing it in a field as low as 13 Gauss. Many other types of pacemaker are affected by fields of 20 to 30 Gauss but many models have not been reported on. This extreme sensitivity is only

466

found in modern pacemakers of the 'demand' type. The older generation of pacemakers had a fixed beat rate which they imposed on the heart. This is known as asynchronous operation. Most modern pacemakers have two operating modes. The normal one is a demand system whereby the pacemaker only supplies a pulse if the natural heart beat is too slow. There is, within the pacemaker, a reed switch which is magnetically activated and this can throw the pacemaker into an asynchronous mode exactly like the older standard system. The field strengths quoted above are those needed to activate this reed switch and hence change the operating mode of the pacemaker. The effect on the patient would generally not be catastrophic and the pacemaker would revert to the demand mode as soon as the magnetic field dropped to below that needed to activate the reed switch. For some models of pacemaker the demand or synchronous operating rate is the same as the asynchronous rate so the change of operating mode would not be felt by the patient. Despite this there is always a potential hazard in affecting so sensitive a system as the heart, so pacemaker exposure to even these low magnetic fields should be avoided as far as possible.

The effects on the reed switch are usually the lowest field effects observed on cardiac pacemakers but are by no means the only possible effects. At high field strengths it is theoretically possible to get torque on the pacemaker itself and cause it or its attachment leads to twist within the soft tissue of the chest. NMR apparatus, and particularly NMR imagers, use time-varying and radio-frequency magnetic fields. At certain frequencies these varying fields may well be capable of causing electromagnetic interference with pacemaker operation, especially if the frequency is close to that which is being monitored by the demand-type pacemaker. This could cause considerable disruption of normal operation.

The considerable variation in sensitivity of pacemakers has led to the suggestion that individuals using these devices should not be investigated by NMR imaging procedures. It is also considered wise to prevent any possibility of approach of pacemaker wearers close to an operating magnet and all magnet laboratories should have prominent notices warning pacemaker users of the hazards.

Effects on metallic implants

Metallic implants vary in size from very small aneurysm clips or steel sutures to the massive structure of a hip prosthesis. Joint replacement is becoming increasingly common so the larger implants are widespread in the population, presumably including medical and laboratory personnel as well as hospital patients. A patient who has undergone hip replacement will normally be aware of the presence of a foreign body, but the presence of a steel suture or clip is often not known by its wearer, although these are in common use. It is also possible that a patient will be unaware that an implant such as a heart valve may be ferromagnetic.

There are basically two ways in which these implants can be affected by NMR conditions. Firstly, if subjected to magnetic fields of sufficient strength and gradient, ferromagnetic implants can move either longitudinally or rotationally within the field. Secondly, if subjected to high rates of change of magnetic field or high levels of radiofrequency field, conductive implants become heated and can burn the surrounding tissue.

The possibility of sufficient longitudinal force or torque being induced in a ferromagnetic implant is related to field strength, gradient and the size and shape of the implant. Tests have been carried out on a large number of different types of clips and sutures and the majority have been found to twist significantly in the level of field encountered at the entrance to a standard medium field imaging magnet. Fields within the poles of many laboratory magnets would be even higher, although access is more difficult. It has been demonstrated than an aneurysm clip can be twisted right off an artery (in a rat) by moving it into a strong magnetic field and this, of course, could be fatal if it occurs, for example, in the human brain where steel clips are frequently used. Non-magnetic clips do exist and a variety of non-magnetic forms of stainless steel are available for manufacture of implants. Since there will always be the possibility of not knowing that a patient has a steel implant, the main drive to avoid this hazard should come from the manufacturers of the devices. In the case of an operation on someone who is known to be exposed to magnetic fields, e.g. a worker in NMR imaging or in a magnet laboratory, the surgeon should be reminded of the possible hazards of magnetic implants and where possible any potential implants checked for ferromagnetism.

Heating by time-varying magnetic fields and radiofrequency fields is related to the field frequency and to the size of the implant. Only in very extreme cases would an object as small as an aneurysm clip be heated significantly, but a hip prosthesis offers a large induction loop so heating will be proportionally greater. The irregular shape of most prostheses make calculation of the loop radius, and hence the amount of current induction, very difficult. In one test, however, it was found that two hip replacement prostheses, placed together in a 600 ml bath of saline and subjected to a changing magnetic field (unspecified rate or extent of change) caused an increase of nearly 6 °C in the temperature of the saline. It is possible that these conditions were extreme but they do suggest that problems could arise in certain laboratory conditions. Radiofrequency heating of implants is also a significant factor but the radiofrequency power needed to produce a dangerous heating level is outside that allowed by the exposure regulations of most countries.

Quenching of superconducting magnets

Superconducting magnets have the unique potential to cause one group of hazards arising from the possibility of 'quenching'. A superconducting magnet operates because certain alloys, e.g. niobium-titanium and niobium-tin, lose all electrical resistance when chilled to very low temperatures such as by immersion in liquid helium (4 K). Unfortunately, if anything goes wrong with the system, e.g. shorting or a local temperature rise (which is most likely to occur through bad routine maintenance allowing a drop in level of the coolant), the alloy wire which forms the magnet winding immediately reassumes its electrical resistance and since current is flowing through it it heats up. This boils off liquid helium and the progressive effect spreads through the entire set of windings. The energy held in the magnet is dissipated as heat, resulting in total loss of the helium as a gas or vapour. This is termed 'quenching'.

Unexpected quenching of a cryomagnet is potentially hazardous in several ways. The most obvious way is the venting of the helium gas. A given weight of helium occupies a volume about 700 times greater as the gas than as the liquid. Most cryomagnets are designed to vent this gas easily since the quenching is by no means instantaneous, and the outer casing of the magnet is designed to support the quench (which is occasionally performed deliberately). Hazard can arise, however, if the venting is not controlled and the gas is allowed to escape into the laboratory. Helium is not, in itself, poisonous but in a small laboratory it could displace sufficient of the air to lead to breathing trouble. Free venting of the gas/vapour mixture could cause severe cold burns if it was not directed away from laboratory workers. Care should, therefore, be taken to ensure that the vents of the magnet are not directed into the working area of a room (in NMR spectrometers these are usually directed upwards) and that the laboratory volume is sufficient to eliminate air displacement problems. Venting of large superconducting magnets such as those used in NMR imaging should be examined in much more detail. They must be connected to the outside air by piping that is adequate in diameter to take the flow (the total volume to be vented is very large indeed) and which will not be affected by the extreme cold of the venting gas. The outlet of this vent must be placed where it cannot be a hazard to passers-by.

Other potential hazards associated with quenching are related to the sudden drop in the field. For a short period the immediate vicinity will be subjected to a changing magnetic field and this will induce eddy currents in conductive materials. This is particularly the case if anybody is close to or inside the magnet when it quenches. The human body provides a very suitable conductive loop for eddy current induction, as we will see in a later section. In fact this is unlikely to be a major hazard because of the methods of manufacture of most superconducting magnets. The superconducting alloy wire is generally in bundles embedded in a copper matrix. When the alloy bundle goes 'critical' the copper carries the current to some extent and absorbs the energy release for a short period. This slows the entire quenching process down so that a large cryomagnet will take up to 30 seconds to drop its field completely. This normally would be sufficient to bring the rate of change of field to well within safe limits.

Recommendations to avoid indirect hazards

1. Measure the fringe fields round each magnet so that the extent of any potential problem is realized.
2. If fields over 5 Gauss occur in any public area this should be closed off or warning notices put up. The magnetic field will pass through a wall and may extend outside a building. Planting of a dense shrub border round the building would keep people away.
3. Warning notices should be placed wherever the field exceeds 10 Gauss to prevent entry of people wearing pacemakers.
4. If the field is high enough to attract objects, a barrier should be erected and entry restricted to trained personnel or people who have been questioned and searched.
5. Anyone approaching the magnet should be warned (preferably by means of a large notice) that the field can affect metallic implants and erase credit cards.
6. If anyone shows discomfort or pain they should be removed immediately from the vicinity of the field and a check made for metallic implants.
7. Superconducting magnets should be serviced regularly and the coolant level checked frequently.
8. Superconducting magnets should only be placed in large, well-ventilated rooms or they should have a special venting system to carry away the helium during quenching. The venting system needs to be of cold-resistant material.

BIOLOGICAL EFFECTS OF MAGNETIC FIELDS

The three types of magnetic field encountered in NMR imaging, namely static, time-varying and radiofrequency, are all capable of interacting with the human body. Not all of these interactions imply hazard to the person concerned, especially at the relatively low exposure levels used in even high-field NMR imaging or TMR. We will, however, consider the variety of different effects since in extreme cases some may represent safety problems. Normal laboratory NMR will only have to consider static field effects and these are minimal at fringe field strengths if one is considering the direct biological effects of the magnetic fields. Other work involving magnets (e.g.

operation of large particle accelerators) will involve exposure to one or more of the three categories to be considered here.

The literature, especially for the 1950s and 1960s, contains a large mass of contradictory reports on observed effects of exposure to magnetic fields. Many of the reports of those decades were anecdotal or of badly controlled experiments and it is difficult to sort the good from the bad work. Problems of this type tend to confuse many 'safety' studies and because of this the following discussion will be oriented towards possible mechanisms for inter-action of field and tissue rather than a list of reported findings of varying scientific value.

Static or main fields

NMR studies are performed over a wide range of field, from the earth's field of about 50 micro Tesla used by one worker looking at body fluid pools, to greater than 10 Tesla used for high-resolution NMR spectroscopy. In this latter case the laboratory worker is only subjected to the magnet's fringe fields which are much lower than the internal operating field and in reality, for NMR work, we can regard the limits of NMR imaging as being the limits of exposure. These range from the 0.04 Tesla of the Aberdeen Mk I spin warp imager to 2.0 Tesla used in the new generation of NMR imagers and in some TMR systems. Some instruments have been designed to use higher fields but only over parts of the body.

There are various ways in which strong static fields might affect the living body, but the one of greatest importance is the induction of flow potentials. When a conductive fluid such as blood flows through a vessel which is oriented perpendicular to a magnetic field, an electric potential is generated across the diameter of the vessel. This is known as magnetohydrodynamic induction and is the basis of several systems for measuring flow rate. The size of this flow potential E, is given by:

$$E = BdV$$

where e is in volts, B is field strength in Tesla, d is vessel diameter in metres and V is velocity in metres per second. It is seen that the larger the blood vessel the greater the flow potential across it so that the great vessels around the heart, and possibly the heart itself, are likely to show the biggest effect. It has been found experimentally, using squirrel monkeys, that flow effects can produce an electrical potential of about 0.07 mV/Tesla which can be observed superimposed on the T wave of the normal ECG signal (Figure 20.2). The great vessels in the human are larger than those of the squirrel monkey and it is to be expected that the generated potential will be larger. The mean peak aortic velocity in the human is about 0.63 metres per second and the aorta diameter is in the order of 0.025 metres so the theoretical

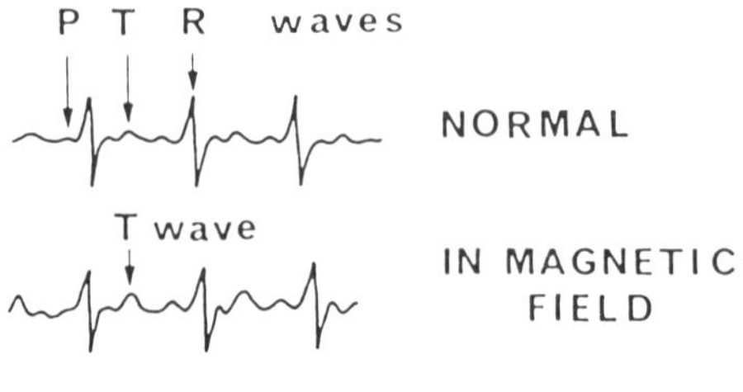

Figure 20.2 Effect of flow potential induced by a magnetic field on recorded ECG

generated potential would be about 15.7 mV/Tesla. This, however, would only be the case for vessels perpendicular to the magnetic field and maximum exposure in NMR imaging at the moment would only produce one-fifth of this electrical potential. The quoted value is across the entire diameter of the vessel, but the important aspect from the point of view of cell function would be the potential across any one cell, and this is very much lower. The experiment with monkeys showed that during an exposure of 10 minutes duration to a field strength of 10 Tesla the flow potential was observed but there was no change in heart rate and no arrhythmia. Recent studies with rats, dogs and monkeys have suggested that the abnormal ECG is observed at field strengths as low as 0.3 Tesla but in no species was there any change in heart beat or in the aortic blood pressure. It seems, therefore, that even if NMR imaging fields are pushed up higher than 2 Tesla, there is little likelihood of danger to normal individuals from induced flow potentials.

It has been suggested that other effects such as Faraday induction due to the pulsatile flow of blood through the chest wall or viscosity changes in the blood due to the pressure pulses in the arteries might affect ECG or aortic pressure but such effects would be minor compared with the magnetohydro-dynamic potential induction and would be no more harmful.

Other possible interactions of the main static magnetic field with living systems include orientation changes of magnetically susceptible cells or groups of macromolecules and also the possibility of effects on nerve conduction. At very high magnetic field strengths it is, in theory, possible to change the orientation of structures such as the retinal rods or of certain bacteria which have a strong and anisotropic diamagnetic susceptibility. The effects due to fields of up to 2 Tesla appear to be very small and no ill effects have been reported. Nerve conduction effects are also likely to require much stronger magnetic fields than are currently used in NMR imaging. The basis of these effects is that the nerve acts like a conducting wire in the magnetic field. In such a case there is an effect on the moving charge which causes a distortion which is perpendicular to both the magnetic field and the direction

472

of charge movement. This results in a reduction in charge velocity through the wire, or in conduction velocity along the nerve. Theoretical predictions suggest that a field of 24 Tesla would be required to produce a 10% reduction in nerve impulse conduction velocity.

Time-varying magnetic fields

Time-varying magnetic fields are of minimal importance to workers with conventional NMR spectroscopy but they play an important role in NMR imaging since they are generated by the switching of the gradients which provide the spatial information about the spins. The peak field strength is small compared with the main magnetic field but the important aspects are the total field change experienced by the subject and the rate of change (dB/dt where B is field and t is time). There is a well-known physical mechanism whereby a time-varying magnetic field can affect a biological tissue, which is by the induction of eddy currents. Biological tissues, containing considerable quantities of ions in water, are highly conductive and the various surfaces and interfaces in the body can constitute conductive loops for eddy current induction.

In a simple annulus of conductive material, as for example, the outer surface of the head, the eddy current (i) induced by a changing magnetic field (dB/dt) is given by:

$$i = \sigma \cdot \frac{dB}{dt} \cdot \frac{r \cdot dr \cdot h}{2}$$

where σ is the conductivity of the annulus, r is the radius of the loop, dr is the radius of the annulus material and h is the thickness of the slice (See Figure 20.3). If effects on the human body are to be considered, the main factor will be the density of current at any place on or in the body. Because of all the

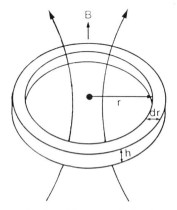

Figure 20.3 Conducting annulus for eddy current induction

473

variations in shape and the many meetings of surfaces it is virtually impossible to calculate this accurately. A figure can be obtained if a simple annulus of material is considered of the same conductivity as most body tissue. In this case the current density is given by:

$$\frac{i}{dr \cdot t} = \frac{\sigma r}{2} \cdot \frac{dB}{dt}$$

So for a radius of 10 cm (roughly that of the outer region of the head) and a tissue conductivity of 0.2 Siemens/m with a rate of change of field of 1 Tesla/s, the induced current density will be $1\,\mu A/cm^2$. Membrane ion currents are in the order of $1\ mA/cm^2$ and it would need a rate of change of field of 1000 Tesla/s to generate an equivalent eddy current.

The problems already mentioned have led workers to follow an observational rather than a theoretical route in seeking to estimate safe levels of exposure to varying magnetic fields. There has been general agreement that high rates of field change are needed to produce an observable effect (as predicted) but it has also been suggested that the threshold levels are frequency-dependent. Most studies have used directly applied electric currents rather than ones which were magnetically induced, and typical findings have shown effects such as the induction of visual phosphenes (flashing lights) at AC current levels as low as 0.01 mA if the AC frequency is 20 Hz. Above and below this frequency a greater applied current is required. 20 mA at 60 Hz is required to inhibit breathing by thoracic tetanization whilst it requires up to 100 mA at 60 Hz to induce ventricular fibrillation.

Magnetically induced effects have been observed at high field change rates, e.g. twitching is seen in the body wall of rats exposed to a pulse of damped sinusoidal shape of period 0.33 ms. A similar pulse shape and frequency delivered through a surface coil to the human fore-arm could induce muscle contraction at a threshold level of 2100 Tesla/s. It was estimated that the induced current density over the largest loop available was in the order of $5\ A/cm^2$. Surface coil studies with rats appear to suggest that the muscular twitches are the earliest effects one can expect to see, occurring at lower field change rates than ECG disturbance. Exposure to changes in the order of 60 Tesla/s has no effect on the ECG of the rabbit.

RF magnetic fields

The RF fields needed to induce changes in the spin angle are able to penetrate tissue very well. The penetration depth is frequency-dependent, the absorption dropping with frequency. There is much debate in the literature about effects of RF fields but the only well-substantiated effects are associated with tissue heating. It has been calculated that an RF source putting out a peak power of 30 W over 10 ms, with a duty cycle of 0.1 will present 2.5 mW/cm^2 average power density to the head. The amount of power which is absorbed will be considerably less than this, for example, at 10 MHz and a power density of 1 mW/cm^2 the absorption will be about 1 mW per kilo body weight. The possibility of hazard from heating at this level should be considered by comparison with the basal metabolic rate (BMR) which is approximately 1 W/kg. Few imaging systems are likely to use suffi-cient RF power to approach the BMR heating level but even if power was delivered at the level of 1 W/kg it would take an hour to raise the body temperature by 1 °C, even assuming no heat loss. From this point of view NMR imaging methods would seem to be quite safe. There are, however, some operations which require fairly high power levels, e.g. spin decoupling in certain TMR studies. In these cases there may be concern about heating of certain organs such as parts of the eye which have no blood supply to help them dissipate the excess heat.

Safety recommendations

NMR imaging is a technique of considerable medical importance and its mode of operation has attracted the attention of safety standards boards in several countries. Recommendations for exposure limits have been made by organizations such as the Bureau of Radiological Health (Food and Drug Administration) of the United States and the National Radiological Protec-tion Board (NRPB) in Great Britain. In general, the recommended maximum levels of exposure suggested by these organizations are similar and in neither case do they impose severe limitations on the development or use of biomedi-cal NMR procedures. Indeed, if the recommendation of the NRPB are compared in their publications over the past few years it can be seen that there has been a fairly considerable relaxation as progress in both NMR imaging techniques and in investigation of potential hazards has demon-strated the low hazard level associated with exposure to magnetic fields.

The latest guidelines produced by the NRPB (December 1983) are listed below as an indication of the limitations:

Static magnetic fields – should not exceed 2.5 Tesla to the whole or a substantial part of the body of those exposed to the imaging procedure. Operating staff should not have long-term exposure to more than 0.02 Tesla to whole body or 0.2 Tesla to the limbs.

Time-varying magnetic fields – for periods of magnetic flux density change exceeding 10 ms, exposure should be restricted to less than 20 Tesla per second rms for all persons. For periods of change less than 10 ms the relationship $(dB/dt)^2 t < 4$ should be observed where dB/dt is the rms value of the rate of change of the magnetic flux density in any part of the body in Tesla per second and t is the duration of the change of magnetic field in seconds.

Radiofrequency fields – acceptable exposure should not result in a rise in whole body temperature of more than 1 °C or more than 1 °C in any mass of tissue not exceeding 1 g.

As well as these guidelines on specific exposure, the NRPB also suggests that patients with cardiac pacemakers should not be exposed, that imaging procedures should be stopped if patients with large metallic implants feel any pain or discomfort and that women in the first trimester of pregnancy should not be exposed.

Although some of the exposure figures underlying these recommendations may be open to debate, the recommendations as a whole provide a reasonable framework within which NMR procedures can be undertaken and in which workers in magnet laboratories can have reasonable confidence about the lack of short-term effects of their exposure. It is, therefore, suggested that similar limits be adopted in any magnet laboratory.

LITERATURE TO BE CONSULTED

Athey, W.T., Ross, R.J. and Ruggera, P.S. (1982). Magnetic fields associated with a nuclear magnetic resonance imaging system. *Mag. Res. Imag.*, 1, 149-154

Budinger, T.F. (1981). Nuclear magnetic resonance (NMR) *in vivo* studies: known thresholds for health effects. *J. Comput. Ass. Tomogr.*, 5, 800-1

Budinger, T.F. and Cullander, C. (1983). Biophysical phenomena and health hazards of *in vivo* magnetic resonance. In Margulis, A.R., Higgins, C.B., Kaufmann, L. and Crook, L.E. (eds.) *Clinical Magnetic Resonance Imaging*. (San Francisco: Radiological Research and Education Foundation), pp. 303-320

Kaufmann, L., Crooks, L.E., Margulis, A.R. and Proseus, J.O. (1983). Siting. In Margulis, A.R., Higgins, C.B., Kaufmann, L. and Crooks, L.E. (eds.) *Clinical Magnetic Resonance Imaging*. (San Francisco: Radiological Research and Education Foundation), pp. 321-324

McRobbie, D. and Foster, M.A. (1984). Threshold for biological effects of time-varying magnetic fields. *Clin. Phys. Physiol. Meas.*, 5, 67-68

Mansfield, P. and Morris, P.G. (1982). Biomagnetic effects. In *NMR Imaging in Biomedicine*. (New York: Academic Press), pp. 297-332

National Radiological Protection Board (1983). Revised guidance on acceptable limits of exposure during nuclear magnetic resonance clinical imaging. *Br. J. Radiol.*, 56, 974-977

New, P.F.J., Rosen, B.R., Brady, T.J., Buonanno, F.S., Kistler, J.P., Burt, C.T., Hinshaw, W.S., Newhouse, J.H., Pohost, G.M. and Taveras, J.M. (1983). Potential hazards and artifacts of ferromagnetic and nonferromagnetic surgical and dental materials and devices in nuclear magnetic resonance imaging. *Radiology*, 147, 139-148

Pavlicek, W., Geisinger, M., Castle, R., Borkowski, G.P., Meaney, T.F., Bream, B.L. and Gallagher, J.H. (1983). The effect of nuclear magnetic resonance on patients with cardiac pacemakers. *Radiology*, 147, 149-153

Polson, M.J.R., Barker, A.T. and Gardiner, S. (1982). The effect of rapid rise-time magnetic fields on the ECG of the rat. *Clin. Phys. Physiol. Meas.*, 3, 231-234

Saunders, R.D. (1982). Biological Hazards of NMR. In Witcofski, R.L., Karstaedt, M.B. and Partain, C.L. (eds.) *Proceedings of an International Symposium on Nuclear Magnetic Resonance*. (Winston Salem, US: Bowman Gray School of Medicine), pp. 65-71

21 Laser Safety

A.L. McKenzie

LASER HAZARDS

Laser accidents have occurred regularly since the device was invented in 1960. Accidental exposures to the eyes, in particular, can be traumatic – one account by an accident victim describes 'a distinct popping sound' in the back of his eyeball and his subsequent horror as his vision filled with streams of blood[1]. The early literature has frequent descriptions of incidents of this kind, but, as the reports lost their novelty value, and since little biological information can be gleaned from the circumstantial nature of such cases, the incidence of such publications has declined over the last decade. This should not be interpreted as a reduction in the number of such accidents – indeed it may be a disadvantage that less attention is being drawn to such catastrophic laser accidents.

Eye damage is by no means the only hazard associated with the use of lasers. There is a greater risk of accidental injury to the skin than to the eye, simply by virtue of the larger area of exposed skin than eye, and the consequently higher probability of inadvertent laser exposure, although, of course, it is much easier to live with a skin burn which will probably heal completely, than with irreparable damage to the vision. Apart from causing personal injury, any laser which delivers a CW ouptut of more than about 500 mW may, when focused, ignite inflammable materials. This is of particular concern in the presence of inflammable gases. The majority of lasers use high voltage to excite the active medium – either directly or by driving an optical pump lamp. In experimental systems, particularly, great care should be taken when working with such electrical circuits. Some lasers use toxic gases as an active medium – some thought must go into the pumping and extraction of these gases.

SAFETY STANDARDS

Several national standards exist controlling the safe use of lasers[2]. In the UK, for example, there is the BSI[3] standard and, in the USA there is the ANSI[4] standard and the BRH[5] standard. These are fairly similar to each other in philosophy and in detailed recommended limits for maximum permissible exposure (MPE) to eyes and skin. While it would be possible to apply these rules and levels without understanding the principles behind them, such an approach leaves no room for interpreting the rules in the light of local requirements and for accommodating to new circumstances as they arise. Therefore, we present below an account of the risks to the eye and skin at various wavelengths and pulse durations, with an indication of hazardous levels of irradiation and radiance. In later sections we shall give examples of calculations to determine safe levels for the eye and to prescribe appropriate eye protection in various circumstances. We shall then consider the other types of laser hazard mentioned above, and how to deal with them.

THE HAZARD TO THE RETINA

Damage to the retina – the light-sensitive layer at the back of the eye – can be catastrophic (Figure 21.1). In general, a laser beam lesion will be manifest to the victim as a blind spot which may only be revealed when staring at a blank screen. However, damage to the foveal area of the retina would result in a very annoying blind spot in the centre of vision, so that the victim would be forced always to look to the side of anything he wished to examine. Even more disastrously, an injury to the optic nerve could totally wipe out the vision of that eye.

The principal site of radiation absorption in the retina is not the sensory part of the retina but a layer of cells called the pigment epithelium which lies

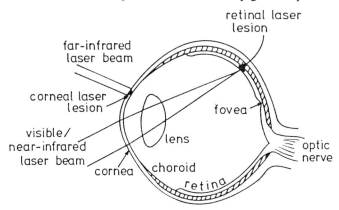

Figure 21.1   Laser lesions in the eye

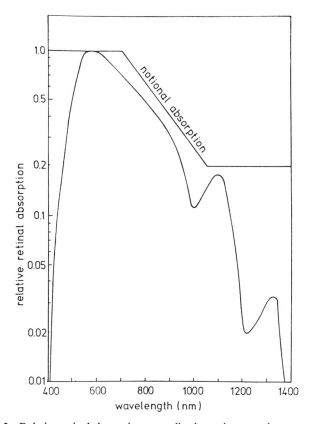

Figure 21.2 Relative retinal absorption normalized to unity at maximum

deepest in the retina. These cells contain highly pigmented melanin granules which absorb over a wide range of visible wavelengths. The heat generated at these sites spreads to the sensory retina, and, at sufficiently high temperatures, will render the cells functionless. Very high-power, short-pulse lasers, such as a Nd YAG mode-locked laser, may generate a momentary ball of plasma causing hydro-dynamic shock waves which will mechanically disrupt the retina irreparably and probably cause haemorrhage into the vitreous – the clear gel which fills the eyeball. Such mechanical damage accounts for the 'popping sound' described at the beginning of this chapter.

At longer wavelengths than red, the pigment epithelium becomes a less efficient absorber of radiation and so the effect of exposure is less concentrated. Furthermore, the ocular media (cornea, aqueous, lens and vitreous) which are transparent to visible light, begin to absorb strongly beyond 700 nm. From 700 nm to 1400 nm, that is, in the near-infrared, radiation is absorbed progressively by the ocular media so that, beyond 1400 nm, virtually no radiation reaches the retina. Figure 21.2 shows the relative amount of radiation absorbed by the retina[6], and also the notional absorption used by national standards in determining maximum permissible exposure limits. Because the retina absorbs less radiation in the near infrared, the levels which have been fixed for visible radiation are relaxed by the reciprocal of this notional absorption, at wavelengths between 700 nm and 1400 nm.

INTRABEAM EXPOSURE AND SMALL SOURCES

A direct exposure to the eye by a laser beam is called intrabeam exposure, and is made particularly hazardous at visible and near-infrared wavelengths, because the relaxed eye can focus the beam into a very small spot on the retina. The power falling within unit area is called the irradiance, and is measured in W m^{-2}. The concentration of power by the curved refracting surfaces of the cornea and lens result in a high optical gain, so that the irradiance at the retina may be many orders of magnitude greater than that entering the eye (the corneal irradiance). On a simple model, if the image of the laser beam were focused into the smallest possible spot (only a few microns in diameter[7], according to physical optics) the optical gain would be found by taking the ratio of the pupil area to image area. Larger pupils would admit more light into the tiny image, and so one would calculate a correspondingly higher gain. However, in practice, larger pupils tend to produce more scattered radiation within the eye, and there is also a tendency for the retinal image size to increase, with the result that the optical gain is, for practical purposes, a constant 10^5. The relation between corneal irradiance, E_c, and retinal irradiance, E_r, may be summarized by the equation

$$E_r = 10^5 E_c.$$

VIEWING EXTENDED SOURCES

Viewing the radiation diffusely reflected from surfaces irradiated by lasers can also be hazardous, particularly if the laser is a high-power device, and if the surface has a high reflectivity for the illuminating wavelength. An extended source cannot be imaged onto a diffraction-limited spot, as may be the case with intrabeam exposure; rather, it illuminates a finite area of the retina. It is insufficient simply to specify MPE values for diffuse radiation in terms of the total irradiance at the cornea, because account has to be taken of the area of the retina which is being illuminated. This is done by using the quantity radiance, defined in terms of irradiance per unit solid angle (W m^{-2} sr^{-1}). The retinal irradiance may be found from the radiance, L, of the source from the following relation:

$$E_r = \pi L d_p^2 / 4 f_e^2$$

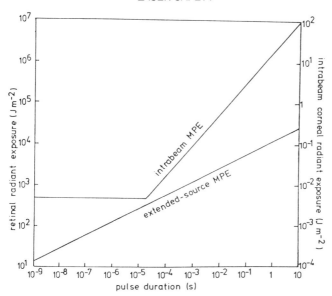

Figure 21.3 MPE levels for visible radiation

Here, d_p is the pupil diameter and is assumed to be 7 mm, the largest normal size found in practice. The nominal focal length of the eye, f_e, is taken to be 17 mm. It is sometimes easier to determine the radiance at the eye from a diffusely reflecting source. Since the radiance at the eye is the same as the radiance of the source, the radiance at the eye may be substituted for L in the above formula.

MPE FOR RETINAL IRRADIANCE

The philosophy behind maximum exposure (MPE) limits is that an exposure of the eye or skin to radiation below the MPE level should involve a negligible risk of damage to the organ. Safe levels of exposure have been determined using both human eyes, prior to enucleation for disease, and eyes of trained monkeys. Wide ranges of exposure were used, both in intrabeam experiments and extended-source experiments, so that the threshold power or dose, which has a 50% probability of inducing a burn, could be determined. The MPE is set at a level where the probability of damage is acceptably low, and is generally a factor of 10 or so lower than the threshold levels.

Figure 21.3 shows MPE values for visible light for pulse durations ranging from 10^{-9} s to 10 s. The MPEs are quoted in terms of retinal radiant exposure for both intrabeam exposure and extended-source exposure. In the intrabeam case, where exposure is related simply to ocular or corneal exposure, through the optical gain factor, the corresponding corneal MPEs are also indicated in the diagram. The same scale cannot be used for extended-source viewing, because corneal MPEs would then need to be in terms of radiance, and not irradiance.

The general trend of the retinal irradiance MPE graphs may be understood from consideration of thermal diffusion in the retina[8]. In the first place, it is natural that the graph for extended-source viewing lies below that for the intrabeam case, because heat cannot diffuse so easily from the larger areas corresponding to extended-source images as from the smaller spots of direct beam irradiation. Therefore, damage will take place at lower values of power or energy per unit area in the extended images. This reduced potential for heat diffusion out of the region also goes some way to explaining the lower gradient of the extended-source results compared with the intrabeam points, at least for exposures greater than 10^{-5} s.

The sloping section of the intrabeam MPE graph exhibits a $t^{0.75}$ dependence. This is consistent with rough thermal arguments, since a given amount of heat can dissipate more completely during longer exposures, and, therefore, retinal exposure thresholds should be higher for longer pulse durations. However, the dependence on time must be sublinear, because direct proportionality between energy input and time would imply the same power input for all threshold exposures, regardless of duration. Below 10^{-5} s, there is virtually no time for heat to diffuse out of the target, and so the intrabeam MPE becomes independent of pulse duration at very short exposure times[9].

NEAR-INFRARED RETINAL MPEs

As we have indicated, the PMEs in the wavelength range 700–1400 nm are relaxed by the reciprocal of the notional retinal absorption indicated in Figure 21.2. Of course, this means that energy is delivered increasingly to the more anterior structures of the eye at longer wavelengths. The near-infrared region has been indicted in the production of lens cataracts, but the MPE levels for the retina are well below those levels believed to be cataractogenic for either short or chronic exposures.

RETINAL EXPOSURE LIMITS – LONG EXPOSURE TIMES

When exposure times are longer than about 10 s, photochemical injury begins to become important for visible wavelengths (between 400 nm and 700 nm). At shorter times the allowed retinal exposure is restricted by thermal injury, but, during longer exposures, while heat may diffuse away harmlessly, photochemical damage tends to be cumulative and predominates over the thermal hazards[10]. Blue light has a far greater potential for inducing photochemical damage than red, and, as a consequence, the MPE for intrabeam viewing of

400 nm light over extended times may be as low as 10^{-2} W m^{-2} compared with 1.8 W m^{-2} at 700 nm. In practice, of course, steady intrabeam viewing for long periods of time does not occur, and the extended-source viewing limits are of greater interest, corresponding to laser light diffusely reflected in a room which a worker may occupy for several hours. The long-term MPE for wavelengths between 400 and 550 nm (covering the argon-laser wavelength range, for example) is 21 W m^{-2} sr^{-1} compared with 3.7×10^{3} W m^{-2} sr^{-1} at 700 nm.

RETINAL EXPOSURE LIMITS FOR VERY SHORT EXPOSURE TIMES

Very little data exists for ultra-short exposure times, of less than 10^{-9} s, and so the MPE is specified in terms of a power which, if applied continuously for 10^{-9} s, would deliver the radiant exposure (in J m^{-2}) corresponding to the MPE for 10^{-9} s. Evidently, such a power, applied for less time than a nanosecond, cannot do more damage than if it were applied for the full nanosecond. For visible lasers, the limiting power is 5×10^{6} W m^{-2}, which implies a maximum exposure dose of 5×10^{-3} J m^{-2} in 10^{-9} s.

THE CHOICE BETWEEN INTRABEAM AND EXTENDED-SOURCE MPEs

Since MPE tables exist for the two separate conditions of intrabeam and extended-source viewing, there has to be a criterion for deciding which table to use in given circumstances. When viewing an extended source it could be quite safe to use the intrabeam tables to determine the appropriate MPE for the corneal irradiation, but this would be too conservative, since the intrabeam tables assume that all the power is concentrated into a small area on the retina, whereas it is spread more thinly in an extended image. Hence the extended-source tables would legitimately permit a higher total corneal irradiance than the intrabeam tables in this case. However, smaller sources subtend smaller angles at the eye so that, for a given source radiance, L, the total corneal irradiance is less. The question is, what is the smallest angle, α_{min}, above which it is advantageous to use the extended-source data? The relation is given by[11]:

$$\alpha_{min} = \left(\frac{4\,E_c}{\pi\,L} \right)^{\frac{1}{2}}$$

where E_c and L are the tabulated intrabeam and extended-source MPEs respectively. Since E_c and L vary with exposure times in different fashions (illustrated by the graphs in Figure 21.3), α_{min} must also be a function of the exposure time, and ranges from a minimum of 1.5 mrad at around 20 μs to 24 mrad at 10 s and greater. Notice that, at these angles, the retinal image is far from a minimal spot – the purpose of α_{min} is not to determine retinal spot sizes, but simply to indicate the point where it is advantageous to use the extended-source data.

FAR-INFRARED RADIATION – CORNEAL AND LENS IRRADIATION

At wavelengths greater than 1400 nm, far-infrared radiation is absorbed in progressively anterior parts of the eye. Beyond 2 μm it is the cornea which is primarily at risk. A corneal burn may be manifest as a surface irregularity or a white opacity. A minor lesion, restricted to the outer cellular layer of the cornea, the corneal epithelium, will probably heal and disappear within 2 days, which is the regeneration time for these cells. Deeper burns may cause permanent damage. Since there is no question of the eye focusing this radiation as there was for the visible spectrum, the permitted corneal ir-radiances are higher than for the visible range, and apply equally to intra-beam and extended-source conditions. For example, the intrabeam MPE for a 1 s exposure to visible radiation is 18 Jm^{-2} which is to be compared with 5600 Jm^{-2} for a far-infrared exposure of the same duration.

CORNEAL AND LENS IRRADIATION – UV

Hazards to the eye from UV sources are considered elsewhere in this handbook. However, UV-emitting lasers can deliver powers which are much greater than those normally encountered from other sources, and it is worth noting that, between 315 nm and 400 nm, for pulse durations of less than 10 s, the main hazard is thermal damage, and the same MPE is applied as for the infrared region. At longer times than 10 s, however, photochemical damage becomes more important than thermal effects, since the heat can diffuse away. At shorter wavelengths, photochemical effects become increasingly important, and, from 302.5 nm down to 200 nm, MPE tables take no account of thermal damage, even for very short pulses, but specify a maximum permissable dose of 30 J m^{-2}.

Since the ocular media absorb too highly to allow UV laser beams to be focused onto the retina, the same MPEs are used for extended source viewing as for intrabeam viewing.

HAZARDS TO SKIN

We have already pointed out that a skin burn should give rise to less concern than eye damage. However, while the eyes may be protected, it is not practical to cover all of the skin, and a laser burn to exposed skin is, therefore, a relatively common accident. For visible and infrared radiation the damage mechanism is thermal rather than photochemical, whereas for the UV, the erythematous reaction – reddening of the skin – attests to the photochemical nature of the injury.

Beyond 1400 nm in the far-infrared, and in the UV, the MPE is taken to be the same as that for the cornea. At visible and near-infrared wavelengths (from 400 nm to 1400 nm), although the damage mechanism is the same as that for the far-infrared case, the radiation diffuses more deeply into tissue, so that heating is more diffuse, and less localized. As a consequence, the MPE levels for the visible and near-infrared spectrum are relaxed to twice the allowed levels for the far-infrared range.

PULSED SOURCES – SHORT PULSE DURATIONS

If individual durations of pulses in a train are less than 10^{-5}s, then, if the pulse repetition frequency is F, the MPE which would apply to a single pulse should be reduced by a factor $\sqrt{F}$. For example, the MPE for a visible light pulse lasting 1 μs is 5×10^{-3} J m^{-2}. In a train of 100 such pulses per second, the MPE per pulse would be reduced to 5×10^{-4} J m^{-2}. If the pulse repetition frequency is greater than 278 Hz, the reduced MPE is taken to be 6% of the single-pulse MPE.

It may be, however, that the pulse repetition frequency is so high that the total exposure dose of the whole train of pulses, each with the permitted reduced MPE, actually exceeds the MPE for a single pulse of the same duration as the pulse train. For example, a 0.25 s exposure to the eye of the train cited in the above example would have an MPE of $25 \times 5 \times 10^{-4}$ J m^{-2} = 1.25×10^{-2} Jm^{-2}, which is much less than the MPE for 0.25 s (6.4 J m^{-2}). However, suppose that the pulse repetition frequency of the 1 μs pulses had been 10^5 Hz. In that case, the MPE per pulse would be $0.06 \times 5 \times 10^{-3}$ J m^{-2} = 3×10^{-4} J m^{-2}. An exposure of 0.25 s would contain 2.5×10^4 pulses, giving an MPE of $2.5 \times 10^4 \times 3 \times 10^{-4}$ J m^{-2} = 7.5 Jm^{-2}. This just exceeds the MPE for a single pulse of 0.25 s duration, and so the MPE which should be used would be the lower figure of 6.4 J m^{-2}, corresponding to 2.56×10^{-4} J m^{-2} per pulse.

PULSED SOURCES – LONGER PULSE DURATIONS

If the individual pulse durations are longer than 10^{-5} s, the correction factor is not used, and, instead, the MPE is first determined for an exposure time which is the total of all pulse durations in the pulse train. This is then divided by the number of pulses in the train to derive the MPE for each and every pulse.

LIMITING APERTURE

In deciding MPE levels in practical situations, particularly for intrabeam exposure, it should be kept in mind that the irradiance of a laser beam is not uniform, but will vary across its diameter. The question is – over how large an area may the power be averaged, when calculating the irradiance due to a laser beam? Obviously, the larger the area, the less the irradiance, but then this may give a false indication of safety, whereas the irradiance on the beam axis may exceed the MPE for the wavelength and exposure time in question.

For far-infrared and ultraviolet radiation (wavelengths greater than 1400 nm or less than 400 nm) the largest area which may be used, the limiting aperture, is a circle 1 mm in diameter. For visible light and near-infrared radiation, since, in the worst case, any radiation entering a 7 mm pupil will be focused onto the retina, regardless of whether it enters the centre of the pupil or the periphery, the limiting aperture is taken as a 7 mm diameter circle.

LASER CLASSIFICATION

Lasers are internationally classified according to the hazard they represent to the eye. There are four classes (Table 21.1) and class I constitutes the most innocuous category. A class I laser is of such low power that it cannot exceed the MPE for the eye, and such devices are, therefore, safe to view without eye protection.

Table 21.1 Classification of CW lasers

Class I	Powers not to exceed MPE for eye
Class II	Visible laser beams only; powers up to 1 mW; eye protected by blink reflex time of 0.25 s
Class IIIa	Relaxation of Class II to 5 mW for visible radiation provided beam is expanded so that eye is still protected by blink reflex
Class IIIb	Powers up to 0.5 W; direct viewing hazardous
Class IV	Powers over 0.5 W; extremely hazardous

The class II category is reserved only for lasers with a visible output between 400 nm and 700 nm. This allows a class to be defined where protection is afforded by the blink reflex of the eye, taken conservatively to be 0.25 s in duration. The MPE for this time is 6.4 Jm^{-2}, which, averaged over a 7 mm pupil, is produced by a 1 mW laser, which, therefore, sets the upper limit to the power in this category.

Class III lasers represent the range of powers between the 'safe' lasers and the highly dangerous ones. This class may be subdivided into classes IIIa and IIIb. Class IIIa relaxes the class II limit of 1 mW for CW lasers and, instead, allows up to 5 mW, provided that, wherever the output beam is accessible, it is so diverged that a total power greater than 1 mW cannot enter the 7 mm pupil. Class IIIa extends to infrared and ultraviolet sources also, provided that these comply with class I requirements. In other words no special protection is needed for the eye against class IIIa products, and the blink reflex will be adequate against visible radiation. Optical viewing of class IIIa beam may, however, be hazardous, since the objective of the instrument will be greater than the pupil of the eye in area.

Class IIIb lasers are more powerful and may reach a maximum of 0.5 W CW or 10^5 J m^{-2} pulsed (pulse duration under 0.25 s). Direct viewing of the beam will probably exceed the MPE for the eye and is, therefore, to be considered hazardous, but the beam may be observed using diffuse reflection off a surface, provided that the eye is more than 50 mm from the viewing area, and that the diameter of the image is at least 5.5 mm and a limit of 10 s is set for the observation time.

Lasers which are too powerful to fall within the class III category are class IV lasers, which are extremely hazardous. It is the manufacturer's responsibility to classify a laser, and, if a laser is designated higher than class I, then certain precautions have to be taken by the user.

With a class II laser, care should be taken not to aim the direct beam, or its specular reflection at the eyes. Warning signs should be posted where access to the beam is possible.

In addition, if the product is a class III or class IV laser, consideration should be given to interlocking the device to a barrier such as a door into the laboratory. In this way the unexpected entry of personnel into the room would disconnect the power to the laser. The laser should be activated by a key which may be removed to render the equipment inoperable. A beam attenuator should be incorporated which diminishes or blocks off the output when required. There should be an indication, either audible or visible, that the beam is 'on'. Visible warning, such as an illuminated notice with the words 'laser emission', should be sited conspicuously, and as close to the output aperture as practicable.

EYE PROTECTION

For class IIIb and class IV lasers, since the MPE for eyes may be exceeded, the user must wear eye protection when such lasers are being used. Most suppliers of lasers are able to provide goggles or spectacles for use with their product. Goggles are preferable to spectacles since the latter do not easily fit over prescription spectacles. Also, the goggles usually fit more snugly around the eyes, protecting them from radiation entering from the sides. Goggles with separate filters generally afford poor peripheral vision, lack of which can be dangerous in a laboratory.

When ordering goggles from a supplier, three factors have to be considered. First, the wavelength range over which protection is required should be determined. Second, the attenuation, or optical density needed to ensure that the MPE for the eye is not exceeded, should be calculated. Third, the durability of the eyewear should be assessed[12]. If the wavelengths of the laser are in the infrared or ultraviolet, then the protection filters will probably be transparent to visible light. On the other hand, a filter designed to absorb in the red (e.g. He-Ne laser radiation) will appear blue-tinted, and, for blue or green laser light (e.g. from an argon laser) orange-tinted filters are used.

The optical density is found by taking the ratio of the highest possible eye irradiance or radiant exposure to the MPE for the eye, and then taking the logarithm of the result. As an example, suppose that a 3 W CW argon laser is to be used in a laboratory, and that there is a danger of reflection of the beam into the eye. The maximum irradiance would then be 3 W divided by the area of a 7 mm pupil – the limiting aperture for visible radiation. Hence,

maximum irradiance $= 3/(\pi/4\ (0.007)^2)$ W m^{-2}
∴ maximum radiant exposure in 0.25 s $= 19.5 \times 10^3$ J m^{-2}

This must be reduced to at most the MPE for the eye for visible light for a pulse duration of 0.25 s (the nominal blink reflex time). The appropriate MPE is 6.4 J m^{-2}. Hence

ratio $= 19.5 \times 10^3/6.4$
$\quad\quad = 3 \times 10^3$
so optical density $= \log_{10}(3 \times 10^3)$
$\quad\quad\quad\quad\quad\quad = 3.5$

There is a simpler way of deriving the necessary optical density in the case of visible radiation. In the above example the aim is to reduce the beam to the equivalent of a class II laser, which may have a maximum CW power of 1 mW. Hence, to reduce a 3 W beam to the class II level requires an attenuation of

attenuation $\quad = \quad$ 3 W/1 mW
$\quad\quad\quad\quad\quad = \quad 3 \times 10^3$

Hence the optical density is 3.5, as before.

It is wise to increase the optical density by unity, when specifying eyewear, provided that the filters do not become so dark as to prevent ordinary viewing in the laboratory. The eyewear should be of rugged construction, and goggles should be fitted with ventilation outlets to prevent steaming up when worn. It is wise to test the filters of the eyewear by directing the laser beam at the filter edge to see what damage is produced by the deliberate exposure. Manufacturers of eyewear are generally unwilling to state the maximum permissible designed input of their filters, but such a test will provide an indication.

A recurrent problem with protective eyewear for visible beams is that the filters can be so effective that the beam is totally invisible. This can not only be a nuisance; it can be dangerous. In the case of orange-tinted filters for protection against the blue-green argon beam, a fluorescent screen may be used, so that the position of the beam is indicated by the yellow fluorescence, visible through the filters. This solution is not available for red beams, since any fluorescence they produce would be at an even longer wavelength, and, therefore, still invisible through blue-tinted filters. An alternative approach is to reduce the power of the beam emitted from the laser while alignment takes place. The insertion of an attentuator could reduce the beam to below 1 mW, and the beam, at this class II level, would be safe even for momentary intrabeam viewing.

OPTICALLY AIDED VIEWING

The point about a telescope or microscope is that it collects light with a large objective lens and concentrates it through a small circle, the exit pupil, which is approximately coincident with the pupil of the observer's eye (Figure 21.4).

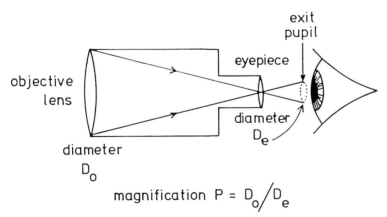

$$\text{magnification } P = D_o / D_e$$

Figure 21.4 Optically aided viewing

From the geometry of the optics, it can be shown that there is a relation between the diameter, D_o, of the objective lens, that of the exit pupil, D_e, and the magnification, P:

$$P = D_o/D_e$$

Because of the concentration effect, the irradiance at the exit pupil – the corneal irradiance – is increased by the ratio of the areas of the objective to the exit pupil:

$$\text{increase in corneal irradiance} = (D_o/D_e)^2 = P^2$$

However, the retinal image dimensions are also increased by the magnification P, and so the retinal image area will be a factor of P^2 greater than the image without magnification. Hence, surprisingly, the retinal irradiance is not increased by using a microscope or telescope to view an extended source.

If, however, the optical instrument is used to view the direct laser beam, then the image may well be diffraction-limited, so that the area is not noticeably increased. In that case, the retinal irradiance is increased by the square of the magnification.

SAFETY CALCULATIONS

Intrabeam exposure

It is generally unnecessary to perform calculations to determine whether or not direct exposure of the eye or skin to a laser beam is dangerous. This is because, if the laser has been categorized as a class IV laser, then it is definitely dangerous, and the appropriate eyewear should be used. The exception to this is where the beam is divergent from some optical component, so that the irradiance falls below the class II level at some distance from the optics.

Diffuse exposure

Small sources

It is frequently the case that the direct beam of a laser is enclosed behind panels which are interlocked to the laser, and is therefore inaccessible, but that some of this radiation leaks as scattered radiation into the room. One might then ask whether such radiation constitutes a hazard, either to eyes or skin. Take an extreme case where the laser beam is focused onto a matt-surfaced material, and where the spot may be observed by the light diffusely reflected. If we make the assumption that the surface is an ideal diffuser – a

Lambertian surface – so that there is no specular component, then the irradiance at a distance r from the reflecting spot is given by:

$$E = \frac{P\rho \cos \theta}{\pi\, r^2}$$

where θ is the angle between the normal to the surface and the line from the spot to the point of measurement (see Figure 21.5), ρ is the reflectivity of the

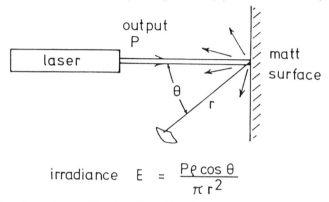

$$\text{irradiance} \quad E = \frac{P\rho \cos \theta}{\pi\, r^2}$$

Figure 21.5 Irradiance from a diffusely reflected laser beam

surface and P is the beam power. The maximum irradiance occurs when $\theta = 0$. For example, suppose a 1 W argon laser beam is focused onto a surface. How far must the eye be from the surface before viewing is safe without protective eyewear?

We assume that this is a case of intrabeam viewing, since the radiation is focused into a small spot. The irradiance a distance r from the spot is:

$$E = \frac{1\ \text{W} \times 1 \times 0.1}{\pi\, r^2}$$

where $\theta = 0$ and a reflectivity of $\rho = 0.1$ has been assumed. If we assume that the experimenter wishes to stare at the spot continuously for 60 s, the appropriate MPE, from tables, is 100 J m^{-2}, delivered in 60 s = 1.67 W m^{-2}. For safety, this irradiance has to be greater than the calculated irradiance:

$1.67 \geq 0.1/\pi r^2$
$\therefore r \geq 0.14$ m

Hence the spot must be viewed from a distance no closer than 140 mm for a period of 1 min, or there is a hazard to the eye. With such a system, it would be prudent to wear eye protection, because, if the focused spot can be seen by diffuse reflection, then, in practice, the direct beam is probably accessible.

Extended sources

In some systems the direct, focused laser spot cannot be seen, but some radiation 'leaks' around corners, having been scattered twice, or more. Such systems may be designed for use as a class I system, by being totally enclosed, so that protective eyewear need not be worn. However, there may be concern over the radiation which is scattered out, and it is useful to be able to show that this radiation is, in any event, not hazardous.

Suppose that the enclosed laser is a 1 W argon system, and that the diffused radiation is observed as being scattered from a circular area 100 mm in diameter. Is there an eye risk for a worker, say 1 m from the scattering surface, over extended periods of time? At a distance of 1 m, the angle subtended by a 100 mm circle is 5.7°. For time periods greater than 10 s, the limiting angular subtense, which separates intrabeam conditions from extended source viewing, is 24 mrad ($= 1.4°$). Hence we have an extended source, and the MPE corresponding to continuous viewing at argon wavelengths is 21 W m^{-2} sr^{-1}. There is a simple relation between the irradiance from a surface (in W m^{-2}) and its radiance (W m^{-2} sr^{-1}) and which may be derived[13] from equation (1):

$$L = E/\pi \qquad (2)$$

where L is the radiance of the radiation diffusely reflected from the matt surface. Returning to the problem, the worst possible case is for the scattering surface to be directly illuminated by an expanded 1 W beam, in which case, taking a reflectivity of 0.1, the irradiance of the surface is:

$$\text{irradiance} = \frac{1 \times 0.1}{\frac{\pi}{4}(0.01)^2} = 12.7 \text{ W m}^{-2}$$

and so, from equation (2), the radiance is

$$\begin{aligned}\text{radiance} \quad &= \quad 12.7/\pi \text{ W m}^{-2} \text{ sr}^{-1}\\ &= \quad 4 \text{ W m}^{-2} \text{ sr}^{-1}\end{aligned}$$

This is below the MPE for continuous viewing (21 W m^{-2} sr^{-1}) and so the laser is safe. In practice, the reflectivity may be higher, but then not all of the 1 W will be incident upon the scattering surface, since we have assumed secondary scatter, and so the true radiance will probably be even further below the MPE than this calculation suggests.

VIEWING DIFFUSE RADIATION THROUGH A MICROSCOPE

It has been mentioned that the increase in corneal irradiance when using an optical instrument increases as the square of the magnification of the instru-ment. In some circumstances this increase may exceed the MPE where unaided viewing would be safe. Suppose a sample is irradiated with a beam focused to 0.1 mm on the surface of the sample. At a distance of 100 mm, the angle subtended by the diffusely reflecting spot is 1 mrad, which is well below the 24 mrad upper limit for intrabeam viewing. (In practice, the unaided eye would have to view from further back, as 100 mm is less than the standard least distance of distinct vision). At 100 mm, the maximum irradiance from the spot illuminated by a 3 W laser is, assuming a reflectivity of 0.1, using equation (1),

$$\text{irradiance} = \frac{3 \times 0.1}{\pi (0.01)^2} \text{ W m}^{-2}$$

$$= 9.5 \text{ W m}^{-2}$$

Over a period of 10 s, this is 95 J m^{-2} which is just below the 100 J m^{-2} MPE for visible light in a 10 s exposure. Hence, viewing this spot with the unaided eye is not hazardous. However, if a microscope is used to observe the sample, so that its objective lens is 100 mm distant from the target, the angle subtended by the spot is greater by a factor equal to the magnification, which, typically, is around 7.0. In the present case this would mean an angular subtense of 7 mrad, still well below the extended-source criterion. The ir-radiance at the exit pupil is increased by the square of the magnifiation, giving rise in this instance to 4660 J m^{-2} in 10 s viewing – some 46 times greater than the MPE for intrabeam viewing.

Obviously such a situation is hazardous and requires precautions, such as inserting a neutral-density filter into the microscope, in order to reduce the irradiance below the MPE.

THE SPECTROSCOPY LABORATORY

In some laboratories access to hazardous class IV laser beams is prevented by having interlocked panels which switch off the laser when they are removed. However, the spectroscopy laboratory is one environment where this is not always practicable. In particular, if the work is research-orientated rather than routine, say within a Raman spectroscopy unit at a university, laser beams will have to be aligned and samples placed correctly into the beam path. In such circumstances the greatest care must be exercised. Protective eyewear worn while aligning a visible beam and inserting a sample – for example, a highly reflecting glass or a test electrode – into the beam, is impracticable, because the experimenter is simply unable to see the beam through the eye filters. The safest procedure is either to turn down the laser power or to attenuate the beam with a neutral-density filter, and then to make all adjustments very slowly so that no unexpected reflection can enter the eye. If necessary, final adjustments can be made with closed doors by observing the required signal from a photomultiplier/monochomator and optimizing the apparatus to achieve the highest signal.

Such laboratories, like all areas where class IV lasers are used, must be designated 'laser controlled areas', and entry should be restricted to essential personnel. Warning signs must be posted outside the door, and it is a good idea to leave appropriate eyewear on a table beside the door. Consideration should also be given to interlocking the door so that the laser power is cut off when the door is opened. Experience in working in such environments counts for a great deal. Since, in practice, new research students will frequently use the equipment, they should receive training and familiarization with the laser system before being allowed to work unsupervised in the laser controlled area.

LASER SAFETY IN THE OPERATING THEATRE

Lasers are being used increasingly in hospitals, and the laser worker may find himself advising on safety in such environments. Some situations arise, however, which are characteristic of the medical use of lasers[14,15]. For example, operating microscopes which view the treatment site and will transmit a powerful flashback through the optics of the operator's eye, must be protected by an automatic filter which is interposed electromechanically before the therapy exposure. Examples are the 'slit lamp' used in opthalmology or the endoscope used in conjunction with a visible argon beam. Near-infrared Nd YAG laser radiation is more easily dealt with by using a filter which is transparent to visible light but absorbs in the near-infrared. The manufacturer of these instruments will supply the necessary filter, and the user simply has to satisfy himself that the filter has been incorporated into the instrument.

As with all class IV lasers, eye protection should be worn whenever a clinical therapeutic laser is being used. It may be considered impracticable to interlock the laser to the theatre doors, as this could upset treatment.

Anaesthetic tubes pose a particular hazard when working in the vicinity of the nose and throat. If a tube is pierced, it can catch fire. The tube should be protected by reflecting aluminium tape, or covered by metallic tubing. A fire extinguisher should be available in the theatre, or immediately outside.

POWER METERS

Unlike the health physicist attached to a nuclear processing plant or atomic power station, there is no need for the laser safety officer to monitor the environment for possible background laser radiation. If a class IV laser is being used, then, quite simply, there is a hazard, and the appropriate measures described in this chapter should be taken. If, despite this, the safety officer feels the need to measure laser power, there will almost certainly be available in the laboratory power meters appropriate for the power and wavelength range in question. However, most situations encountered in practice may be handled by simple calculation to determine whether exposures are above or below the relevant MPE limit.

INCIDENTAL LASER HAZARDS

At the beginning of this chapter it was observed that other hazards exist apart from the danger of personal injury to the eye or skin. The risk of fire in connection with anaesthetic gases has been mentioned already, but, of course, all inflammable materials are at risk in the presence of a class IV laser. A common accident is to persuade a new laser to lase by adjusting the mirrors while standing at the end of the device, so that, at the onset of lasing, the clothes are burnt. Scientists with a small round hole burnt in their tie belong to an exclusive but identifiable club! Laser beams should be terminated by a non-inflammable material such as a brick. There should always be a CO_2 fire extinguisher at hand in a laser laboratory.

The chemicals used as active medium in some lasers can be hazardous if the tube is not sealed. For example, if a He-Cd laser is connected to a vacuum system, then the exhaust gases from the pump should be taken outside by a pipe, avoiding contaminating the laboratory with cadmium vapour. The dyes which are the active medium of tuneable dye lasers require periodic changing, either because they become exhausted or because a change of wavelength is required. Care should be taken when handling the dyes, since the effect of long-term skin exposure is not well understood, particularly with dyes used for infrared laser beams. In any case, dye is so messy that gloves would normally be worn, if only to avoid unsightly stains.

Since lasers require high-voltage electrical supplies, there is an inherent risk when using a home-made system as distinct from a commercial package. The precautions appropriate for electrical work are to be found elsewhere in this book.

ACTION SUBSEQUENT TO ACCIDENTAL LASER EXPOSURE

By the nature of the hazard, a laser exposure to the eye is over before any measures can be taken to minimize it. In a severe case the victim may be shocked, and should be treated accordingly until medical assistance arrives. All accidental eye exposures must be reported as soon as possible to a doctor who will arrange for an opthalmic examination. Meanwhile, the circumstances of the accident must be investigated and the cause determined. In some countries a central agency collects data relating to such accidents and so the information should be forwarded to the appropriate authority.

POLITICS AND PRACTICE OF LASER SAFETY

The practice of laser safety is frequently regarded by laser workers as a nuisance, and by administrators as a set of rules to be applied absolutely without regard to local circumstances. Neither view is justified, of course, but, as long as the laser worker is sensible in his approach to safety, and avoids accidents, he will be giving administrators less incentive to interpret the rules harshly. In the final analysis it is probably very difficult to make progress in a laser laboratory which is foolproof, but then, laser workers are not by nature foolhardy, and the best advice must be to work with foresight and to take the necessary precautions without so obstructing the work that it is impossible to accomplish the original task.

References

1.   Decker, C.D. (1977). Accident victim's view. *Laser Focus*, **13** (8), 6
2.   Sliney, D.H. and Wolbarsht, M.L. (1980). *Safety with Lasers and other Optical Sources*. (New York: Plenum)
3.   British Standards Institution (1989). *Radiation Safety of Laser Products*. BS 7192
4.   American National Standards Institute (1976). *Safe Use of Lasers* Standard Z-136. (New York: ANSI)
5.   US Department of Health, Education and Welfare (1975, revised 1978). *Performance Standard for Laser Products*, 21 CFR 1040. (Washington: FDA/BRH)
6.   Geeraets, W.J. and Berry, B.S. (1968). Ocular spectral characteristics as related to hazards from lasers and other light sources. *Am. J. Opthalmol*, **66** 15-20
7.   Gubisch, R.W. (1967). Optical performance of the human eye. *J. Opt. Soc. Am*., **57** 407-15
8.   Sliney, D.H. (1980). Laser Safety: past and present problem areas. In Hillenkamp, F., Pratesi, R. and Sacchi, C.A. (eds). *Lasers in Biology and Medicine*. (New York: Plenum)
9.   Mainster, M.A., White, T.J., Tipe, J.H. and Wilson, P.W. (1970). Retinal temperature increases produced by intense light sources. *J. Opt. Soc. Am*., **60** 264-70
10. Ham, W.T., Mueller, H.A. and Sliney, D.H. (1976). Retinal sensitivity to damage from short wavelength light. *Nature*, **260** 153-4
11. Carruth, J.A.S. and McKenzie, A.L. (1986). *Medical Lasers: Science and Clinical Practice*. (Bristol: Adam Hilger)
12. *The Protection of Eyes Regulations* Schedule 3. (London: HMSO)
13. McKenzie, A.L. (1987). Optical parameters in laser safety. In *Medical Laser Safety*, Report No 48. (London: IPSM)
14. Carruth, J.A.S. and McKenzie, A.L. (1982). The argon laser in dermatology: safety aspects. *Clin. Exp. Dermatol*., **7** 247-54
15. Carruth, J.A.S., McKenzie, A.L. and Wainwright, A.C. (1980). The carbon dioxide laser: safety aspects. *J. Laryngol. Otol*., **94** 411-17

22 Precautions to be Taken by Field Workers Relating to Specimens Collected for Final Analysis in the Laboratory

G. E. Chivers and R. Toynton

The whole issue of laboratory-based technical staff moving out to work in the field is very important in the context of health and safety at work. While this chapter will focus on the hazards associated with the collection of samples (including observational, measuring and recording activities), many of the problems considered are relevant to laboratory workers moving into the field for any purpose.

This is particularly the case if 'the field' is taken to include work in both the built-up environment and the natural environment. Laboratory staff are frequently expected to operate in both environments, whether the task is collecting product samples in a process plant for quality control purposes or river water samples for pollution monitoring work. Clearly, health and safety considerations will vary depending on whether the field work to be carried out relates to the built-up environment or the natural environment, in the sense that greater control is possible over the built-up environment. However, there are a number of general considerations relevant to the health and safety of workers operating outside their laboratories which can be considered in the first part of this chapter before beginning to differentiate between the built- and the natural environment. Subsequently, some special considerations in the natural environment are outlined later in this chapter.

General hazards faced by laboratory workers moving out into the field

Some of the main hazards include:

1. Travel and transport hazards
2. Entering an unfamiliar environment
3. Difficulties of access to the work site
4. Approaching and working in close proximity to unrecognized or disregarded hazards
5. Working alone
6. Poor communications
7. Working in confined spaces
8. Working in hazardous positions
9. Working in awkward or cramped conditions
10. Bringing equipment or chemicals on site
11. Lack of back-up preventative safety facilities
12. Lack of equipment and facilities for use in emergencies
13. Remoteness from the emergency services
14. Unfamiliarity with work systems in operation
15. Unfamiliarity with established safety systems on site
16. Unfamiliarity with personal protective equipment and protective clothing to be utilized
17. Difficulties of observation, measurement or sampling
18. Hazards of the samples themselves
19. Natural hazards such as wind, rain or cold (which can affect work in both the built-up environment outdoors and, of course, are of great significance in the natural environment)
20. Working overseas.

Some discussion is needed in regard to these general hazards and their control before moving on to consider specific field environments.

Travel and transport hazards

For most people the journey by car or bike to work each day represents a greater prospect of a serious accident than daily tasks in the laboratory. It follows that any requirement to travel during the working day to carry out field work will itself increase the risk of accidents. This risk is frequently compounded by the need to transport equipment, and the likelihood of using an unfamiliar vehicle, usually bigger than normally driven. This is not the place to discuss the high level of general traffic accidents in today's society, but, certainly, precautions should be taken to avoid further increasing the risks. It is essential that proper planning is undertaken in connection with travel and equipment transportation. Vehicles should be purchased, hired, designed or modified with close regard to the intended use or range of uses for field work. Many accidents have arisen from unsuitable vehicles being utilized, for example, the carrying of hazardous chemicals in a standard car where vessels have broken open, or the overloading of small vans with heavy equipment which has upset road performance.

If laboratory workers are expected to drive vehicles to the field, they must be trained to a satisfactory standard of driving competence in such vehicles rather than being expected to jump into them at short notice and drive off. Wherever possible, clear instructions on the destination and what to do on arrival should be provided. Travel routes should be chosen with safety and convenience in mind rather than purely with regard to time saving. Loading and unloading of vehicles often generate hazards and staff required to do this and to carry equipment should be well trained in kinetic handling techniques. Clearly, it is essential to maintain vehicles in good working order, and this needs special care where the vehicle is used by several workers.

Entering an unfamiliar environment

This is a common problem in field work. Clearly, wherever possible, staff should be accompanied at all times by other workers who are familiar with the site and its hazards. This may be impractical, especially if a great deal of the field work is to be carried out, or of course where nobody is familiar with the site (for example, investigations in poorly explored regions of the natural environment, or investigations in old sewer systems or mine workings which are not marked on existing plans).

When a visit is to be made to an established site where work is in progress but the staff member is unfamiliar with the site, formal arrangements are necessary for the reception of the visitor by an experienced site worker. This is often a company rule for entry to manufacturing and processing plants, for various reasons, including safety. However, there may be no established reception procedures in regard to working around the perimeter of such plants, or for entry to farmers' fields, let alone the natural environment.

In addition to any prior training received by the employee, the site worker receiving the visitor should carry out a full briefing and orientation on the site. Attention should be drawn to key hazards, and the safety rules and procedures in force to combat these. Any protective clothing, equipment or facilities to be provided by the site operator should be handed over or indicated with detailed explanations as to their use. At the same time, the staff member should go over the work to be done on site, what this will involve, in detail, and any hazards which can be envisaged (bearing in mind that the field worker may be generating hazards for normal site workers or the plant in carrying out the sampling).

Wherever possible, field workers should try to fit into the existing safety systems, if any, of the site visited. These will have been thought out in detail and tested over a period of time. However, there may be situations where this is not possible or where the work is unique and no existing safety systems are relevant. In such cases, it is essential for the field worker to plan the operation with those fully familiar with the hazards on the site. A system for carrying out the work at minimum risk (as far as reasonably practicable) must be found and written down, copies being held by all concerned. The plan must be communicated to all site workers whose own tasks could be adversely affected by the sampling activity, or who could cut across the activities of the field worker and create hazards.

Once such a system is established and made operational the staff may proceed to the sampling area under the supervision of an appropriate site worker, perhaps a first line supervisor.

Clearly, such an approach is not possible when entering a site where there are not site workers. Nevertheless, there may be personnel with knowledge of the site who can accompany the field worker, help in the planning of a safe system of work and generally provide advice and support. Often sites to be entered are owned by organisations which carry details of the site at head-quarters, and it is necessary to liaise with headquarters staff over the question of availability of experts on the site, known hazards or rules for work on site.

For an undertaking in the natural environment, or indeed in abandoned built-up environment areas (from derelict buildings to old mine workings or waste tips), there may be no information available from site owners. In such cases any records held in the public domain should be sought, for example, in land office registers or historical records. Checks can be made with the Meteorological Office over expected weather conditions, or with agencies such as the local water authority or the Coast Guard over other environmental conditions.

Where conditions on site are not well understood it is essential that personnel with experience of such sites accompany the field worker, and, where necessary, a thorough investigation of the site be undertaken before the work itself is planned out.

Difficulties of access to the work site

This is by no means an uncommon problem in regard to observational, measurement or sampling work in the field. Wherever possible, the need for such tasks should be taken fully into account at the design stage for building, plant and general site developments. Very often field workers are subjected to quite unnecessary hazards by the lack of forethought of designers who locate sampling access points (if any) in extremely awkward or inaccessible places. This may necessitate climbing considerable heights, entering confined spaces, crawling through pipes or under structures, reaching, twisting, leaning and so on. One possibility is to design remote sampling facilities, automatic monitoring systems and telemetry links into the plant. If this is not feasible every effort should be made to design out hazards to workers when simply gaining access to sampling points.

An example of one such problem arose in the railway industry some years ago where there was a need to investigate a number of parameters associated with the performance of a new type of railway carriage under expected operational conditions. This involved setting up measuring equipment on the outside roof of the carriage and checking or adjusting it while the train was moving at high speed. Since the tests had to be carried out at night, to avoid normal daytime rail traffic, there was a great added danger of operating in the dark! Clearly, such hazardous work should be designed out wherever possible, in this case by automatic systems for the adjustment of measuring equipment on the train roof and for transmitting information electronically back into the carriage.

The designing out of such hazards is less feasible in the natural environment, or where the future need for sampling was simply not envisaged at all at the design stage. However, even in regard to the natural environment, steps can be taken to introduce automatic sampling or improve access to sampling points where repeat sampling is to be carried out. Thus, automatic sampling and analysis plant has been located on river banks with telemetry links to remote recording equipment. Alternatively, sampling stations have been built into river banks which can be utilized with minimum risk of workers falling into deep or fast flowing waters.

An example of extremely difficult access for sampling, which was not anticipated when structures were designed, concerns extensive programmes of investigation of modern tower blocks. Many of these very tall blocks of offices (or apartments), built in the 1960s, are already suffering extensive deterioration. This is leading, in some cases, to serious worries about complete collapse of the building and, in other cases, to worries about masonry or ornamental features falling off the buildings and crashing to ground level (the latter events are already far from uncommon). These problems necessitate thorough investigation of the outside of the buildings at levels much higher than can be reached by standard elevated platforms. Samples of deteriorating concrete are needed, as are observations of the extent of deterioration, and photographs. To deal with such problems the companies concerned with sampling have had to employ experienced rock climbers and train them to climb the buildings. As these staff usually have no previous relevant technical qualifications they have needed training in the sampling to be done. Although by no means a fully satisfactory outcome this is clearly preferable to attempting to train personnel to climb up tower blocks.

Many analogous problems could be cited in the natural environment, where samples must be taken from high cliff faces, from the bottom of mine shafts, or from the ocean bed. Again, experts at gaining access to the sampling points must be employed and given sufficient training to carry out the sampling. This approach was very successful in obtaining samples from the moon. In some cases, of course, staff may have a combination of technical expertise and expertise in working in the difficult environment, and are employed for this reason.

There is an ever-increasing range of equipment which allows laboratory staff ready and safe access to high sampling points, and which has been developed for maintenance work at heights. Similarly, special vessels have been designed to allow access to many different kinds of difficult waterways, for example, bogs and wetlands, deltas and estuaries. For the future, some of the remaining problems of difficult and hazardous access will surely be resolved by the increasing adaptation of robot technology. Already, robot crawlers have been developed to approach suspect bombs, carrying television cameras which transmit pictures back to observers sitting at a safe distance away. Similarly, mechanical 'pigs' have been developed to push television cameras right through sewers and drains to investigate their condition or locate blocks, where, at one time, workers would have been required to enter them under cramped and hazardous conditions.

Approaching and working in close proximity to unrecognized or disregarded hazards

Clearly, the approach outlined above for entering sites will go a long way to resolving such problems. Where sampling hazards in the built-up environment are significant, planned safe systems of work may be further formalized into 'permit-to-work' systems. Such permits are commonplace in connection with maintenance work and can ensure that hazardous machinery is locked off, electrical systems closed down, atmospheres checked for flammable or toxic substances (or for absence of oxygen) and so on. Wherever possible, hazardous equipment which must be approached by personnel in order to take samples, should be switched off and safely locked off, for example by a personal padlock, the unique key being held by the person using the equipment. Where this is not possible, the plant and work system must be designed to minimise risks to the worker taking samples. Machine guards will normally eliminate hazards from moving machinery, but may not always be applicable. Thus, it may not be desirable to either guard or switch off stirrers or pumps in open tanks in process plants where samples must be taken from the surface of liquids. In such cases, well designed barriers and supports must be incorporated to ensure that personnel do not slip into tanks while taking samples, and drown in the liquid, or sustain injury by its very nature, or by moving parts such as stirrer blades.

Clearly a full account of standard industrial hazards and their control is beyond the scope of this chapter, and these matters are well covered elsewhere. The key issue to bear in mind is the naivety of personnel when they go into unfamiliar plants. It must always be borne in mind that they may be putting plant workers at risk, for example, by placing equipment where it could fall from a height, or by bringing non-flameproof equipment into a potentially flammable environment.

The natural or 'semi-natural' environment will throw up a range of hazards to the sampler that are not controllable by the procedures developed for in-plant maintenance work. The very fact of working out-of-doors introduces climatic considerations ranging from heat and cold to high winds and even lightning. The field worker may be investigating rock samples which prove to be toxic, plants which prove to be poisonous, domesticated animals which are less than friendly, and so on. These hazards will be considered in detail later, but clearly, where the hazard cannot be eliminated by design or control of the environment, even greater emphasis must be placed on safe systems of work, protective equipment, clothing and training.

Hazards of the built-up environment which cannot be readily reduced by switching off plant include fast moving vehicles where sampling or measuring must be carried out at the roadside or by rail tracks., or where the work is taking place near to high voltage electricity transmission systems. These particular situations have given rise to the deaths of many workers, including staff involved in inspection or sampling work. Again, workers in the field should fully investigate the safety procedures which have been developed for maintenance workers who have to face such hazards. Such procedures, which may cover formal legal requirements in statutory regulations, industry codes of practice, company codes or safety rules, should be used as a basis for the development of safe systems of work for sampling activities. Generally speaking, the deaths of maintenance workers in these high risk situations have arisen from ignorance or disregard for well-established procedures. The complacency which is sometimes the cause of blatant disregard of safety procedures in roadside or trackside maintenance working is unlikely to be shown by laboratory staff. The bigger worry here is that inexperienced workers show poor judgement in regard to the distance away or speed of approach of fast moving vehicles. High voltage electrical cables and equipment are a great menace however, since they give no visible sign of danger, are often regarded as 'safe by position' (in the air or below ground), are not heavily guarded or protected, and exhibit characteristics which are not comparable with familiar mains voltage equipment. Staff must be trained in regard to high voltage hazards where there is any possibility of the sampling work bringing them close to such cables or equipment; staff required to work repeatedly in the field should enter into a longer training programme to familiarize themselves with a very wide variety of potential hazards.

Staff increasingly find themselves requested to go out into the field to test potentially hazardous atmospheres, or collect samples of suspect substances. This may occur on a one-off basis or involve regular testing and monitoring. Clearly, the minimum amount of work should be carried out on site, where safety facilities are poor. Generally, the toxicity of atmospheres, other than in confined spaces (see below) will be at sub-acute hazard levels. The bigger worry concerns repeated exposure to lower levels of hazardous substances, where there may be potential long-term health hazards. The classic current example is asbestos monitoring, where staff are frequently required to monitor atmospheres which are suspected of containing significant quantities of asbestos particles, or collect samples of deposited dust which could contain asbestos. Clearly, work should be planned so as to minimize exposure to the asbestos threat, in terms of time spent in the environment, and the collection of dust samples without disturbance of heaps. However, unless the levels of asbestos (or other harmful substance) are known to be insignificant with regard to short-term exposure, then full protective clothing should be worn and appropriate, effective respiratory protective equipment employed (ranging from an approved face mask to full positive pressure breathing apparatus).

Portable systems to provide local exhaust ventilation are available and may be appropriate where some work is required on site which could generate toxic dusts or fumes (e.g. cutting off samples from metal work, concrete or natural rocks).

Working alone

From the above discussion it is clear that lone working by laboratory staff in the field should be avoided as far as possible. For inexperienced staff it should be avoided completely, with an experienced site worker (or a field worker experienced in that type of natural environment) constantly in attendance. As staff gain experience at a site, local management will probably seek to reduce the involvement of a support worker. This is an increasing problem today, with staffing levels in organizations being continually reduced to lower costs.

One approach to this problem is to designate a limited area of the site where personnel will be fully trained as regards actual or potential hazards. Within this limited area, the worker will be deemed competent to be left alone. Should the task require operating at any time outside this limited area, contact should then be re-established with experienced site workers. Where the lone worker on site runs any risks higher than those common to 'lone workers' in the home, the office, or perhaps even the laboratory, then systems should be set up to monitor their safety. Systems vary from the unsophisti-cated (and desirable) checking by site workers or security staff at periodic intervals (of say 30 minutes), to telephone checking, through whistles and flares for use in emergencies, to the wearing of alarms by lone workers which can be set off by touch or automatically when they fall down following accidents.

It is important to know where lone workers are planning to operate as well as what they are planning to do, so that they can be located in emergencies (not just those they cause, but say, following a bomb threat and site evacu-ation order).

Lone working in the natural environment is highly undesirable, even for experienced staff. Close checking by other personnel, as described above, may not be possible (although telephone checking could be substituted by a periodic radio check-in procedure). Where individual workers, or even groups, are going into the natural environment, detailed information must be left at base, covering all plans, locations, movements and expected time of reporting back to base. If the environment to be entered is likely to be significantly hazardous (in terms of possible weather changes, the possibility of getting lost and so on) then the police and possibly other emergency services should be informed of the work programme. (See Figure 22.1)

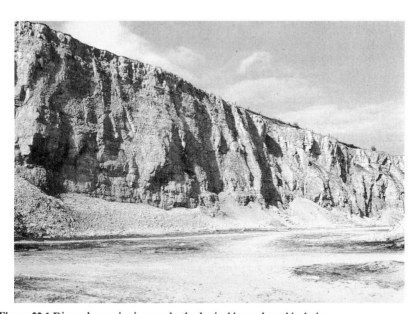

Figure 22.1 Disused quarries impose both physical hazards and isolation

Poor communications

The issue of poor communications is an important one for personnel to consider when going into the field. This problem is less significant on an industrial site, but takes on much greater significance when staff are planning to work in the natural environment (or semi-natural environment such as at a reservoir). Firstly, if the journey is long and the work site remote, staff must plan to cover all their needs from within their own resources. This is true for general aspects of the work and, additionally, for the welfare of the staff. It is particularly significant in regard to safety information and equipment, both of a preventative nature and for dealing with emergencies. The absence of appropriate safety equipment can lead to staff taking unnecessary chances because of their unwillingness to return to base to obtain the equipment. The absence of first aid or other equipment required for use in emergency situations may lead to accidents which although not too serious under normal circumstances could be extremely serious on site (broken legs for example).

Perhaps the most important facility lacking at many sites is running water, a commodity which is taken for granted by most laboratory-based workers. Clearly, removal of corrosive liquids from the skin, or the washing of wounds become much more difficult in the absence of substantial quantities of water. Even normal hygiene precautions such as the washing of hands before eating food may not be possible, a highly significant point if the handling of potentially toxic or infectious material is being contemplated.

While most hazards which could be envisaged are unlikely to give rise to problems on any one site expedition, it is far better to be pessimistic at the planning stage, and to take equipment to cover all foreseeable eventualities, than just to hope for the best.

Groups of workers operating at remote sites should keep in regular touch with base as far as possible, and should be aware at all times of the nearest house, the nearest telephone point, the nearest hospital and so on, so that the best response to any emergency is possible.

Working in confined spaces

Sampling requirements frequently involve entry into, and work within, confined spaces. Such confined space operations are notoriously hazardous, whether consisting of tanks or vessels within industrial plants, or caves and pot-holes in the natural environment. The overriding problem concerns the atmospheric situation, where the absence of significant air ventilation can readily lead to an absence of oxygen, or the presence of toxic or flammable gases or vapours. Many workers have been killed or suffered serious ill-health effects (such as severe brain damage) as a result of being overcome by toxic gases (or absence of oxygen, or both) on entering confined spaces. Common problems are the build-up of toxic hydrogen sulphide and flammable methane from anaerobic decomposition of biodegradable wastes and the flow of dense carbon dioxide gas or chlorinated solvent vapours into confined spaces below ground level.

It is essential that entry to confined spaces in the industrial plant environment is controlled by a 'permit-to-work' system. This in turn should involve the switching off and securing of all relevant mechanical and electrical systems, the blocking off of all routes whereby hazardous vapours could enter the confined space (ranging from pipes to drains), the thorough checking of the atmosphere for oxygen levels, and the absence of any flammable gases or vapours, or predictable toxic gases or vapours. Unless the atmosphere is satisfactory and certain to remain so, any staff entering the confined space should wear breathing apparatus. It should be noted that the very act of walking through sludge at the bottom of a tank may disturb dense toxic vapours. In many cases it is necessary for staff to wear a lifeline to assist in hauling them from the confined space (for example a tank or effluent pit), should he or she be overcome despite all precautions. Frequently, the worker is not expected to work in the confined space but is present to test the atmosphere before other staff enter. Wherever possible, this must be done from outside the confined space using appropriate sampling equipment. Even the act of putting one's head into the confined space to take a sample (of the air itself or the other substances present) can be dangerous. Personnel have been overcome by fumes when putting their heads down into manholes over drains, or even by bending down close to such openings to take samples. Again, it is very important to have a second worker present in case of emergencies, who must also be trained in emergency procedures, and told specifically not to enter the confined space without precautions if the first worker collapses. (Several workers have died one after the other in a number of incidents by going to the aid of a workmate in this way).

Confined space hazards in the natural environment cannot be so readily controlled as in the built-up environment, but many of the same precautions apply. Here, the risk of trips and falls, working in very poor light, lack of knowledge of the actual site and other problems must be added to the problems of potentially hazardous atmospheres. As the hazards increase, for example, entry to pot-holes or disused mines, then experts must be employed to take the samples. Wherever possible, systems of work should be developed (or designed-in) so that confined space entry for sampling purposes is not required. The increasing sophistication of measuring instruments and remote or automatic sampling equipment is of great help in this respect.

Working in hazardous positions

Clearly such work should be avoided as far as possible. Where this cannot be avoided, then back-up precautions must come into play to minimize risks. Common examples of sampling work in hazardous positions include working at heights, working where there is a risk of objects falling on staff, working over or adjacent to water courses or working over or adjacent to open vessels. In the built-up environment, platforms, gantries, walkways, stairs, handrails, barriers and kicking boards should be utilized to achieve safe access to all necessary areas of buildings or plants. In such cases, common risks remaining involve unguarded machinery, unprotected live electrical wiring and equipment, especially at heights. Such equipment has frequently been regarded as 'safe by position' on the argument that workers do not need access to the high level installation. Thus it is essential to check for such equipment and ensure that it is switched off and isolated before approaching the area for sampling purposes. Classic examples of accidents arising from this type of problem involve overhead cranes in tall workshops where the high level mechanical equipment is unguarded and the downshop electrical wiring is unprotected.

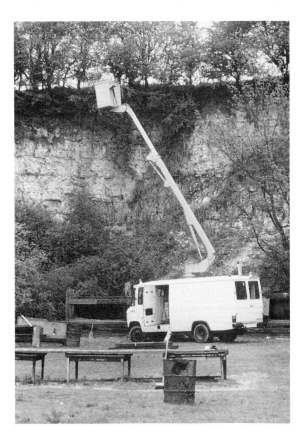

Figure 22.2 Mobile elevating platforms avoid dangerous scree-slopes to reach quarry faces

Where no lifts or stairs are available it is frequently possible to utilize purpose-designed mobile elevating platforms so that staff (and their equipment) can stand on a flat surface with no strain involved in getting up to higher levels. Such platforms (Figure 22.2) are much preferable to using either cradles pulled up by ropes or ladders, especially if any sampling equipment must be carried up. Platforms must be operated in strict accord with the code of safe working supplied by the manufacturer.

In the natural environment it is sometimes necessary to employ ropes and cradles to get to the sampling point and to work there. Obviously, staff must be well trained to utilize such equipment, and the equipment itself must be carefully and regularly checked by a competent person.

All precautions that can be taken to avoid objects falling from heights should be taken. Where this problem could still arise during sampling, the area below the sampling point must be closed off, signposted and access prohibited. All site workers should wear safety helmets to minimize the severity of head injuries from falling objects. Non-slip footwear is another important feature of protective clothing, in the context of avoiding slips and falls at heights.

Working by or over water courses is a major hazard for technical staff employed by the water authorities and others. It is crucial to recognize that even adults have drowned in a few feet of water, where a slip has led to a fall and consequent head damage to unconsciousness. Many inexperienced workers also underestimate the depth of natural water courses, the strength of currents or tides, the unevenness of the river bed, dangers of floating objects, pollutants and other hazards which make natural water courses much more dangerous than swimming pools, even for strong swimmers.

Again, systems of work should be developed to minimize the risk of workers falling into water courses while taking samples. Where any residual risk remains, then a second person must be in attendance, life-jacket worn, a lifeline attached, the emergency services alerted, and so on, according to the degree of risk involved. Only strong swimmers should undertake the work because of the immediate panic which weak swimmers or non-swimmers experience on unexpected immersion in deep, flowing water. The second person must be fully trained in lifesaving and resuscitation procedures.

Working in awkward or cramped positions

Here, the issue is less related to sudden death but more to long-term injury (often to the back or knees), ill-health problems if the work takes place repeatedly over long periods, and to the quality of working life generally. Wherever possible, such work should be designed out, and where it is still necessary, fit staff should be selected, suitable protective clothing provided, and the job rotated to minimize harm to any one worker. Sometimes, such ergonomically undesirable working conditions are combined with serious hazards such as working at heights or by deep water, and can lead to serious accidents as staff become fatigued. In the natural environment, cold and dampness often contribute to the enhanced risk of accidents.

Bringing equipment or chemicals on site

Bringing chemicals on site should be avoided wherever possible. If it is necessary to carry out tests *in situ* using chemicals, then the least hazardous substances possible should be employed in minimum quantities. Full precautionary measures must be utilized, with special reference to eye protection and the provision of eye-wash bottles. The limitations on washing facilities in the field must be kept in mind at the planning stage, and thick polythene lined securely fastening bins (or similar) employed to hold used containers. In transporting chemicals to and from site, considerable thought is needed to ensure that containers are suitable and that effective segregation of incompatible substances is achieved. Many countries have specific regulations on the transportation of hazardous substances, even in small quantities, and this is certainly true for the UK.

Equipment brought on site may present hazards simply by virtue of its weight, and individual loads should be planned taking into account the capacity of each worker to lift and carry the load over a distance without excessive strain. Often, strain results as much from the awkward shape or size of equipment as from its weight. Containers and carrying straps should be designed and utilized to assist the task. Wherever possible , mechanized or hand-pushed trolleys should be used to convey heavy equipment.

Another hazard which can arise with equipment is the possibility of it providing a source of ignition, from electrical contacts or even friction sparks where metal contacts stone, in the presence of a flammable atmosphere. While this will be most likely to occur in a confined space, it is possible to find pockets of flammable gas in open air environments, both natural and built-up. Such a possibility should always be borne in mind, and especially where it is planned to light matches for cigarettes, lamps or fires.

Electrical and mechanical equipment is often taken into the field to power tools and instruments. While well-guarded machines will not usually present extra mechanical hazards, electrical equipment can prove considerably more hazardous in the field. Dampness can give rise to corrosion and shorting problems, and wet hands make much better electrical contact with faulty equipment. Equipment brought into the field periodically is inevitably much more likely to be subjected to damage to cables, wiring and protective casings. While robust equipment should be designed and selected, regular visual inspection and basic electrical testing is essential to ensure the equipment is not deteriorating in use. Many safety conscious organizations require all electrical equipment to be checked in this way after every return to store following field use. A further precaution is to use low voltage equipment wherever possible (in the UK this means portable electrical equipment operating at 110 volts rather than the mains 240 volts). While this approach is valuable, one should never forget that 'it is the current that kills', not the voltage, and it is possible for large storage batteries to be dangerous in terms of the current passed through the body if the skin is wet and good electrical contact is made.

Lack of back-up preventative safety facilities

For much field work it is just not possible to provide the same level of preventative safety facilities, either in terms of software or hardware, that is normal in laboratories today. There is a wide range of portable equipment, such as small local exhaust ventilation systems, which can help in this case, provided electrical power is available. Inevitably, however, there is a need to focus on increased use of personal protective equipment. This topic is discussed later.

One possibility is to take a mobile laboratory out into the field, which does provide some limited safety services. Variations on this theme include converted buses, purpose designed trucks or caravans, and a variety of floating laboratories on boats and ships. It is even possible to transport light-weight prefabricated laboratory units to the site of work, where the extent of activity can justify this.

Lack of equipment and facilities for use in emergencies

A range of portable equipment for use in emergencies is available, ranging from lightweight first aid boxes to eye-wash bottles and small fire extinguishers. However, the field situation will often not offer the facilities which can usually be drawn on in a well-planned laboratory.

Planning of the field work must take this into account, and some practical response must be planned for all emergency situations which can be envisaged. Such planning will focus attention on the emergency equipment which is needed for the field work. It will also alert the field work team to the capabilities which will be expected from them in the field, from first aid to fire fighting. Any necessary training can be obtained to ensure that the field team can provide the emergency response needed to meet any foreseeable eventuality.

Remoteness from the emergency services

Problems which can arise in field work due to difficult communications have been stressed above. Again, where the work is to be carried out in locations remote from the emergency services, this problem should be kept well in mind when planning the work so that high risk operations are avoided. Alternatively, if the sampling work is vitally important, the work team can be enlarged to include medics and other specialists. In any case, the appropriate emergency services should be informed in detail of the work to be done and advice sought as to possible problems and appropriate action to be taken in emergencies. First aid capabilities may need to be enhanced, since standard first aid training assumes the prompt intervention of the professional medical services, rather than periods of hours (or even days) when the first aider will have to provide further treatment and nursing.

Unfamiliarity with work systems in operation

A number of key issues in this regard have been covered before in the context of site entry. While laboratory staff are under the supervision of experienced site staff the problem will be minimal. However, the longer the laboratory staff member spends on site the less supervision is likely to be provided. Sometimes, work systems which operate for a number of days are then changed as the work to be done changes. It is essential that site management ensures that laboratory staff on site are kept closely informed of any changes in work systems which could affect the safety situation. Thus, waste-water sampling in an electroplating plant may not involve significant risk where the waste-water contains low levels of toxic metals, but this becomes a different proposition on the days when plating work involves the use of sodium cyanide solutions which is rinsed off into the effluent plant. Similarly, sampling work in a little-used quarry may involve little risk except on the days of the month when blasting work is taking place. Frequent meetings between the site staff and the laboratory staff to discuss such matters will minimize such problems.

Unfamiliarity with established safety systems on site

If laboratory staff are to spend any time on site unsupervised, they must be informed about all the relevant safety systems including the emergency procedures. The provision of key documentation is necessary, and durable pocket cards listing the essential safety rules and details of what to do in emergencies are invaluable. Some companies operate formal safety training programmes for contractors' workers coming onto the site, and laboratory staff may benefit from attending such programmes. They should demand basic site safety information if not initially provided by the site management, and refuse to start work if dissatisfied in this regard.

Unfamiliarity with personal protective equipment and protective clothing to be utilized

Staff members are familiar with a certain range of personal protective clothing, but not always with the full range which may be necessary for site or field work. Often, the most worrying issue is the need to wear respiratory protective equipment of some kind. The selection of such equipment is a task for an occupational hygienist or a similarly qualified person. While a full discussion of such equipment is beyond the scope of this chapter, some key points are listed below.

Key considerations in the selection of respiratory protective equipment for field work

1. The initial choice is between ventilated helmets, face masks and positive pressure breathing apparatus with its own air supply.
2. Unless the atmosphere is certain to contain normal levels of oxygen at all times, positive pressure breathing apparatus is essential.
3. Breathing apparatus is heavy and cumbersome, restricts movement and communication, is expensive, requires extensive training and can generate its own hazards.
4. Ventilated helmets (of the Airstream type) are normally designed to draw ambient air through a filter and over the head and face of the worker. As such, they offer modest protection against dusts. They are not suitable for use with very harmful dusts (such as asbestos) and are of course ineffective against toxic gases and vapours.
5. Ventilated helmets are relatively comfortable to wear, offer built-in head protection, provide a cooling draft of air and can be operated by battery in the field.
6. Face masks can offer a high level of protection in the field, but must be of an appropriate type and make a very close fit to the face.
7. Training in their use is required to ensure that staff fit them properly.
8. For protection against dusts, the higher the standard of protection required, the better the filter system, and the more difficult it will be for the wearer to breathe normally.
9. For canister respirators against gases and vapours it is essential to use the correct type of canister. A respirator containing an ammonia gas removing cartridge is of no value where the atmospheric danger suspected is, say, hydrogen sulphide gas.

10. Canister respirators can provide protection only against low levels of the toxic gas for short periods – once the absorbent substance in the canister has been used up, the toxic gas can reach the nose in full force.
11. The shelf-life of canister respirators is quite limited, often 3 or 6 months, and it is essential to check this before taking canisters out into the field.
12. Respirators are not appropriate where toxic substances likely to be present in the atmosphere cannot be predicted, or where more than one toxic substance could be present.
13. Taking into account points (1) and (12), together with worries over effectiveness (especially fit to face), possibilities of wrong selection and other limitations of respirators, there is an increasing trend towards the use of positive pressure breathing apparatus, even in the field.
14. No respiratory protective equipment will provide protection unless strict hygiene protocols are employed to avoid toxic contamination of the inside areas of equipment. Similarly, it must be maintained to a high standard and carefully protected to take into the field.

Protective clothing in the field will include types familiar to staff, such as face masks, safety goggles and gloves. Overalls and rainproof coats are likely to replace laboratory coats, and safety helmets and footwear will frequently be needed. The suitability of footwear for the field terrain and tasks to be performed must be carefully considered, with a selection being needed where the field visit involves, say, walking first through boggy areas and then climbing up steep slippery paths or ladders.

For work in the open air staff will need to give full consideration to the choice of warm, waterproof clothing to protect them against the elements. This is especially the case for work in the natural environment, remote from cover, where cold, wet conditions can cause exposure, reducing work efficiency and ultimately causing hypothermia (and in extreme cases death). For prolonged periods of work in the field in inclement weather, several changes of clothing should be supplied for each individual, with plenty of towels, so that all can keep dry and warm between work periods.

Fortunately, there has never been such a wide selection of warm, weatherproof, light and flexible clothing as is currently available. Manufacturers and consultants can advise on a suitable choice of clothing for almost any climatic condition.

Difficulties of observation, measurement or sampling

Such difficulties in field work tend to arise from problems of access to the sampling or measuring point, as described earlier. Many accidents to staff have occurred from leaning and stretching in hazardous areas in order to take samples or measurements. Wherever possible, the hazards should be designed out so that standard sampling or measuring equipment can be used in the usual way. Alternatively, the equipment can be modified to reduce the risk. Where repeat samples or measurements will be needed on a continuing basis, automatic systems should be considered, ranging from remote sensing and telemetry to robotics. Where intermittent grab samples suffice, or one-off determinations are needed in a survey, simple measures can often be utilized to reduce risk levels. Thus, many of the cases of workers falling into tanks while taking samples in process plants or sewage works arise because a sample bottle has to be held under the tank liquid. The worker leans or hangs over the tank in a bent position, possibly holding a wet handrail for support, and slips while stretching out and down to obtain the sample. Attaching the sample bottle securely to a chain or rod can completely avoid this risk at minimal cost. Similarly, rock or dust samples can be safely picked up at a distance by tools attached to hand-operated extendible arms operated by the trained worker.

Observational work can sometimes be carried out at a distance by tele-scope or by the use of remote cameras, TV monitors and similar devices which do not require staff to approach the hazard area. Again, the emphasis must be on prior planning of systems of work to obviate risk taking on site.

Where there is no alternative to staff taking samples in a precarious situation, emphasis must be placed on such devices as secure safety harnesses with support ropes, lifelines and life-jackets, or other emergency back-up equipment, as appropriate.

Hazards of the samples themselves

While in many cases the samples to be obtained involve no significant risk, there are cases where the samples themselves are potentially harmful. Generally, this is because the sample contains toxic (or radioactive) substan-ces or potentially infectious micro-organisms. On occasion, samples may contain flammable or even explosive substances. Field work may involve the collection of poisonous plants or insects or, in some cases, large harmful creatures, ranging from stinging fish to poisonous snakes. Field workers who have protected themselves against hazards in collecting the samples must be aware of the need to transport and deliver the samples in such a way that others are not put at risk. This means designing or choosing suitable, secure containers, clearly labelled as to their contents. There are many cases of samples being delivered to laboratories for examination and analysis in leaking containers, or containers giving no indication on the outside that the contents are potentially harmful. Examples have ranged from small packages (even some delivered through the post) which arrived leaking suspect blood onto the hands of delivery staff and the recipient laboratory staff, to un-marked containers which, on opening, flicked toxic dust onto unprotected workers or stabbed them with 'sharps' such as broken glass. While laboratory based staff expecting to receive packages of potentially harmful samples should develop safe systems of work to protect themselves, the onus remains with the field workers to minimize risks at the outset by taking well designed and labelled containers into the field.

Natural hazards

Problems due to exposure to the elements were mentioned previously. To wet, wind and cold should be added excessive sunshine and heat and lack of water. Ice and settled snow will fundamentally change the nature of the outside environment from the safety viewpoint and may well require a variety of specialized equipment (and transport). High winds or driving rain may make some sampling operations unsafe.

To such obvious problems can be added hazards of flash floods, hurricanes, volcanic eruptions, lightning and similar natural phenomena. Local knowledge is invaluable in anticipating such hazards, as with tidal phenomena, quicksands, hidden pot-holes (or man-made but disused mineshafts or wells), areas prone to avalanches or rockfalls and the like. Where such hazards have arisen in the past, they are likely to occur again at some time, and multiple fatalities have arisen from over-optimistic assumptions about current favourable conditions prevailing indefinitely.

Drawing on past experience and predicted weather reports, taking sensible decisions about where to camp, proceeding cautiously, observing old rules such as not standing under trees during lightning storms; all these techniques and others can be employed to minimize risks from natural hazards. More specific risks from natural hazards will be discussed later in this chapter under specialized sampling activities.

Working overseas

From time to time laboratory workers are required to travel abroad to carry out field work or collect samples. Where this involves just short distance land movement across a border, the extra problems are the usual political, diplomatic, cultural, language, documentation and currency concerns. However, if the visit involves long distance travel, say by plane, to a totally different continent (hence overseas) there can be very considerable extra hazards for workers. Obviously problems arise from the very different customs, geography, climate, water, food and living conditions in the country visited. Field trips into remote areas will obviously require even more detailed planning than in the home country. Disease is a frequent threat, varying from mild stomach disorders due to dietary changes, through to serious polluted water-

516

related illnesses like cholera, or insect borne diseases such as malaria, in hot developing countries.

Despite information and warnings, it is by no means unknown for technical workers to become very ill from drinking water from suspect mains systems, or even direct from natural sources. Even medical students carrying out field work have contracted serious illnesses from drinking water from streams in hot countries. Any water to be used for cleaning (especially the teeth) should be sterilized with disinfectant tablets and only bottled drinks imbibed.

Diseases of contagion can often be combated by prior inoculation and taking of prescription drugs, and such precautions should be redoubled for field workers who will often be exposed to greater risks than normal business visitors or tourists. Knowledge of disease symptoms for the more common local diseases should be given to the field team, with details of how to treat afflicted individuals and how to get emergency assistance.

A threat to field workers that can exist in some countries arises from wild animals. While such threats are often greatly exaggerated, they are undoubtedly very real in some cases. Whether the threat arises from wild bears, poisonous snakes, sharks or any other creature, staff are ill-advised to ignore warnings, and should take suitable precautions as advised by the local authorities.

The infrastructure support for field work in many developing countries is weak, and it may be necessary to take many pieces of equipment, articles of clothing and materials which could be readily purchased in an advanced country. Wherever possible, an overseas major group work activity should be preceded by a planning visit by group leaders to investigate local conditions. Scientists and technicians with laboratory experience and local field experience are to be found in most countries, and visiting staff are usually well advised to contact these local experts for support as consultants. In addition to advising on all natural hazards, such local technical staff can be a great source of knowledge on local politics, local officials and regulations (what it takes to get equipment and samples through customs), and perhaps more importantly in these unsettled times, local crime problems or terrorist threats.

SPECIALIST SAMPLING WORK IN THE FIELD

Introduction

While it would be impossible to cover all specialist areas of field work sample collection, consideration of some specialist areas can throw further light on the generality of problems discussed above.

As earlier discussion has been orientated somewhat towards the built-up environment and the work of chemists, this part of the chapter will focus on field work sampling by geologists and biologists. Analogies can then be drawn with scientists and technologists facing similar hazards, such as archaeologists, agriculturalists and land surveyors.

Health and safety implications of geological sampling in the field

Many of the hazards typically faced by geologists in the field have already been discussed: remoteness and poor communications; lone working; climatic problems; difficulties of the terrain, including disused man-made sites; problems of transporting equipment; working near deep water or underground; utilizing chemicals and so on.

Here, some more specific hazards faced by geologists in the field can be added.

Hazards of tools

In geological sampling the collection of specimens may require the use of geological hammers, chisels or rock-drills. These hammering, cutting and drilling implements are themselves potentially hazardous, being heavy with sharp edges and points. In contact with rock or each other they become far more dangerous. Tools should be of high quality, hammers having secure heads, chisels with sharp edges and non-burred heads (to avoid pieces of the chisel head breaking off under impact from the hammer). A geological hammer with a chisel point should not be used as a chisel and hit with a second hammer since this may cause dangerous splintering. Whenever hammers or drills are used on rocks, goggles should be worn, since many rocks can send particles flying into the face. Where highly siliceous rocks are concerned, such as quartzite or chert, but particularly in the case of flint, (Figure 22.3) it is also wise to wear thick protective gloves and a face mask. Shards of flint can inflict deep cuts on the hands without warning.

Noise and vibration hazards

The use of equipment other than that needed for the simplest methods of specimen collection should not be allowed underground, and this only after advice from someone who knows the current state of the workings. Any raised noise or vibration levels could bring down the roof of underground workings. Similar problems can arise under cliff faces in natural environments or in quarries, or by scree banks, where noise or vibration can bring about rock falls. Impact noise and vibrations from hammering are especially likely to give rise to these serious results.

The physical removal of samples combined with the noise and vibration

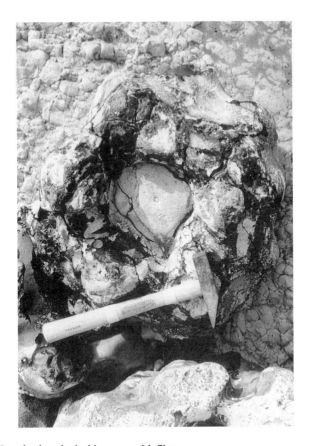

Figure 22.3 Standard geological hammer with flint

involved may cause serious instability if these are taken from a cliff or quarry face, or even just beneath an earth bank.

Vibration effects on the body

The shock on the wrist and arm from hammering, and the vibration, if excessive, when using drills can cause injury and can lead to long-term deformity or physical handicap if carried on frequently over the years.

Occupational deafness hazards

High noise levels can be generated when hammering or drilling against rock,

519

and when undertaken over any length of time require the use of appropriate ear-defenders.

Dust hazards

The use of the above equipment on rocks may give rise to hazardous dust particles which may be inhaled or accidentally ingested. While the open air situation is helpful in regard to inhalation problems, confined spaces or low level areas sheltered from air movement can result in hazardous dust built-up in the atmosphere. Mines and quarries, of course, may have high levels of dust in the environment due to work in progress. As discussed above, dust masks should be worn wherever there are significant levels of any dust in the environment, while special respirators are called for where siliceous dusts are involved, as is common for many rock working operations. Any possibility of encountering asbestos dust demands full precautionary measures.

Naturally toxic substances

Rocks and other natural materials of geological interest are in effect chemical compounds. While most are relatively harmless, there are a minority which are toxic. Of the 200 toxic materials listed by Puffer[1], many are so rare, or so disseminated through their host rocks or other minerals, that they pose no real threat. There are, however, around 40 minerals which are common enough to be a toxic risk. All but four or five of these are outside the usual list of common, or relatively well-known minerals, and this is both a danger and an aid. On the one hand it means that these are not often encountered, while on the other it means that they may more easily be encountered unknowingly.

The largest single group of toxic minerals are those containing arsenic. The most frequently encountered dangerous arsenic containing minerals are Annabergite: [$Ni_3(AsO_4)_2. 8H_2O$], Erythrite: [$CO_3 As_2 O_8.8H_2O$] and Pharmacolite: [$4(CaHA_s)_4.2H_2O$]. Mercury minerals such as Calomel: [$Hg_2 Cl_2$] need to be treated with caution, as do those containing cobalt, cadmium and thallium. Most of the lead minerals which may be toxic are those which also contain these above elements.

Although these minerals are toxic enough for inhalation hazards to be considered a risk, it is much more likely that any poisoning will be via accidental ingestion. This may occur from placing the contaminated fingers to the mouth, smoking (particularly hand-made cigarettes or pipes), and especially by eating contaminated food. Clearly the absence of hand washing facilities is a major cause of the problem, but hand wipes can be provided, and food and water kept covered and well away from the potentially toxic rock samples.

Finally, the risks of hazardous dusts and toxic gases are greatly enhanced when working underground, due to the lack of ventilation. Beyond any problems already outlined, in areas of granite rocks or rocks derived originally from granite (e.g. arkosic gritstones) there may be risk of radon build-up if ventilation is insufficient. Any entry into a previously sealed underground area must take this possibility into account, and radioactivity measurements should be undertaken.

Health and safety implications of biological sampling in the field

In most developed countries and many developing countries large areas of the 'outdoors' are no longer devoted to uncontrolled nature, but are given over to farming or forestry. Therefore, biologists are faced with a range of both natural and man-made hazards such as pesticides used in farming. Indeed, biologists are increasingly involved in sampling work in and around the built-up environment, whether for example on the verges of motorways or on top of mining spoil tips which are being developed ecologically for conservation reasons.

Some of the hazards faced by field workers across this range of environments have now been outlined, and this section will focus on some hazards more specific to biological sampling.

Hazardous plants

Hazardous plants, both wild and cultivated, can present significant risks to biological field workers. Hazards range from the toxicity of plants (1) via ingestion of sap from hand contamination (or indeed the plant if eaten in error) (2) via skin penetration or skin contact, across to physical injury from thorns or barbs, and to plant wounds allowing entry of pathogenic bacteria.

Skin irritation from contact with plants is a common hazard and can give rise to very unpleasant rashes, or even swelling or blistering. The stinging nettle *Urtica dioica* for example, is covered with stinging hairs which penetrate the skin on contact and inject a poison which causes blistering of the skin coupled with intense burning or itching. The most effective and well-known plants in terms of causing skin irritation are those of the family Anarcardiaceae, for example, poison ivy *Toxicodendron radicans*. However, the sap of common cultivated flowers such as daffodils, hyacinths and tulips is irritant and can cause painful lesions around and under the fingernail as well as an itching type of dermatitis in some cases. Euphorhiaceae have extremely irritant sap which causes severe burning of the mucous membranes, and is dangerous if it gets into the eyes.

The effects of contact with irritant plant material vary considerably from person to person and with the season. Indeed, some people seem immune from particular plant irritants, and their effects will vary greatly from one individual to another. Nevertheless, a sensible precaution is to wear gloves wherever possible. If it is impractical to wear gloves, a barrier cream containing sodium perborate can be used. Eye protection should always be worn where there is any chance that sap may spray out into the face during work with plants. Hands and gloves should be washed carefully before other parts of the body are touched and before eating and drinking. Irritated skin can be soothed with cold water, antihistamines or anti-burn creams.

Other parts of the body should be protected against stinging by wearing overalls, headwear and strong shoes, which will also minimize the chance of physical damage from branches, thorns or even stems and leaves of plants such as grasses. Even the fruit of trees can give rise to hazards if it is heavy, ripe and falls from heights onto the unprotected heads of field workers.

The most significant infection risk following deep puncture wounds from plants (or other sharp objects in the environment) is the entry of *Clostridium tetani* possibly leading to tetanus. For this reason, anyone working with their hands in the field should take a course of anti-tetanus injections, boosted periodically to retain immunity. Any wounds should be thoroughly cleaned, treated with antiseptics and covered.

Allergens

Plant materials which are small enough to inhale may produce allergies, such as 'farmer's lung'. Allergic syndromes can be developed from fungal spores, soil algae and pollen grains. While individuals will vary greatly in the extent to which they develop allergies, the concentration of allergens in the atmosphere will influence the incidence and severity of allergic reactions. Wherever possible, work should be planned to minimize the discharge of allergens into the air, to provide ventilation, and, if necessary, to utilize respirators. Workers developing allergic responses despite precautions should be withdrawn from the work if possible, especially where potentially asthmatic staff are involved. In the worst cases, serious lung damage can result from persistent exposure to allergens.

Animal hazards

The hazards of wild animals were referred to briefly above in the context of deliberate attacks on workers. Usually, animals will not attack unless threatened or rabid, very hungry or in some other way troubled. Sometimes when workers are deliberately attempting to catch free-living animals, or their young, defensive action from the animal is likely in terms of biting, pecking, clawing, goring or scratching. Generally, workers engaged on such tasks will be aware of the dangers and protect themselves accordingly.

Greater dangers can arise where animals are inadvertently disturbed, or where accidentally stepped on or touched. A wide range of shellfish create hazards of the latter type and can inflict nasty cuts from sharp shells or spines. Molluscs and Crustacea can inflict painful pinches and abrasions which can become infected. Protective footwear will avoid many of these hazards, and any wounds should be treated with a disinfectant. Reptiles and fish can also give a painful bite, sometimes leaving teeth in the skin which can increase the risk of infection. Again, protective clothing will minimize such risks.

Some animals and insects can bite or sting and at the same time secrete venom, or toxic chemicals. Again, individuals vary greatly in response, but in the worst cases, such poison bites or stings can cause serious adverse reactions, and at the extreme, even death. While poisonous bites and stings normally cause only local swelling, pain and itching, more systemic reactions indicate serious poisoning (including for example breathing problems, sickness, abdominal pains, fever, cramps or even paralysis). Such serious systemic effects indicate the need for urgent medical attention. Particularly hazardous are venomous bites or stings in or near the eyes, nose, mouth or throat. These can lead to severe swelling and respiratory difficulties, even asphyxia or serious eye damage, and certainly require urgent medical care. Again, prevention is better than cure, and the use of close-weave fabrics closed at the throat, wrists and ankles, gloves, boots and head protection will obviate most problems, mosquito netting being available to cover the face and keep off insects. Field workers often refuse to wear such protective clothing due to appearance or discomfort (especially in hot weather). However, some slight discomfort in the field is much to be preferred to severe pain from animal bites or insect stings. Even midges or ticks repeatedly biting on large skin areas can cause considerable suffering over subsequent days. Animals can carry diseases hazardous to man, and rabies was mentioned earlier. Britain is fortunately free of this problem, but there is the danger of Weil's disease which is transmitted by rats.

Agricultural pesticide hazards

The problems of hazardous chemicals in the field have already been discussed earlier in this chapter. However, such chemicals are widely used in farming and forestry today as pesticides, herbicides and fungicides. While such toxic substances should be used with great care, there have been many incidents of workers being contaminated with them. Biological workers may be deliberately entering an environment where such chemicals have been used, in order to investigate the outcome. In this case they will be aware of the hazards and can take appropriate precautions. Greater dangers arise where biologists enter agricultural or forestry areas not knowing that chemicals have been sprayed. This should be avoided by always checking carefully with local management before entering. Incidents have occurred where spraying has been carried out in areas where workers are present, or where wind has carried the spray from one area to another.

Again, close liaison with local management should obviate this risk. In any case, if the wind is more than a gentle breeze (say more than 5 km/h) spraying should not take place.

CONCLUSIONS

Staff entering the field for sample collection place themselves at greater risk than by remaining in the laboratory. However, provided this is recognized, and such trips are not treated as 'joyrides' or 'days off', but are carefully planned in line with the work to be done and the hazards to be faced, then the risks can be kept to an acceptable level. There is no substitute for local knowledge and experience, and, wherever possible, field work of the type discussed here should be a team effort between technical sampling experts and field experts. Over a period of time, either group can learn the work and gain the experience of the other so that all are finally fully competent in all respects. This is the ideal to be sought, and with continual implementation of safe systems of work can lead to very low residual risks.

LITERATURE CONSULTED

American National Standards Institute. (1977). *Safety Code for Portable Wood Ladders*, **14.1a** (New York: ANSI)

American National Standards Institute. (1977). *Safety Code for Portable Metal Ladders*, **14.2a** (New York: ANSI)

Arscott, A. and Armstrong, M. (1976). *An Employer's Guide to Health and Safety Management*. (London: Kogan Page)

Collins, C.H. (ed.). (1985). *Safety in Biological Laboratories*. (Chichester: Wiley-Interscience)

Duffus, J.H. (1980). *Environmental Toxicology*. (London: Arnold)

Flecknell, P.A. (1986). Exotic Animals. In Pearce, N.H. and Evans, S.E. (eds.), *Animals, Humans and Safety, IUSO Symposium Proceedings Number 3*. (Bristol University for Institute of University Safety Officers)

Forsyth, A.A. (1986). *British Poisonous Plants, Bulletin No 161*, Ministry of Agriculture, Fisheries and Food. (London: HMSO)

Gloss, D.H. and Wardel, M.G. (1984). *Introduction to Safety Engineering*. (New York: Wiley)

Health and Safety Executive. (1980). *Poisonous Chemicals on the Farm*. (London: HMSO)

Health and Safety Commission. (1984). *Approved Code of Practice on the Classification and*

Labelling of Substances Dangerous for Supply and/or Conveyance by Road. (London: HMSO)

Health and Safety Commission. (1987). *The Road Traffic (Carriage of Dangerous Substances in Packages etc.) Regulations 1986.* (London: HMSO)

Hickling, E.M. (1985). Selection and use of respiratory and other personal protection – review of ergonomic factors. In Pearce, N.H. and Evans, S.E. (eds.). *Identification and Control of Occupational Health Hazards in Research and Education, Symposium Proceedings Number 4.* (Bristol University for Institute of University Safety Officers)

Howie, F.M.P. (1987). Safety Considerations for the Geological Conservator. *Geological Curator*, **4**, No 7, 379–401

Kinghorn, A.D. (ed.). (1979). *Toxic Plants.* (New York: Columbia University Press)

Lynch, P. (1982). Matching protective clothing to job hazards. *Occupational Health and Safety*, **51**, 30–34

Nichols, D. (ed.). (1983). *Safety in Biological Fieldwork – Guidance Notes for Codes of Practices*, 2nd Edn. (London: Institution of Biology)

Puffer, J.H. (1980). Toxic minerals. *Min. Rec.*, **11**, 5–11

Tampion, J. (1977). *Dangerous Plants.* (Newton Abbot: David and Charles)

Wray, J.D. (1975). Safety and the hazards of using living organisms or material of living origin, *J. Biol. Ed.*, **9**, 3 and 140

References

1. Puffer, J.H. (1980). Toxic minerals. *Min. Rec.*, **11**, 5–11

23 Safety Measures to be Taken when Moving to a New Laboratory

W.E. Green and D. Donaldson

INTRODUCTION

This chapter has been written with the hindsight of our experiences of moving into and opening a new comprehensive division of pathology, consisting of four major departments on a new hospital site. Previously, the clinical chemistry and haematology departments were situated in one hospital, and the microbiology and histopathology departments in a second hospital. These hospitals were 10 miles apart.

During the period between the planning stage in 1976 and completion of the new hospital in 1983, a code of practice[1], directives from the Department of Health and Social Security, and other legislation were introduced. Changes to the design and services, therefore, had to be made both during the building and after the commissioning period.

It is essential that, before actual work is undertaken in a new laboratory, extensive safety checks are carried out. The move to a new laboratory must likewise be planned for maximum safety. To achieve this it is useful to regard the move as being in five phases, each of which will be discussed in the following pages.

PREPARATION FOR AND PLANNING OF THE MOVE

The preparation for and planning of the move takes place over a period of time during the commissioning period; it must be the responsibility of the most senior scientific or technical officer of the establishment. It is important, therefore, that an office is set up on the new laboratory site as soon as possible. This should be at the beginning of the commissioning period, in order that there can be ready contact with engineering and works staff. Immediate notice can then be brought about any items which need rectification, a record kept of them and a check made that corrective action has been taken. During this period it is essential that the officer identifies those parts of his normal duties which can be delegated to his deputies, so as to avoid unnecessary travelling between sites. Moreover, this should allow maximum time to be spent on the new site. A complete set of plans must be obtained. These should give details of each departmental laboratory, e.g. clinical chemistry, haematology and blood transfusion, microbiology, and histopathology with cytology; offices and other facilities must be included. Details on the plan should include the services, i.e. gas, water, electricity, telephone points, deionized and distilled water supply points, compressed air and vacuum outlets, extraction, ventilation, air conditioning, safety cabinets and work stations. The siting of major free-standing equipment such as centrifuges, chemical analysers and blood cell counters should also be included. The plans should be kept readily available for immediate reference on a table or bench, together with the data pack which gives details of all planned services, equipment and special provisions for lighting, electricity loadings, etc. A computer printout giving details of all equipment to be purchased or transferred is also of value.

Having obtained the plans, and after carrying out the foregoing procedures, a timetable is drawn up for the move; this should state approximate dates for the removal of each department, which should not all be transferred at the same time, as unforeseen safety problems may arise which could affect other sections, e.g. the ventilation may transmit smells or other environmental hazards. The move will inevitably include major equipment such as free-standing clinical chemistry analysers, centrifuges and counters for measuring radioactivity. Whenever possible, specialist firms which carry out regular maintenance on this type of equipment should be employed. They should be responsible, after decontamination by the scientific staff, for dismantling the equipment on the old site, then transferring, re-installing and testing on the new site. This procedure ensures that the greatest possible safety measures will be employed, using skilled persons; it must, therefore, be included in the timetable. A specialist removal firm should also be used for other smaller equipment, such as water-baths, incubators, refrigerators, bench centrifuges, glassware and stores. They will provide personnel for loading and unloading, packing cases, and trolleys for transportation. All items to be transferred should be identified with an adhesive label.

CHECKING THE NEW PREMISES PRIOR TO THE MOVE

It is useful to formulate a safety check-list for each department in the new premises prior to the move. This should be compiled from the plans and the data pack which provide the details of the special provisions required for each laboratory. The following check-lists serve as illustrations. They are not meant to be full and comprehensive, as requirements may differ from department to department. These lists can also be used as a basis for future safety audits.

Table 23.1 General check-list: all departments

Item	Safety check
Benches	Fixing, surfaces
Natural gas outlet	Operation, leakage
Electrical power	Fixing, permanent wiring, polarity
Sinks, wastes, water supply outlets	Connections, leakages, colour coding of taps
Compressed air and vacuum outlets	Connections, pressures, colour coding of taps
Handwashing facilities	Siting, towel dispenser, disposal sack
Eyewash station, coat hooks, personal lockers	Provision, siting
Fire equipment	Siting, correct type, colour coding
Safety signs	Correct positioning
Chemical storage	Siting, correct category storage
Gas cylinders	Storage, electrical fittings, securing
Lighting	Correct output
Floors	Construction materials
Shelving	Fixing
Refrigerator and incubator rooms	Temperature control, alarms, door locks
First aid cabinets	Siting and contents

1.   *General check-list applicable to all departments* (Table 23.1)
     (a)   *Benches*. All benches should be securely fixed[2]. They should be examined to ensure that all surfaces are impervious, smooth and resistant to disinfectantsr[3–5].
     (b)   *Natural gas outlets*. These must operate easily between the 'off' and 'fully on' positions and must be tested for leakage[6].
     (c)   *Electrical power points*. Supply points must be firmly fixed into the service ducts. Some items of equipment which are not moved during normal use are connected to the electrical supply by permanently installed wiring and have separate isolated switches. These should be tested for operational safety, and their polarity must also be checked[7].
     (d)   *Sinks, waste outlets, hot and cold water supplies*. All these items should be checked and tested to ensure that they have been connected correctly and that there are no leakages.
     (e)   *Deionized water outlets*. These are usually installed over a sink, most likely next to an ordinary water supply. There should be a colour coding on the control tap. The connection between the

529

control tap and the deionized water supply must be checked to ensure that it has been installed correctly.

(f) *Compressed air and vacuum outlets.* It is usual for most laboratories to have a compressed air supply and a vacuum line. These are usually sited together and should both be colour coded with a different type of connector for each service. A safety check must be made to ensure that these have been properly connected. The pressures and vacuum level should also have been checked[8,9].

(g) *Handwashing facilities.* Each work area should have handwashing facilities in close proximity, with both hot and cold water supplies[2,10–12,37]. A paper towel dispenser and disposal sack holder should also be provided[11].

(h) *Eyewash station.* Some safety advisers advocate the provision of an eyewash station, particularly in chemistry laboratories[13,19]. This should be sited in close proximity to the handbasin.

(i) *Coat hooks.* Coat hooks should be provided for protective clothing. These should be near the entrance to the laboratory area[14,15].

(j) *Personal lockers.* Provision should have been made for an area to house personal lockers and coat hangers, so that outdoor clothing is not taken into the laboratory working areas[14].

(k) *Fire hoses and extinguishers.* Each laboratory working area should have a water fire hose and fire extinguishers within easy access[16-18]. The types of extinguisher which should be available are: carbon dioxide - coloured black, powder - coloured blue, and if there is no fire hose available, water - coloured red (Table 23.2).

Table 23.2   Fire extinguishers

Type of extinguisher	Electrical	Solvents	Chemicals which react with water	Paper, rags, wood, etc.	Remarks
			Fires for which suitable		
Water (red)	No	No	No	Yes	
Carbon dioxide (black)	Yes	Yes	Yes	Yes	Do not use in confined space
Powder (blue)	Yes	Yes	Yes	Yes	Not for small fires in delicate machinery

(l) *Safety signs.* Check that all safety signs are correctly positioned, indicating hazardous areas and emergency exits. These should include emergency exit, fire exit, containment level III accommodation and prohibition signs, e.g. 'No smoking, eating, drinking'[20].

(m) *Chemical storage areas.* Storage rooms for flammable solvents and toxic chemicals are best situated away from the main laboratory building, preferably outside. They should comply with safety regulations[16, 81,82].

(n) *Gas storage area.* Gas cylinders must be stored in special well-ventilated stores which should have flame-proofed electrical fittings. Cylinders must also be stored vertically in segregated groups and secured with safety chains. It is mandatory for the storage area to have both warning and 'No smoking' signs[16,21,84,85,86].

(o) *Lighting.* Laboratory lighting must not cast shadows over working benches and should have a 200/300 lux output[21-23]. All fluorescent light tubes must be of the colour-matching type.

(p) *Floors.* All floors should be constructed of non-slip materials; surfaces containing graphite are used for most laboratory areas, while terrazzo is desirable in cleaning and preparation areas[10,24].

(q) *Shelving.* All shelving must be checked to ensure safe and secure fixing. This particularly applies to 'spur-type' shelving.

(r) *Refrigerator and incubator rooms.* All refrigerator and incubator rooms should have a temperature control alarm system which is wired to a fault indicator panel with audible alarm[48]. The door lock should be checked for opening from inside, so that it can easily and safely be opened in cases of accidental closure.

(s) *First aid cabinets.* Each laboratory area should have a first aid cabinet in a readily accessible position; small, medium and large sterilized unmedicated dressings, triangular bandages, adhesive wound dressings, adhesive plaster, absorbent cotton wool, sterilized eye pads, bottles of common salt, Epsom salts (magnesium sulphate), 1% acetic acid and a tablespoon should be some of the items contained in the cabinet[25,26].

Table 23.3 Check-list: clinical chemistry department

Item	Safety check
Autoanalysers	Wastes, electrical and water supplies
Radioimmunoassay	Compressed air supply for some gamma counters, benches, floors, electrical supply for centrifuges
Piped gases	Colour coding, valves, leakage, special requirements
Atomic absorption spectrophotometer	Gas pressure, air extraction
Distilled water apparatus	Electrical loading, connections for water supply, waste
Fume cupboards	Controls, extraction rate, wastes
Douche shower	Siting, operational safety

2. *Check-list applicable to a clinical chemistry department (Table 23.3)*
   (a) *Autoanalysers.* Most free-standing clinical chemistry analysers have waste outlets. These should be connected to the main under-floor waste pipe which should be resistant to corrosive acids, solvents, etc. A continuous water supply is needed for some equipment – e.g. Technicon SMA plus – which must be run at the correct pressure[27]. It is also advisable to have an electrical supply suspended from the ceiling service duct to avoid the safety hazards caused by electrical cables extending across the floor.
   (b) *Radioimmunoassay laboratory.*
      (i)   Gamma counters. Some older type gamma counters need a piped compressed air supply. This should be checked for correct function, pressure and safety.
      (ii) *Workbenches and floors.* Both of these items must conform to the safety regulations for radioisotope laboratories[28,29]).
      (iii) *Centrifuges.* These are often free-standing and have a fixed electrical supply with a separate isolated switch. This should be checked for correct operation.
   (c) *Piped gases.* Argon, hydrogen and nitrogen are used in gas chromatography, acetylene in atomic absorption spectrophotometry, and propane in flame photometry. The on/off valves for all these gases should be checked for correct labelling and the outlets checked for correct colour coding. All the pipelines must be checked for leakage. Storage cupboards for the piped gases should be outside the building and must have louvred lockable doors. The doors should have warning signs affixed. Acetylene needs special piping and must not be allowed to come into contact with copper or any alloy containing more than 70% copper[9,16,21,30,46,62].
   (d) *Atomic absorption spectrophotometry*
      (i) The acetylene gas reducing valve should be set to the correct pressure, as required by the safety regulations[9,16,21,30,46,62]
      (ii) The extraction unit together with the inverted funnel hood must be checked for leakage and operational safety.
   (e) *Distilled water apparatus*
      (i) The electrical supply should be checked for correct output load.
      (ii) The water inlet for distillation and cooling, and the waste outlet with overflow should be checked for correct connections.
   (f) *Fume cupboards*
      (i) The controls for fume cupboards must be fitted on the outside[4].

(ii) All fume cupboards should be tested and labelled to show the category of performance. When the hazard is moderate there should be a minimum flow rate of 0.43 m s^{-1} at a sash opening of 600 mm. The minimum flow rate should be increased to 0.71 m s^{-1} at a sash opening of 600 mm when working with volatile highly toxic compounds[21,31]

(iii) The drain waste and any other waste entering the same drain should be checked to see that there is a sealed trap.

(iv) Special water sprinklers should be fitted to fume cupboards for washing the surfaces when carrying out work with perchloric acid[32].

(g) *Douche shower.* A check should be made to see that the shower is operational; any electrical sockets or switches should be shielded from water splashes.

Table 23.4 Check-list: haematology and blood transfusion department

Item	Safety check
Blood cell counters	Effluent wastes
Cell counting room	Temperature, ventilation
Blood bank refrigerators	Temperature controls, high- and low-temperature alarm systems
Automatic blood grouping machines	Effluent wastes

3. *Check-list applicable to a haematology and blood transfusion department (Table 23.4).*

(a) *Haematology blood cell counters.* Provision must be made for the effluents from automated blood cell counters to be discharged directly into the waste plumbing system. A drip cup in the bench is the most commonly used method. A safety check should be made to ensure that the wastes have been correctly connected. Polypropylene waste pipes should be installed, as sodium azide is sometimes used as a preservative for cell counting solutions[33,34].

(b) *Ventilation.* A check should be made that the cell counting area is adequately ventilated, as room temperatures of 30 °C or over cause malfunction of the microprocessor controlling the equipment.

(c) *Blood banks.* A thorough safety check on the blood bank temperature control and alarm systems should be made to ascertain that they have been correctly installed.

(d) *Auto-blood grouping machines.* The effluents from these should be discharged into polypropylene drip cups; polypropylene waste pipes from these should feed directly into the plumbing system as

sodium azide is frequently used as a preservative in blood grouping sera and other reagents[33,34].

Table 23.5 Check-list: microbiology department

Item	Safety check
Containment level III accommodation	Door fittings, notices, cabinets, ducts, fans, controls, air flow
Gas cylinders	Safety fixings
Centrifuges	Microbiological safety requirements
Reception	Restriction notice, benches
Cleaning and sterilizing rooms	Sink and machine wastes, mains water and deionized water connections, autoclave tests, hot air sterilizer tests, recorders, warning signs, floors
Plate pouring machine	Autoclave safety tests, deionized and mains water connections
Laminar flow cabinet	Type, operational safety

4. *Check-list applicable to a microbiology department, including reception, cleaning and sterilizing areas* (Table 23.5)
    (a) *Containment level III accommodation.* Each clinical laboratory has containment level III accommodation which is normally located within the microbiology department. It is essential that the safety of this room is scrupulously checked. The door to the room must have the warning sign 'Danger of infection' within the bio-hazard symbol displayed on the outside. A glass panel must also be fitted, but should there be no input ventilation, a louvre is required[15]. At least one exhaust protective cabinet (class 1) will be fitted and this must be checked for the correct fitting of a high-efficiency particulate filter. The passage of air into the cabinet must also be checked for safety with a vane anemometer. The flow of air must be at least 0.75 m s^{-1}, but not in excess of 1.0 m s^{-1}. Other safety measures such as exhaust fan, audible warning and airflow indicator must be passed for safety[35–37,43].
    (b) *Gas cylinders.* Cylinders of carbon dioxide/hydrogen for anaerobic cultivation and carbon dioxide for incubators are frequently used in a microbiology laboratory. For safety purposes the cylinders must be strapped, chained or clamped vertically in the position in which they are to be used, or alternatively gas cylinder stands must be provided[10,21,38].
    (c) *Centrifuges.* A safety check should be made to ensure that all centrifuges in the department have sealed buckets, so that there is adequate protection from category B1, B2 and C micro-organisms and agents.

(d) *Reception*. A safety sign restricting entry to authorized staff must be displayed on the door. The sorting benches must be impervious and resistant to disinfectants[3].

(e) *Cleaning and sterilizing areas*

   (i) All wastes from sinks and glass washing machines, and mains water and deionized water supplies, must be checked for correct connections and leakage.

   (ii) Autoclaves must be thoroughly tested before routine use, for safety of operation, using thermocouples placed at the bottom and in the middle of loads. This determines the penetration time, which when added to the exposure time, ensures sterility. The procedure must be repeated with different types of load, e.g. fluids and discard waste. All recorders must be checked for correct operation and accuracy. Wastes from the autoclave to drainage should be checked for correct pipe bore and connections[39–41].

   (iii) Hot air sterilizers and their chart recorders must be checked for safety before use.

   (iv) Mandatory warning signs and autoclave operating instructions must be prominently displayed in these areas[42].

   (v) The floors in these areas should be constructed of terrazzo material; this is very hard-wearing and more resistant to bacterial survival[10,24].

(f) *Plate pouring machine with autoclave*. The autoclave attachment to a plate pouring machine must have an insurance certificate before it is used[40]. The mains water and deionized water supplies should be checked to see that they are correctly connected.

(g) *Laminar flow cabinet*. Media preparation departments often have a laminar flow cabinet installed. This should be checked for safe and correct operation before use[43].

Table 23.6 Check-list: histopathology and cytology department

Working area	Safety check
Cytology processing room	Protective cabinet, door fittings, ducts, notices, fans, controls, air flow
Formol-saline preparation room	Air extraction, door fittings, floor, electrical fittings
Block storage area	Fire precautions
General working area	Douche shower, operational safety
Slide staining and mounting area	Bench level extraction
Cutting-up room, specimen mounting room	Siting of sink disposal unit, bench level extraction, electrical fittings, window glass, operational safety

535

5. *Check-list applicable to a histopathology and cytology department (Table 23.6)*
    (a) *Cytology processing room*
        (i)   An exhaust protective cabinet (class I) is normally fitted in this room. Safety checks, as already described for cabinets in microbiology, should be carried out[36,43,44].
        (ii) Hooded air extraction at bench level must be checked for safety as toxic solvents such as xylene are used when mounting cover slips over specimens on microscope slides[21,47,49].
    (b) *Formol-saline preparation room*
        (i)   As formaldehyde vapour may be present in this room there should be both high- and low-level air extraction with a louvred grill in the door. The correct rate of extraction should be checked so that formaldehyde vapour does not enter other working areas[21,47,49,52].
        (ii) The floor in this room should consist of terrazzo material together with a drain in case of formaldehyde spillage[10,24].
        (iii) There should be no electrical points in this room and the lighting connections must be flashproof in order to avoid explosions[17,50]
    (c) *Storage of paraffin blocks.* As paraffin blocks of prepared material are a fire risk, a safety check should be carried out to ensure that fire precautions are adequate[51].
    (d) *Bench level extraction with hoods.* Hooded air extraction at bench level must be provided in the specimen cutting-up room, specimen mounting room and over the slide staining and mounting bench. This must be checked for operational safety[21,47,49,52].
    (e) *Sink disposal units.* These are usually fitted to sinks in the cutting-up and specimen mounting rooms. They are used to dispose of small pieces of tissue after processing. A check should be carried out to ensure that the tissue has been safely ground up (without leaving residual formaldehyde vapour in the sink area) and discarded into the drainage system.
    (f) *Douche shower.* A check should be made to ensure that both the shower and drainage are operational.
    (g) *Cutting-up and processing room*
        (i)   A check should be made that the window of this room has translucent glass, particularly if it can be overlooked from other buildings.
        (ii) Paraffin wax and solvents used in the processing of tissues are great fire risks in this area. Careful safety checks should, therefore, be carried out on all electrical and electronic equipment, plugs, and sockets to avoid the possibility of sparking and consequent explosion[21,47,48,51].

THE MOVE

After all the pre-move safety checks have been carried out on accommodation, services, fittings and safety equipment, including the special requirements of each department, the actual move should then follow in four phases.

Secondment of senior staff to the new premises

The role of the most senior scientific or technical officer on the establishment changes at this stage to that of co-ordinator and trouble-shooter, but at the same time retaining links with the contracting engineering and works staff. At this juncture there will also be hospital engineering and works staff on the site. It is, therefore, essential that the most senior scientific or technical officer of each department is seconded to the new site and that part of his or her normal duties is delegated to deputies. A list of new and transferred equipment should be given to the officer whose duties will be to supervise the installation and to carry out the operational and safety checks. Any malfunctions or safety problems should be notified to the co-ordinator who will take the necessary corrective action.

Delivery of new equipment direct to the new laboratory site

Delivery of new equipment for the laboratories will usually be made to a central hospital store. The storekeeper should notify the co-ordinating officer who will arrange for the equipment to be transferred, with the delivery note, to the laboratory. The contents of each consignment should be meticulously checked in order to avoid subsequent problems with the suppliers about non-deliveries and short-deliveries.

The departmental senior officer, having positioned the equipment in its allocated place, will then carry out the installation and necessary safety checks. If the installation is to be undertaken by a contractor the officer should be present to supervise the work.

Transfer of existing equipment from old site to the new site

When the majority of the new equipment has been installed and checks have been carried out, it is advisable to run samples in parallel on both new and old equipment. This procedure often highlights problems in operating new instruments, and these can therefore be rectified before the move takes place. The departmental senior officer, having made certain that all installations in the new department are operating satisfactorily and safely, should next arrange a date for transfer of equipment and work from the old department. The move is best achieved over a weekend when the workload is usually lower than during the week. Specialist firms should be engaged to move the large pieces of equipment, and the opportunity taken to have major maintenance carried out at the same time. Equipment which has been used for testing biological materials must be disinfected and made safe before being dismantled or disconnected in preparation for the transfer[53,54]. To avoid confusion at the time of the move, all equipment, boxes of materials and other items for transfer should have an adhesive label. This method will assist any contractors carrying out the move.

Transferred equipment should be checked for operational safety after installation on the new site. These checks should include: examination of compressed air connections to old type gamma counters and flame photometers; piped gas supplies to atomic absorption spectrophotometers, gas chromatographs and flame units; drainage from free-standing chemical analysers; and all electrical connections, fuses and insulation[7-9,16,21,27,30,46,62].

Special care must be taken when packing glassware to avoid breakage during transit. A large number of items such as pipettes, test tubes, measuring cylinders and flasks will still be in the same packaging as that in which they were received from the suppliers. They can be safely transported without further packing, but 'With Care' labels should be attached to the boxes. Likewise, items which have been in daily use should be packed in similar manner. Pieces of glass apparatus should be carefully placed in boxes, surrounded with polystyrene packing, secured and labelled with a list of contents, not forgetting 'With Care' labels, and any other hazard warning notices.

The transfer of chemicals will present the most hazardous problem, particularly if the new laboratory is some distance from the old one and public roads have to be used. In clinical laboratories the following categories of chemicals, which must always be treated with the utmost care, are commonly used[55]:

1. Highly reactive chemicals; strong acids, strong bases, halogens, etc.[63]
2. Flammable chemicals; acetone, benzene, ethanol, methanol, toluene, xylene, etc.
3. Toxic chemicals; carbon tetrachloride, cyanides, formaldehyde, mercury, silver nitrate, etc.
4. Carcinogens; naphthylamines, benzidene, o-tolidene, chromates, etc.[56,57,64]
5. Unstable chemicals; acetylene, sodium and potassium chlorates and perchlorates, titanium chloride, picric acid, hydrogen peroxide, etc.[58,59,63]

Under the Health and Safety at Work Act (1974), suppliers are required to warn of dangers and to indicate safety precautions. This is done by the use of standard hazard warning symbols and by further written information on the label (Figure 23.1). Additional regulations are in force which state requirements for the transport, packaging and labelling of dangerous substances[60]. Vehicles must always carry the appropriate hazard warning signs and fire extinguishers. Protective equipment for personnel handling chemicals and driving vehicles must also be provided in case of accident or spillage, e.g. rubber or plastic gloves, face shields or goggles, rubber boots, all-purpose respirator, brush, rubber dustpan and large polythene bucket – the latter for holding broken glass[61].

Flammable chemicals are often supplied in 23 litre drums. These should be checked to ensure that they are safely sealed before transporting them between sites.

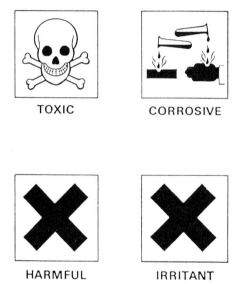

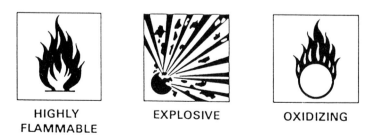

Figure 23.1   Chemical hazard warning symbols

539

Large Winchester bottles containing flammable, toxic and highly reactive chemicals should be transported singly with extreme care, in plastic carriers with tightly fitting screw lids, such as 'Safe Pak' containers[65,66]. Other dry chemicals should be carried in stout, sectioned cardboard boxes. Groups of toxic, highly reactive and flammable chemicals must always be separated for transportation in case of accidents.

Transfer of staff from old site to new site

The final stage of moving a laboratory from an old site to a new site will be the transfer of personnel. Some persons are resistant to change and may even be resentful. It is, therefore, important that all staff are taken round the new premises in small groups during the commissioning period in order to familiarize them with their new surroundings and obtain their views on the environmental working conditions. The opportunity should be taken on these visits to explain alterations in working practices, particularly those which will be introduced as safety measures in the new situation. All staff should attend fire lectures and drills on the new site in order to acquaint them with fire-fighting equipment, emergency procedures and layout of the building in which they will be working.

ENSURING THAT VACATED BUILDINGS ARE MADE SAFE

After the laboratory departments have been moved to the new site and all work on the old site has ceased, the vacated accommodation must be kept locked until it has been made safe for other persons to enter the premises. The accommodation will most likely be used for a completely different purpose, such as offices or stores. It will, therefore, be necessary to remove all old laboratory fittings such as cabinets, ducting, sinks, wastes and benches (Table 23.7).

Table 23.7 Safety of vacated buildings

Safety aspect	Safety procedure
Microbiological	Disinfection of safety cabinets, ducts, switchgear, benches, sinks, wastes, hazardous waste
Chemical	Treatment of sinks and wastes Disposal of waste chemicals Radioactivity checks

Microbiological safety

1. All safety cabinets and associated ducting, fans and switchgear must be disinfected with formaldehyde according to an approved method[43,67,68].
2. Benches on which biological materials have been examined must be washed down with suitable disinfectants such as clear phenolics or hypochlorite (2.5% Chloros)[69].
3. Sinks and wastes must be disinfected with 250 ml of hypochlorite (2.5% Chloros) before any plumbing work is undertaken[54].
4. Any hazardous waste materials must be put into suitable containers or biological hazard bags and autoclaved before disposal[70].

Chemical safety

1. Sodium azide is used as a preservative for serum and in biological test solutions. In many old laboratories there may be metal waste pipes in some part of the drainage system. It is important, therefore, before any work is carried out, to treat the sinks and wastes with 10% ceric ammonium nitrate solution, in order to destroy any residual azides which may be present[33].
2. Laboratory benching, floors and pipework can be contaminated by picric acid waste from automated analysers. Picric acid and especially its calcium, iron, copper and lead salts can be very explosive when dry, and are readily detonated by impact or heat. The dismantling of metallic drains used for picric acid discharge may in itself be a hazardous operation and it is essential, therefore, to seek expert advice[83].
3. The disposal of waste chemicals is controlled by a number of statutory regulations[71–73]. Harmless solids of all types may be placed in waste bins for collection. Harmful solids must either be rendered harmless before disposal, or submitted as chemical waste, being collected and disposed of according to the regulations. Liquid materials not miscible with water must not be discarded into sinks, drains or gulleys; similarly, flammable materials must not be discarded. Aqueous solutions of inorganic substances and soluble organic compounds should be neutralized and well diluted before disposal by drain. Solutions containing cyanides and chromates must be chemically treated or disposed of in the same way as harmful solids. Care should be taken in the collection of waste solvents to avoid incompatible mixtures; major explosions can readily result. They should be collected in separate drums and disposed of as indicated above[74,75].
4. Radioimmunoassay laboratories must be checked for radioactivity; checks must include sinks and wastes. Proprietary detergents such as

541

RBS25, Decon 75 and Decon 90 are very efficient decontaminants which are generally improved by the addition of a little EDTA. They may also be used for decontamination of paintwork, benches and floors[28,45,76].

When all safety checks and measures have been carried out, a signed safety certificate or similar notification should be issued. This should be posted inside the laboratories to inform other personnel entering the premises that safety checks and procedures have been carried out.

ENSURING THAT OLD DISCARDED EQUIPMENT IS SAFE FOR DISPOSAL

When the move to a new laboratory has been completed, it will often be found that there will be some items of old equipment left behind in the vacated premises. Microbiological, chemical and radioactive decontamination procedures must be carried out to render the equipment safe for disposal. Some of the procedures and items most frequently requiring decontamination are discussed below in separate categories (Table 23.8).

Table 23.8 Safety of discarded equipment

Safety procedure	Item
Microbiological decontamination	Centrifuges, refrigerators, water-baths, lids and racks, autoanalyser equipment
Chemical decontamination	Freeze-drying and vacuum systems, glass apparatus
Radioactive decontamination	Glassware, equipment, metal tools

Microbiological decontamination

1.   Centrifuges which have been used for centrifuging biological materials must be treated with glutaraldehyde at a dilution of 2–3% in 0.3% bicarbonate buffer, as it is most effective at pH 7.0–8.0. The trunnions, buckets and rotor should preferably be autoclaved[69,77].
2.   The inside of all refrigerators in which biological materials have been stored should be cleaned with a suitable disinfectant. Chloros must not be used on metal cabinets. However, the hypochlorite Diversol BX is said to be non-corrosive. Clear phenolics, such as Hycolin, Printol and Stericol, are most commonly used[69].
3.   The interiors, gabled lids and racks of water-baths used in microbiology

or serology should be disinfected with glutaraldehyde or a clear phenolic solution at appropriate dilution[69].

4. Cryostat cabinets must be disinfected with 50–100 ml of formalin BP. After leaving for at least 24 hours with the front closure in place, a beaker containing 10 ml of ammonia S.G. 0.880 should be placed in the chamber and left for 1 hour before removal[78].

5. Autoanalysis equipment, particularly dialyser water-baths, should be treated with a disinfectant before dismantling. A 2% solution of glutaraldehyde is most commonly used for this purpose; this should be allowed to act for at least 30 minutes. Analyser manifolds can be treated with a 4% solution of formaldehyde, which should be allowed to run through the system for about 10 minutes and then thoroughly washed through with water[53,54].

Chemical decontamination

1. Freeze-drying and vacuum systems may be used for processing materials containing sodium azide, which has been added to prevent deterioration caused by micro-organisms, e.g. long-term preservation of biological materials such as quality control sera. Hydrogen azide (hydrazoic acid) is readily lost from acidic and weakly basic materials containing sodium azide under conditions of applied vacuum in freeze-drying systems, and is the source of potential explosive and toxic hazards:

    (a) Hydrogen azide may be found in the waste condensate water of the freeze-dryer, which is usually discharged to drains.

    (b) Hydrogen azide, which is extremely toxic, may be discharged from the vacuum pump exhaust into the surrounding atmosphere – a threshold limit value (TLV) of 0.1 parts per million would be considered appropriate for health and safety[79].

    (c) Hydrogen azide may react with heavy metal components of the freeze-drying system, notably copper, forming shock sensitive azides, which are extremely explosive.

    It is essential, therefore, to seek expert advice in order that such equipment can be made safe[79].

2. The contents of any glass apparatus should be disposed of in accordance with approved safety procedures. It is not sufficient to dispose of the bulk of the contents and to leave the residue in the apparatus. This must be removed, and concise instructions given as to how the apparatus is to be cleaned. It is a safety hazard to leave dirty apparatus in a laboratory. Only inert solvents or detergents should be used for clean-

ing, except in special circumstances when safe instructions should be clearly given[74].

Radioactive decontamination

1. Glassware which has been used in a radioimmunoassay laboratory must be cleaned with scrupulous care. All vessels should be clearly marked and segregated for special attention. The glassware may be cleaned by any of the normal chemical agents, of which a mixture of chromic and sulphuric acids is probably the most useful[80]. As previously described, proprietary detergents such as RBS 25, Decon 75 and Decon 90 are very efficient decontaminants.
2. Metal equipment and tools should be surveyed to detect possible contamination. They may be cleaned with a detergent, followed if necessary by a 10% solution of sodium citrate, or ammonium bifluoride. When all other procedures fail with stainless steel, hydrochloric acid should be used, though this may cause corrosion[80].

References

1. DHSS (1978). *Code of Practice for the Prevention of Infection in Clinical Laboratories and Post-mortem Rooms*. (London: HMSO)
2. Munce, J.F. (1962). *Laboratory Planning*. (London: Butterworth), pp. 127,288
3. DHSS (1978). *Code of Practice for the Prevention of Infection in Clinical Laboratories and Post-mortem Rooms*. (London: HMSO), p. 14
4. DHSS (1972). *Safety in Pathology Laboratories*. (London: HMSO), pp. 28, 52, 87
5. DHSS (1981). *Interim Advisory Committee on Safety in Clinical Laboratories*, Bulletin No. 2. (London: HMSO), p. 4
6. DHSS (1972). *Safety in Pathology Laboratories*. (London: HMSO), p. 8.
7. DHSS (1977). *Electrical Safety Code for Hospital Laboratory Equipment*. (London: HMSO), p. 22
8. DHSS (1972). *Safety in Pathology Laboratories*. (London: HMSO), p. 6
9. DHSS (1977). *Hospital Technical Memorandum*, No. 22. (London: HMSO)
10. DHSS (1972). *Safety in Pathology Laboratories*. (London: HMSO), p. 27
11. DHSS (1978). *Code of Practice for the Prevention of Infection in Clinical Laboratories and Post-mortem Rooms*. (London: HMSO), p. 11
12. Collins, C.H., Hartley, E.G. and Pilsworth, R. (1977). *The Prevention of Laboratory Acquired Infection*. (London: HMSO), pp. 8–9
13. DHSS (1972). *Safety in Pathology Laboratories*. (London: HMSO), p. 3
14. DHSS (1978). *Code of Practice for the Prevention of Infection in Clinical Laboratories and Post-mortem Rooms*. (London: HMSO), pp. 10, 12
15. DHSS (1978). *Code of Practice for the Prevention of Infection in Clinical Laboratories and Post-mortem Rooms*. (London: HMSO), p. 13
16. *The Highly Flammable Liquids and Petroleum Gases Regulations, 1972*, No. 917. (London: HMSO)
17. DHSS (1969). *Hospital Technical Memorandum*, No. 16. (London: HMSO)

544

18. *Portable fire extinguishing appliances*, F.S. Data sheets 6001, 6002, 6003. Fire Protection Association (1968). (London)
19. *The Protection of Eyes Regulations*, 1974. (London: HMSO)
20. DHSS (1978). *Code of Practice for the Prevention of Infection in Clinical Laboratories and Post-mortem Rooms*. (London: HMSO), pp. 10, 13, 16, 32, 52
21. DHSS (1973). *Hospital Building Note*, No. 15. (London: HMSO)
22. *The Factories Act*, 1961, section 5, Lighting. (London: HMSO)
23. Munce, J.F. (1962). *Laboratory Planning*. (London: Butterworth), pp. 129–130
24. Munce, J.F. (1962). *Laboratory Planning*. (London: Butterworth), p. 128
25. DHSS (1972). *Safety in Pathology Laboratories*. (London: HMSO), pp. 2–3
26. *Safety in chemical laboratories and in the use of chemicals*. (London: University of London, Imperial College of Science and Technology), 1977, pp. 51–52
27. *Specification and operating instructions for SMA Plus*. Technicon Instrument Co. Ltd, Basingstoke, UK (1975)
28. DHSS (1972). *Code of Practice for the Protection of persons against Ionizing Radiations arising from Medical and Dental Use*. (London: HMSO)
29. Munce, J.F. (1962). *Laboratory Planning*. (London: Butterworth), pp. 151–154
30. *Safety in chemical laboratories and in the use of chemicals*. (London: University of London, Imperial College of Science and Technology), 1977, pp. 8, 40
31. *Safety in chemical laboratories and in the use of chemicals*. (London: University of London, Imperial College of Science and Technology), 1977, pp. 43–44
32. *Safety in chemical laboratories and in the use of chemicals*. (London: University of London, Imperial College of Science and Technology), 1977, pp. 11–12
33. DHSS Circular DS 302/72, *Danger from explosions in laboratory drains from solutions containing azide*, 1972. (London: HMSO)
34. *Safety in chemical laboratories and in the use of chemicals*. (London: University of London, Imperial College of Science and Technology), 1977, p. 9
35. Collins, C.H., Hartley, E.G. and Pilsworth, R. (1977). *The Prevention of Laboratory Acquired Infection*. (London: HMSO), pp. 25–32
36. DHSS (1978). *Code of Practice for the Prevention of Infection in Clinical Laboratories and Post-mortem Rooms*. (London: HMSO), pp. 63–68
37. DHSS Health Circular (79) 3, Annex II, *Revision of Hospital Building Note*, No. 15, 1979. (London: HMSO)
38. Munce, J.F. (1962). *Laboratory Planning*. (London: Butterworth), p. 289
39. DHSS (1978). *Code of Practice for the Prevention of Infection in Clinical Laboratories and Post-mortem Rooms*. (London: HMSO), pp. 21–22
40. DHSS (1972). *Safety in Pathology Laboratories*. (London: HMSO), pp. 10–11
41. Whitehead, J.E.M. (1978). *Autoclaving practice in microbiology laboratories: report of a survey*. J. Clin. Pathol., **31**, pp. 418–422
42. DHSS (1978). *Code of Practice for the Prevention of Infection in Clinical Laboratories and Post-mortem Rooms*. (London: HMSO), pp. 45–46
43. DHSS (1978). *Code of Practice for the Prevention of Infection in Clinical Laboratories and Post-mortem Rooms*. (London: HMSO), pp. 27–30
44. DHSS (1978). *Code of Practice for the Prevention of Infection in Clinical Laboratories and Post-mortem Rooms*. (London: HMSO), p. 13
45. The Hospital Physicists' Association (1975). *Notes for the guidance of Radiological Protection Advisers and Radiological Safety Officers in Departments where Radioisotopes are used*. (London)
46. DHSS Circular WKO (78)3, *Acetylene Gas Installations*, Health Building Note No. 15. Pathology Department, 1978. (London: HMSO)
47. DHSS (1972). *Safety in Pathology Laboratories*. (London: HMSO), p. 80
48. DHSS (1977). *Electrical Safety Code for Hospital Laboratory Equipment*. (London: HMSO), p. 18, para. 23

545

49. Health and Safety Executive, Pilot Study (1976). *Working Conditions in the Medical Service*. (London: HSE), p. 29
50. Health and Safety Executive, Pilot Study (1976). *Working Conditions in the Medical Service, BS229, Flameproof enclosures of electrical apparatus*. (London: HSE), p. 62
51. Health and Safety Executive, Pilot Study (1976). *Working Conditions in the Medical Service*. (London: HSE), p. 26
52. *Safety in chemical laboratories and in the use of chemicals*. (London: University of London, Imperial College of Science and Technology), 1977, p. 22
53. DHSS (1972). *Safety in Pathology Laboratories*. (London: HMSO), p. 36
54. DHSS (1978). *Code of Practice for the prevention of Infection in Clinical Laboratories and Post-mortem Rooms*. (London: HMSO), pp. 31–34
55. *Safety in chemical laboratories and in the use of chemicals*. (London: University of London, Imperial College of Science and Technology), 1977, pp. 7–25
56. *The Carcinogenic Substances Regulations*, 1965. (London: HMSO)
57. Chester Beatty Research Institute (1966). *Precautions for laboratory workers who handle carcinogenic aromatic amines*. (London)
58. DHSS Circular DS 164/75. *Use of perchloric acid*, 1975. (London: HMSO)
59. DHSS Health Notice HN (Hazard) (81)6, *Danger of Explosion in Laboratory Waste Pipes contaminated by Picric Acid*, 1981. (London: HMSO)
60. *The Packaging and Labelling of Dangerous Substances Regulations*, amended 1983. (London: HMSO)
61. DHSS (1972). *Safety in Pathology Laboratories*. (London: HMSO), pp. 42–43
62. *Safety in chemical laboratories and in the use of chemicals*. (London: University of London, Imperial College of Science and Technology), 1977, pp. 38–40
63. DHSS (1972). *Safety in Pathology Laboratories*. (London: HMSO), p. 39
64. DHSS (1972). *Safety in Pathology Laboratories*. (London: HMSO), p. 44–45
65. *Safety in chemical laboratories and in the use of chemicals*. (London: University of London, Imperial College of Science and Technology), 1977, p. 10
66. DHSS (1972). *Safety in Pathology Laboratories*. (London: HMSO), p. 38
67. DHSS (1972). *Safety in Pathology Laboratories*. (London: HMSO), p. 67
68. DHSS (1978). *Code of Practice for the Prevention of Infection in Clinical Laboratories and Post-mortem Rooms*. (London: HMSO), p. 57
69. DHSS (1978). *Code of Practice for the Prevention of Infection in Clinical Laboratories and Post-mortem Rooms*. (London: HMSO), p. 55–56
70. DHSS (1978). *Code of Practice for the Prevention of Infection in Clinical Laboratories and Post-mortem Rooms*. (London: HMSO), pp. 19–20
71. *The Deposit of Poisonous Waste Act*, 1972. (London: HMSO)
72. *Control of Pollution Act*, 1974. (London: HMSO)
73. *Public Health (Drainage of Trade Premises) Act*, 1937. (London: HMSO)
74. *Safety in chemical laboratories and in the use of chemicals*. (London: University of London, Imperial College of Science and Technology), 1977, pp. 46–47
75. DHSS (1972). *Safety in Pathology Laboratories*. (London: HMSO), p. 42
76. *Radioactive Substances Act*, 1960. (London: HMSO)
77. DHSS (1972). *Safety in Pathology Laboratories*. (London: HMSO), pp. 12, 54
78. DHSS (1978). *Code of Practice for the Prevention of Infection in Clinical Laboratories and Post-mortem Rooms*. (London: HMSO), p. 58
79. DHSS Health Notice (Hazard) (82)10, *Danger of explosion in freeze-drying equipment and vacuum systems used to process materials containing sodium azide*, 1982. (London: HMSO)
80. *Radiation Hazards, Safety and Laboratory Design*, personal communication, Laboratory Health and Safety Course Notes, Radioactive Decontamination Procedures, Loughborough University, 1975, pp. 14–15
81. Health and Safety Guidance Series HS(G)51. 1990 (London: HSE)

546

82. *Fire Safety Data* (Information sheets), Volumes 4 and 6. Fire Protection Association (1989) (London)
83. DHSS Health Notice HN(Hazard)(81)6, Danger of Explosion in Laboratory Waste Pipes contaminated by Picric acid, 1981. (London: HMSO)
84. DOH Circular WKO(85)1, *Code of Practice for the Storage of Medical, Pathological and Industrial Gas Cylinders*, 1985. (London: HMSO)
85. Health and Safety Executive, Guidance Notes CS2 (1979). *Storage of Highly Flammable Liquids*. (London: HSE)
86. Health and Safety Executive, Guidance Notes CS4 (1986). *The Keeping of LPG Cylinders and Similar Containers*. (London: HSE)

Abbreviations used in the references

DHSS: Department of Health and Social Security, Hannibal House, Elephant and Castle, London, SE1 6TE

HMSO: Her Majesty's Stationery Office, Publications Centre (Mail and telephone orders only), PO Box 276, London, SW8 5DT

HSE: Health and Safety Executive, Publications Point, St Hugh's House, Stanley Precinct, Bootle, Merseyside, L30 3LZ

Index